Anaesthetic and Perioperative Complications

Edited by

Kamen Valchanov
Consultant in Anaesthesia and Intensive Care at Papworth Hospital NHS Trust, Cambridge, UK

Stephen T. Webb
Consultant in Anaesthesia and Intensive Care at Papworth Hospital NHS Trust, Cambridge, UK

Jane Sturgess
Consultant Anaesthetist at Addenbrooke's Hospital, Cambridge University Hospitals NHS Foundation Trust, Cambridge, UK

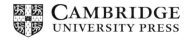
CAMBRIDGE
UNIVERSITY PRESS

CAMBRIDGE UNIVERSITY PRESS
Cambridge, New York, Melbourne, Madrid, Cape Town,
Singapore, São Paulo, Delhi, Tokyo, Mexico City

Cambridge University Press
The Edinburgh Building, Cambridge CB2 8RU, UK

Published in the United States of America by Cambridge University Press, New York

www.cambridge.org
Information on this title: www.cambridge.org/9781107002593

First published 2011

Printed in the United Kingdom at the University Press, Cambridge

A catalogue record for this publication is available from the British Library

Library of Congress Cataloguing in Publication data
Anaesthetic and perioperative complications / [edited by] Kamen Valchanov, Stephen T. Webb,
Jane Sturgess.
    p. ; cm.
Includes bibliographical references and index.
ISBN 978-1-107-00259-3 (hardback)
1. Anesthesia – Complications.   2. Anesthetics – Side effects.   I. Valchanov, Kamen.
II. Webb, Stephen T.   III. Sturgess, Jane.
[DNLM: 1. Anesthesia – adverse effects.   2. Perioperative Care – adverse effects. WO 245]
RD82.5.A57 2011
617.9′6–dc23   2011020617

ISBN 978-1-107-00259-3 Paperback

Contents

Foreword

William T. G. Morton's celebrated demonstration of ether, in Boston, took place in 1846. Very little time elapsed before the first reported death under anaesthesia occurred, that of 15 year old Hannah Greener who was given chloroform for the removal of an infected ingrowing toenail. Of course, the horror of facing the surgeon's knife without anaesthesia was clearly appreciated by patients at that time, so the contribution of modern anaesthesia to improving the lot of mankind was understood. This contribution was encapsulated in Morton's epitaph:

> Inventor and Revealer of Anaesthetic Inhalation
> Before Whom in all time Surgery was Agony
> By Whom Pain in Surgery was Averted and Annulled
> Since Whom Science has control of Pain

Furthermore the risks of surgery in the first two thirds of the 19th century were very high (in part because the importance of antisepsis had not yet been realised), so the balance between the benefits of anaesthesia and its potential risks was acceptable. Since then, the safety of both surgery and anaesthesia has been transformed, but so have the expectations of the public. Progress in anaesthesia has substantially revolved around minimizing and mitigating the risk of complications associated with the perioperative care of patients undergoing surgery, but as the absolute incidence of these complications has reduced, the expectations for measures to avoid them, and for expertise in managing them when they occur, have grown exponentially. Today's patients expect very high standards of care, particularly when things do go wrong. Part of this expectation arises from the fact that anaesthesia today is very safe in fit patients undergoing routine procedures in most high-income countries of the world. However, the truth is that even in these circumstances complications occur from time to time, sometimes with tragic consequences for patients and often also with serious implications for the staff involved in their care. When patients are very young or very old, or have serious co-morbidties, or are undergoing major surgery, the risks are much increased. The situation in some of the less wealthy parts of the world is also much more concerning: Reports suggest that the rate of mortality associated with anaesthesia in parts of Africa (for example) is orders of magnitude higher than in the UK (also for example). *Anaesthetic and Perioperative Complications* is therefore a timely and important contribution to the cause of patient safety.

The strengths of *Anaesthetic and Perioperative Complications* are several. It is clearly and accessibly written. It is sufficiently comprehensive to meet the needs of most busy practitioners without overburdening them with excessive detail. The layout of the book is structured in a way that will make intuitive sense to clinical anaesthetists. And it is written predominantly by practising anaesthetists, including several trainees. This book is not by or for the ivory tower theorist: It is a practical guide by and for clinical anaesthetists at every stage of their career.

The first section of the book provides a brief introduction to the elements of human error and the principles underlying the mitigation of risk, the prevention of complications, and the management of patients when things actually do go wrong. This equips the reader to place the body of the book into context. In the second section, the complications typically associated with anaesthesia are reviewed and discussed. Anaesthetists will intuitively understand the framework of this section: Complications are grouped around airways, the respiratory system, the cardiovascular system, the use of blood products, the administration of drugs, the use of equipment, the provision of obstetric anaesthesia, and so on. These chapters should be mandatory reading for every trainee. For experienced anaesthetists they provide a useful summary of contemporary information about complications related to various aspects of clinical anaesthesia. The third section of the book addresses ethical, legal and practical aspects of complications in anaesthesia. Understanding and managing these matters is a central part of modern anaesthesia, and competency in this area is to be expected of clinicians in all fields of healthcare today.

The editors, Kamen Valchanov, Stephen Webb and Jane Sturgess, have produced a practical and readable book. The ultimate beneficiaries of their work will be the patients whose outcomes will certainly be improved when they are cared for by anaesthetists who have read it, assimilated its information, and put its key messages into practice.

Professor Alan Merry

Contributors

John Andrzejowski
Consultant Anaesthetist, Royal Hallamshire Hospital, Sheffield, UK

Joseph E. Arrowsmith
Consultant Anaesthetist, Papworth Hospital NHS Trust, Cambridge, UK

Sam Bass
Consultant Anaesthetist, Addenbrooke's Hospital, Cambridge University Hospitals NHS Foundation Trust, Cambridge, UK

Clare Bates
Partner in the Healthcare Team in the Litigation Department of Carson McDowell, Solicitors, Belfast, UK

Dominic Bell
Consultant in Intensive Care and Anaesthesia, The General Infirmary, Leeds, UK

David Bogod
Consultant Anaesthetist, Nottingham City Hospital, Nottingham, UK

Tim M. Cook
Consultant Anaesthetist, Royal Bath United Hospital, Bath, UK

Mike Coupe
Consultant Anaesthetist, Royal Bath United Hospital, Bath, UK

Mark Dougherty
Consultant in Cardiothoracic Anaesthesia, Royal Victoria Hospital, Belfast, UK

Derek Duane
Consultant in Neuroanaesthesia and Neurointensive Care, Addenbrooke's

Hospital, Cambridge University Hospitals NHS Foundation Trust, Cambridge, UK

Peter Faber
Consultant Anaesthetist, Papworth Hospital NHS Trust ,Cambridge, UK

Fay J. Gilder
Consultant Anaesthetist, Addenbrooke's Hospital, Cambridge University Hospitals NHS Foundation Trust, Cambridge, UK

Helen Goddard
Consultant Anaesthetist, Norfolk and Norwich University Hospital NHS Foundation Trust, Norwich, UK

Tom Holmes
Advanced Trainee in Intensive Care, University Hospital of Wales, Cardiff and Vale NHS Trust, Cardiff, Wales, UK

Victoria Howell
Specialist Registrar in Anaesthesia, Anglia School of Anaesthesia, UK

James Hoyle
Consultant Anaesthetist, Royal Hallamshire Hospital, Sheffield, UK

Aoibhin Hutchinson
Consultant in Anaesthesia and Intensive Care Medicine, Royal Victoria Hospital, Belfast, UK

Alison Kavanagh
Specialist Trainee in Anaesthesia, Royal Victoria Hospital, Belfast, UK

Andrew A. Klein
Consultant in Anaesthesia and Intensive Care, Papworth Hospital NHS Trust, Cambridge, UK

Nick Lees
Locum Consultant in Cardiothoracic Anaesthesia, St George's Hospital, London, UK

Benias Mugabe
Specialist Registrar in Anaesthesia, Glan Clwyd Hospital, Rhyl, UK

Jurgens Nortje
Consultant Anaesthetist, Norfolk and Norwich University Hospital NHS Foundation Trust, Norwich, UK

Felicity Plaat
Consultant Anaesthetist, Queen Charlotte Hospital, London, UK

Saxon Ridley
Consultant in Anaesthesia and Intensive Care, Department of Anaesthesia, Glan Clwyd Hospital, Rhyl, UK

Andrew Roscoe
Assistant Professor in Anesthesiology, Toronto General Hospital, Canada

Martin Shields
Consultant Anaesthetist, Royal Victoria Hospital, Belfast, UK

Alistair Steel
Specialist Registrar in Anaesthesia, Anglia School of Anaesthesia, UK

Jane Sturgess
Consultant Anaesthetist at Addenbrooke's Hospital, Cambridge University Hospitals NHS Foundation Trust, Cambridge, UK

Rajinikanth Sundararajan
Specialist Registrar in Anaesthesia, Anglia School of Anaesthesia, UK

Kasia Szypula
Specialist Registrar in Anaesthesia, Nottingham City Hospital, Nottingham, UK

Dafydd Thomas
Consultant in Intensive Care, Morriston Hospital, Abertawe Bro Morgannwg University Health Board, Swansea, Wales, UK

Hamish Thomson
Consultant in Anaesthesia and Intensive Care Medicine, St Bernard's Hospital, Gibraltar

Kamen Valchanov
Consultant in Anaesthesia and Intensive Care, Papworth Hospital NHS Trust, Cambridge, UK

A. James Varley
Consultant in Anaesthesia and Intensive Care, Addenbrooke's Hospital, Cambridge University Hospitals NHS Foundation Trust, Cambridge, UK

Stephen T. Webb
Consultant in Anaesthesia and Intensive Care, Papworth Hospital NHS Trust, Cambridge, UK

Matt Wilkner
Specialist Registrar in Anaesthesia, Queen Charlotte Hospital, London, UK

Nick Woodall
Consultant Anaesthetist, Norfolk and Norwich University Hospital NHS Foundation Trust, Norwich, UK

Abbreviations

AAGBI	Association of Anaesthetists of Great Britain and Ireland	ATP	adenosine triphosphate
ABT	allogeneic blood transfusion	AvMA	Action against Medical Accidents
ACEI	angiotensin converting enzyme inhibitor	BAL	bronchoalveolar lavage
		BBV	blood-borne virus
ACS	abdominal compartment syndrome	BChE	butyrylcholinesterase (plasma cholinesterase)
ADP	accidental dural puncture	BIS	bispectral index
ADR	alternative dispute resolution	BMI	body mass index
AF	atrial fibrillation	BPM	beats per minute
AFE	amniotic fluid embolism	CAM	Confusion Assessment Method
AGSS	anaesthetic gas scavenging system	CAM-ICU	Confusion Assessment Method for ICU Patients
AHTR	acute haemolytic transfusion reaction	CC	closing capacity
AI	adrenal insufficiency	CFA	conditional fee agreement
AIH	anaesthesia-induced hepatitis	CIN	contrast-induced nephropathy
AIMS	Australian Anaesthetic Incident Monitoring Study	CK/CCK	creatine kinase
AKI	acute kidney injury	CMR	cerebral metabolic rate
ALA	d-aminolaevulinic acid	CNAS	Clinical Negligence Accreditation Scheme
ALI	acute lung injury	CNB	central neuraxial block
ALS	advanced life support	CNS	central nervous system
ALT	alanine aminotransferase	COPD	chronic obstructive pulmonary disease
ANTS	Anaesthetists' Non-Technical Skills Framework	COSHH	Control of Substances Hazardous to Health
APA	American Psychiatric Association	CPAP	continuous positive airway pressure
APACHE	Acute Physiology and Chronic Health Evaluation System	CPB	cardiopulmonary bypass
		CPP	cerebral perfusion pressure
APL	automated pressure limiting valve	CPS	Crown Prosecution Service
		CRM	crisis resource management
APSF	Anaesthetic Patient Safety Forum	CRP	c-reactive protein
ARDS	acute respiratory distress syndrome	CSE	combined spinal epidural injection
ARF	acute renal failure	CSF	cerebrospinal fluid
ASA	American Society of Anesthesiologists	CT	computed tomography
AST	aspartate aminotransferase	CTP	Child–Turcotte–Pugh Classification
ATN	acute tubular necrosis		

CTPA	computer tomographic pulmonary angiography	HBI	hypoxic brain injury
CV	closing volume	HBV	hepatitis B virus
CVC	central venous catheter	HCV	hepatitis C virus
CVCI	cannot ventilate cannot intubate	HDU	high dependency unit
		HEPM	Healthcare Error Proliferation Model
CVP	central venous pressure	HES	hydroxyethyl starch
CVS	cardiovascular system	HIT	heparin-induced thrombocytopaenia
CVVHD	continuous veno-venous haemodialysis	HIV	human immunodeficiency virus
CVVHDF	continuous veno-venous haemodiafiltration	HMG	3-hydroxy-3-methylglutanyl coenzyme A reductase
CVVHF	continuous veno-venous haemofiltration	HPA	human platelet antigen
		HPA	hypothalamic–pituitary–adrenal axis
CXR	chest X-ray	HR	heart rate
DAS	Difficult Airway Society	HTR	haemolytic transfusion reaction
DC	direct current	IAH	intra-abdominal hypertension
DDS	delirium detection score	ICDSC	Intensive Care Delirium Screening Checklist
DFV	dengue fever virus	ICU	intensive care unit
DHTR	delayed haemolytic transfusion reaction	IDT	intradermal dilutional testing
DIC	disseminated intravascular coagulation	INR	international normalized ratio
		IPH	inadvertent perioperative hypothermia
DLT	double lumen tube	ITR	interthreshold range
DNA	deoxyribonucleic acid	ITU	intensive therapy unit
DVT	deep vein thrombosis	IU	international units
EBP	epidural blood patch	IV	intravenous
ECG	electrocardiography	IVC	inferior vena cava
ED95	effective dose in 95% of patients	IVCT	in vitro contractile testing
		LMA	laryngeal mask airway
EEG	electroencephalography	LAST	local anaesthetic systemic toxicity
EMG	electromyography		
ENT	ear nose and throat	LMWH	low molecular weight heparin
FAW	forced air warming	LOS	lower oesophageal sphincter
FCEs	finished consultant episodes	LSCS	lower segment caesarean section
FFP	fresh frozen plasma	MAC	minimum alveolar concentration
FiO_2	fraction of inspired oxygen	MACE	major adverse cardiovascular events
FNHTR	febrile non-haemolytic transfusion reaction		
FOCUS	focused operative cardiovascular unified systems	MAO	monoamine oxidase
		MAP	mean arterial pressure
FRC	functional residual capacity	MDR	multi-drug resistance
GA	general anaesthesia	MEE	Medical Education England
GABA	γ-amino-butyric acid	MELD	Model for End-stage Liver Disease
GIT	gastrointestinal tract		
GMC	General Medical Council	MEP	motor evoked potentials
GST	glutathione S-transferase		

MH	malignant hyperthermia	PNB	Peripheral nerve block
MHRA	Medicines and Healthcare Products Regulatory Agency	POCD	Postoperative cognitive deficit
MODS	multi-organ dysfunction syndrome	POD	postoperative delirium
		PTP	post-transfusion purpura
MP-NAT	minipool nucleic acid testing	QCC	Quality Care Commission
MRI	magnetic resonance imaging	RA	regional anaesthesia
MRSA	methicillin-resistant *Staphylococcus aureus*	RCA	Royal College of Anaesthetists
NCAS	National Clinical Assessment Service	RIFLE	Risk, Injury, Failure, Loss and End-stage kidney disease
NCEPOD	National Confidential Enquiry in Perioperative Outcomes and Deaths	RNA	ribonucleic acid
		RQIA	Regulatory and Quality Improvement Authority
NGT	nasogastric tube	RRT	renal replacement therapy
NHS	National Health Service	RSI	rapid sequence induction
NHSLA	National Health Service Litigation Authority	RV	residual volume
		SABRE	Serious Adverse Blood Reactions and Events
NICE	National Institute for Health and Clinical Excellence	SAD	supraglottic airway device
NIRS	near-infrared spectroscopy	SAFE	Saline versus Albumin Fluid Evaluation
NIST	non-interchangeable screw-threads	SABRE	Serious Adverse Blood Reactions and Events
NMBA	neuromuscular blocking agent	SALG	Safe Anaesthesia Liaison Group
NMDA	N-methyl-D-aspartate receptor		
NP	neuropathic pain		
NPSA	National Patient Safety Agency	SBAR	situation – background – assessment – recommendation
NRLS	National Reporting and Learning System	SCI	spinal cord injury
NSAIDs	non-steroidal anti-inflammatory drugs	SGA	supraglottic airway
		SGC	Sentencing Guidelines Council
OI	oesophageal intubation		
OPA	oropharyngeal airway	SHOT	Serious Hazards of Transfusion
PA	pulmonary artery		
PALS	Patient Advice and Liaison Service	SNS	sympathetic nervous system
		SPT	skin prick test
PCA	patient-controlled analgesia	SSEP	somatosensory evoked potentials
PCI	percutaneous intervention		
PCT	procalcitonin	SSI	surgical site infections
PDPH	post-dural puncture headache	SV	stroke volume
PE	pulmonary embolus	SVR	systemic vascular resistance
PEEP	positive end-expiratory pressure	TAAA	thoraco-abdominal aortic aneurysm
PEP	post-exposure prophylaxis	TACO	transfusion associated circulatory overload
PHT	pulmonary hypertension		
PMETB	Postgraduate Medical Education Training Board	TAS	transfusion-associated sepsis

TIA	transient ischaemic attack	URTI	upper respiratory tract infection
TMJ	temporo-mandibular joint	UTR	urticarial transfusion reaction
TR-GVHD	transfusion-related graft versus host disease	VAP	ventilator-associated pneumonia
		VCA	vertebral canal abscess
TRALI	transfusion-related lung injury	VCH	vertebral canal haematoma
TRIM	transfusion-related immunomodulation	vCJD	variant Creutzfeldt–Jakob disease
		VF	ventricular fibrillation
TT	tracheal tube	VTE	venous thromboembolism
TURP	transurethral resection of prostate	WCC	white cell count
		WHO	World Health Organization
UFH	unfractionated heparin	WNV	West Nile virus

Preventing complications

Jane Sturgess

'Primum non nocere' – first, do no harm

The phrase 'prevention is better than cure' is never more true than when considering complications. A complication in medicine is an additional problem arising after a procedure, treatment or illness. It may be iatrogenic. The prevention of iatrogenic complications is one of the most important considerations for every physician.

Understanding the causes of errors can help to develop error prevention strategy. James Reason proposed the Swiss cheese model to explain failure (Figure 1.1). He said that the majority of accidents could be traced back to one of four main levels: organisation failure, supervision failure, conditions allowing unsafe acts and unsafe acts themselves. Each of these can be seen as a defence layer. Most often there is a sequence of failures leading to the error, and those failures can be active or latent. Healthcare provision is complex. It has a diverse structure and staff mix, with many interconnections that have to adapt and learn from previous events. The Healthcare Error Proliferation Model (HEPM) was designed as an adaption of Reason's seminal work. It takes the complexity of healthcare into consideration when examining the causes of error.

According to the most recent data from the NHS Information Centre, the number of errors are increasing year on year. Between September 2009 and August 2010 there were 17,051,769 finished consultant episodes (FCEs). A finished consultant episode relates to 'a continuous period of admitted patient care under one consultant within one healthcare provider'. Of these 372,786 were due to a complication. Table 1.1 shows the data relating to those FCEs where the primary cause of admission or clinic referral is 'complication of surgical and medical care' (Figures 1.2 and 1.3). The 60 to 79 age group suffered the most complications. Table 1.2 gives a breakdown of the causes of the complications.

This chapter will consider how to prevent complications from occurring in the first instance, and can be considered under two main sub-headings:

- education and training
- departmental and corporate governance.

Education and training

Education

The Royal College of Anaesthetists (RCA) and the Association of Anaesthetists of Great Britain and Ireland (AAGBI) have led the way in standards and education, and safety,

Anaesthetic and Perioperative Complications, ed. Kamen Valchanov, Stephen T. Webb and Jane Sturgess. Published by Cambridge University Press. © Cambridge University Press 2011.

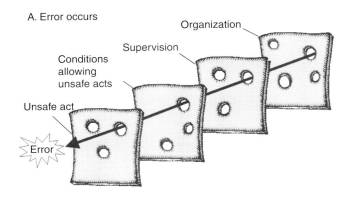

A. Error occurs

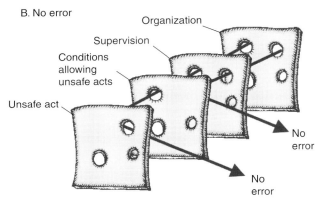

B. No error

Figure 1.1 The Swiss cheese model shows four levels of failure. If there is a defect in any level (or defence) an error is more likely. If there is a defect in each of these defence levels an error will occur as shown in A.

An example of level 4 failure would be organization failure – cut back on staffing and training levels; supervision failure – consultant surgeon or anaesthetist called away leaving junior inexperienced staff to perform case 'out of hours'; conditions allowing unsafe acts – improper communication about the need to proceed and how long the consultant will be delayed; unsafe acts – junior staff proceed immediately with the case.

In B the error is averted as one of the defence layers remains intact. Using the previous example, it can be seen that if proper communication occurred, i.e. if their consultant gave an accurate time frame for their absence the case could be started later with appropriate supervision; alternatively if the team decided the case was non-urgent it could be postponed, and the error would not occur. The next possibility in the given example is the decision by the team to proceed – any member of the team can take the opportunity to delay or at least call for advice.

respectively. The Postgraduate Medical Education Training Board (PMETB) as part of the General Medical Council (GMC), and now Medical Education of England (MEE), have decided to use a competency-based template to guide doctors in training. Many of these competencies will form part of core transferable modules across specialties. This is the training tool anaesthesia, pain and intensive care medicine are familiar with and have been using for many years. During the 'training years' competency is routinely tested. Competence is less formally assessed once practising independently. This may be addressed by the 360-degree appraisal process. Competence (or lack of competence) can be conscious or unconscious. Individuals who are competent or have a conscious lack of competence are more

Table 1.1 Complications of medical and surgical care. Number of finished consultant episodes where the primary cause is complications of medical and surgical care per 1,000 FCEs (by age group) (adapted from HESonline).

	<16	17–39	40–59	60–79	>80
Sep 2009–Aug 2010	9.7	13.4	24.8	29.6	25.0
Sep 2008–Aug 2009	8.9	12.6	23.2	28.0	23.0
Change (per 1,000)	0.8	0.8	1.6	1.6	2.0

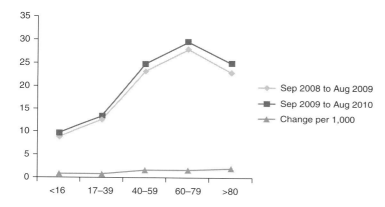

Figure 1.2 Graph to show number of FCEs where the primary cause is complications of medical and surgical care per 1,000 FCEs (x-axis: age/years; y-axis number per 1,000 cases).

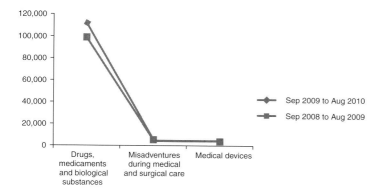

Figure 1.3 Graph to show the primary cause of complication of medical and surgical care (x-axis: cause of complication; y-axis: number of incidents).

likely to act and prevent a complication than those who are unconscious of their lack of competence (Table 1.3, Figure 1.4).

Knowledge

A clear understanding of human physiology and pharmacology, and the changes that occur under anaesthesia or in particular pathological states is a core requirement for anaesthetists. The planned intervention (e.g. surgery, nerve block, ventilation) should also be considered. This knowledge is tested at postgraduate examination. Detailed knowledge relevant to an individuals' practice is likely to be checked during revalidation.

Table 1.2 Number and causative group for FCEs where the primary cause is complications of medical and surgical care (adapted from HESonline).

	Sep 2009–Aug 2010	Sep 2008–Aug 2009
Drugs, medicaments and biological substances causing adverse events in therapeutic use	111,771 (93%)	99,142 (92%)
Misadventures to patients during surgical and medical care	5,404 (4%)	5,184 (5%)
Medical devices associated with adverse incidents in diagnostic and therapeutic use	3,479 (3%)	3,704 (3%)

Table 1.3 Examples of competence.

	Unconscious	Conscious
Not competent	a person who sees no need to continue to develop and alter their clinical practice according to current evidence/guidance	a person who performs landmark-guided regional anaesthetic blocks may be aware of ultrasound-guided techniques and wish to embark on a course
Competent	a person who performs a task well without having to think about the process required to suceed and may even have difficulty explaining exactly how it was achieved (hand writing)	a person who performs a task well, and is able to replicate the task time and time again. This person will understand the technique, have detailed knowledge and be able to teach others to perform the task (central line insertion)

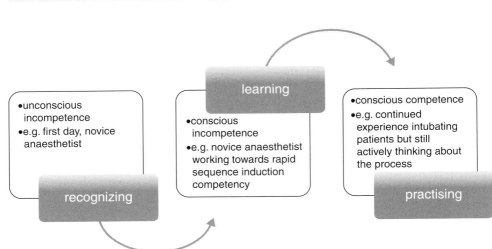

Figure 1.4 The development of competence.

The doctor uses this knowledge to prevent, or at least anticipate and treat, expected complications as they arise. In addition, anaesthetists must be aware of rare or unanticipated complications and prepare strategies to handle them – failed intubation and ventilation, anaphylaxis, malignant hyperthermia. As the clinician becomes more specialized, so the

Table 1.4 Knowledge required to prevent complications.

Types of knowledge
Theoretical
Clinical (including insight into own capabilities)
Environmental – plant and staff
Working of equipment
Available support

Table 1.5 Anticipation of complications.

When are complications more likely to occur?
Tired
Late
Stressed
Task overloaded

knowledge required about specific illnesses increases, for example high-risk obstetrics and cardiothoracic anaesthesia.

Clinical experience complements theoretical knowledge. An awareness of one's own limitations is essential to prevent most complications. Are you able to perform awake intubation or not? Are you aware of the need to be able to perform an awake intubation? Do you need to obtain further training to be able to safely care for your patients?

Good non-technical skills and core clinical knowledge decrease the likelihood of complications. They guide the individual to recognize situations of increased risk and improve resource management. Planning, prioritization and task delegation are just as important to a successful outcome as clinical ability. There are now a number of simulator courses designed specifically to teach non-technical skills; junior doctors are being regularly assessed on them, and they have become part of the medical student curriculum (Table 1.4).

Attitude

The right attitude to work, patient and team is essential. Careful preparation of oneself, the patient and the working environment is important. Knowing when a complication is more likely to happen can also alert you to times of increased risk. This can give the opportunity to delay, or take time to anticipate and prepare. Complications are more likely when you are under time pressure (feeling rushed), when you are task overloaded (supervising more than one operating theatre, have a concurrent non-clinical commitment, in the emergency situation), when you are stressed, when you are tired, when you handover care to another clinician or when you do not have a clear chain of command (tasks become duplicated or are not performed) (Table 1.5).

Behaviour

Individuals may be risk-taking or risk-averse. Human factors training promotes recognition of these intrinsic characteristics, and encourages a change towards risk-averse behaviour.

Maintenance of a logbook can help identify areas of expertise and of deficit. This plays a useful part in directing future training, and can focus discussion during the annual appraisal process to help format an individual development plan.

A professional approach to patients and staff should be maintained. Comments about others' clinical practice must only be given when in receipt of the full facts relating to the clinical incident in question, and only when invited. Comments about patients' illness or treatment plans should not be made in public areas, and notes or data should be stored according to data protection rules. Hospital notes and patient information must not be left in an unsecured area. Complications refer not only to clinical incidents but also to interpretation of those incidents.

If an individual becomes ill they must seek appropriate medical help, report to occupational health and, if necessary, have a risk assessment performed to allow them to either return to work or continue working safely – protecting both themselves and their patients from complications. If you suspect a colleague is ill, you should encourage them to self-report and seek help. If you remain concerned about the effect of ill health on an individual's work performance, you are obliged to report it to your clinical director.

Training and clinical skills

The bulk of training occurs during the foundation and specialist training years, but new skills and knowledge can and should be acquired as a consultant. This should continue throughout a career. Revalidation and recertification will encourage consultants to maintain their breadth of knowledge, and depth, depending on their specialist interest. A learning matrix will guide this. Practitioners should be competent at performing certain tasks (intubation, nerve block, paediatric anaesthesia) and perform them regularly. Learning about the recognized complications and their management (common or serious) is part of task-related training (Table 1.6).

Table 1.6 Foundation and specialist training assessment tools.

Assessment tools for foundation and specialist trainees	Assesses
Mini clinical evaluation exercise (Mini-CEX)	Knowledge, communication and problem solving
Team assessment of behaviours (TAB)	Attitude and behaviour, non-technical skills
Case-based discussion (CBD)	Knowledge, communication and problem solving
Direct observation of procedural skills (DOPS)	Practical and communication skills
Procedural logbook	Clinical case load and experience
Developing the clinical teacher assessment	Teaching, time organization and communication

Safe patient positioning forms part of training. There are cases when the complications of positioning should be discussed with the patient at the pre-operative visit (neuropraxia, visual loss). Attention to detail and knowledge of the potential pitfalls can prevent the complication.

Thorough assessment of the patient guides further pre-operative investigations, e.g. stress echocardiography, coronary angiography, pulmonary function testing. This is best done in advance of admission. Pre-assessment includes planning for the immediate postoperative period. Postoperative care in an appropriate location should be arranged in advance.

As many hospitals move towards a day of surgery admissions policy, pre-assessment of all patients becomes more important. Most pre-assessment clinics have a nurse-led service. Many are moving towards a consultant anaesthetist dedicated to pre-assessment. Considered anaesthetic management by experienced anaesthetists reduces complications in the high-risk patient.

Departmental and corporate governance

To provide a safe service hospitals need the right direction, the right staff and the right facilities.

Each department must communicate effectively about the services it does or does not offer, and how to access them. New services require careful planning and input from each stakeholder to anticipate and prevent complications. For example, anaesthesia within the radiology department requires input from radiologists and anaesthetists to organize facilities, plant and staff that are acceptable to both parties.

Department responsibility

Each department is responsible for ensuring the correct number of staff and skill mix for the safe running of the theatre suite, pain clinic and intensive care unit. This must include nursing staff (theatre and recovery), ancillary staff, anaesthetic assistance and anaesthetists. Staffing numbers must take annual and study leave into consideration.

Departmental guidelines and protocols should be explained at induction for all new staff and be readily available in all clinical areas. Practices for checking and giving of blood are obligatory.

An induction to the department should include orientation to the working environment. Within theatres the location of the blood fridge, difficult airway trolley, resuscitation trolley, dantrolene, fire extinguishers and fire exits must be demonstrated.

Review of previous complications can help to prevent the same problems recurring. Mortality and morbidity meetings discussing clinical incidents and near-misses can highlight areas of risk, and direct training, guidelines or requests for additional equipment. A robust incident reporting system may identify underperforming individuals, and allow early intervention to prevent complications.

Departmental and individual performance should be monitored and benchmarked. Below-average performance should be investigated. Keeping the use of short-term locums to a minimum can prevent complication. Where locum use is necessary, the locum staff should be given the same induction, and subjected to the same standards (including appraisal) as permanent staff.

Clinical processes need to be clear and uniform throughout the working environment. Checklists have been part of the aviation industry for many decades and are widely recognized as contributing to the safety record of the industry. Other high-risk industries, including healthcare, have sought to use checklists to improve their own safety record.

There has been debate about the similarities between medicine (anaesthesia in particular) and aviation. Pilots use simulation exercises, standard operating procedures and checklists. Simulation can help to prepare for uncommon emergencies, but medical simulation has, to date, focused on the individual or teams of doctors. Newer courses are available for the whole theatre team.

Doctors (unlike pilots) do not have standard operating procedures, and they have to diagnose whilst making decisions. Standardized procedures for communication and team responses in the emergency situation should decrease complications (e.g. advanced life support protocols, ALS). Each department must ensure their doctors have up-to-date resuscitation training.

SBAR (situation – background – assessment – recommendation) and SHIFT are communication tools that are an example of standardized information handover. They act as an aide memoir to ensure vital patient information is not missed in handover (Table 1.7).

Table 1.7 Handover tools; SBAR (recommended by the NHS Institute for Innovation and Improvement) and the MPS SHIFT model.

S	Situation
B	Background
A	Assessment
R	Recommendations
S	Status of the patient
H	History to this point
I	Investigations pending
F	Fears of what may unfold
T	Treatment planned until care handed back

The Breslow tape and colour-coded, age-specific resuscitation bags are further examples of standard operating tools that serve to prevent complication in paediatric resuscitation.

Healthcare has adopted the checklist for many areas of practice, e.g. hand washing, central line insertion, administering intrathecal drugs. Checklists have been introduced within the perioperative field. A standard method of checking the patient and documentation on the ward, at the entry to the theatre complex, and before induction of anaesthesia may decrease the risk of complication. The World Health Organization (WHO) checklist has been adopted in various forms throughout the UK, and includes a pre-incision and postoperative check. This check includes clear marking of the surgical site on the ward, checking the mark pre-induction and reconfirming the operation before incision. The aim is to prevent wrong-side and incorrect surgery. Checklists can improve team communication but uptake is not universal.

Corporate responsibility

Corporate responsibility includes a hospital induction programme. Each staff member must be given the opportunity to attend. The expectation is that each staff member will attend. It should include manual handling and a fire lecture. There must be a rapid response fire team to arrange and coordinate safe evacuation in the event of an emergency, and a major incident policy. The hospital is also expected to maintain safe staffing levels for the services it provides, according to the departmental recommendations.

Occupational health services must be provided by the hospital to ensure the health of their staff. There must be a needlestick injury policy in place. National standards are adopted and monitored. Control of Substances Hazardous to Health (COSHH) regulations enforce employers to maintain a set standard in the use and disposal of hazardous substances.

The institution must provide diagnostic support for clinical teams (laboratory, radiology and physiological testing). Reliable information technology systems are essential, including training on any IT programs needed during day-to-day activity within the hospital, and support when the systems fail. Clinicians must be able to both order and review routine and emergency tests. In addition the hospital should ensure satisfactory process and engineering backup for equipment, electrical or plant failure.

Corporate expectations and aspirations for service development and delivery must be realistic and achievable, with robust financial and human resource planning. When changes to either plant or process are expected, the corporation is responsible for providing all stakeholders with timely information on the plans and the anticipated time course. A consultation period should follow, and then a response from the hospital. There should also be a business plan detailing projected costs and income. Management must have a strategy for implementing and monitoring change with patient safety at its heart. Cost reduction should not be at the expense of patient safety. Foundation Trusts have a responsibility to maintain financial governance and are overseen by Monitor.

List of further reading

Academy of Medical Royal Colleges. www.aomrc.org.uk (accessed 15 April 2011).

Association of Anaesthetists. Safety. http://aagbi.org/foundation/safety.htm (accessed 15 April 2011).

Barema. www.barema.org.uk (accessed 15 April 2011).

Department of Health. www.doh.gov.uk (accessed 15 April 2011).

Foundation Programme. www.foundationprogramme.nhs.uk (accessed 15 April 2011).

General Medical Council. www.gmc-uk.org (accessed 15 April 2011).

Health and Safety Executive. www.hse.gov.uk (accessed 15 April 2011).

Medicines and Healthcare Products Regulatory Agency. Safety information. www.mhra.gov.uk/Safetyinformation/index.htm (accessed 15 April 2011).

National Health Service. The Information Centre for health and social care. www.ic.nhs.uk (accessed 15 April 2011).

National Patient Safety Agency. Patient safety resources. www.npsa.nhs.uk (accessed 15 April 2011).

Royal College of Anaesthetists. Professional Standards Directorate. www.rcoa.ac.uk/index.asp?SectionID=3 (accessed 15 April 2011).

Chapter

2

Managing complications

Kamen Valchanov and Alistair Steel

History of anaesthesia and complications in context

Anaesthesia dates from prehistoric times in the form of opium, and the first documented recipes are recorded by the ancient Egyptians. The birth of modern anaesthesia is considered to have occurred in 1846 when William Morton publicly administered ether in Massachusetts General Hospital. His first public demonstration of the use of ether was complicated by a failure to induce anaesthesia. Since then anaesthetic practice has vastly expanded and approximately six million anaesthetics are given in the UK each year. Like all areas of life the practice of anaesthesia is also associated with a variety of complications.

A complication is an unfavourable evolution of a disease process or its management.

We perceive anaesthesia and surgery as a safe process. Indeed, mortality related directly to anaesthesia is now estimated to be less than 1 in 250,000. However, despite the improved safety record, complications will inevitably occur in relation to anaesthesia. Some are related to the anaesthesia alone, some related to surgery, but the majority of complications relate to the complex interaction between anaesthesia, surgery, the patient's condition and human factors. In this chapter we will discuss the general principles of managing complications occurring during anaesthesia.

Complications occurring during anaesthesia are often minor but they can lead to serious health problems, disability and death. The ability to competently manage a complication, however minor, can significantly reduce the risk of harm to the patient. The successful management of a complication relies upon the recognition that a complication has occurred, or is occurring, followed by a series of actions requiring knowledge, technical skills and behaviours that mitigate the consequences of the complication.

Importance of managing complications

Complications occurring during anaesthesia can be due to the deterioration of a patient's condition or errors. Errors can involve human factors, equipment problems, medication errors, technical problems or misjudged severity of the patient's condition. The majority of errors in medical practice are due to human factors. They may result from inadequate training and experience, a challenging working environment, poor team-working, stress and fatigue. However, most complications are multifactorial and it is seldom that a complication occurs due to a single factor. In the UK, healthcare organizations are required by law to have implemented processes to reduce the risks to which patients are exposed. The knowledge

Anaesthetic and Perioperative Complications, ed. Kamen Valchanov, Stephen T. Webb and Jane Sturgess.
Published by Cambridge University Press. © Cambridge University Press 2011.

of how and why complications occur and methods to avoid and manage complications is a powerful tool in the armoury of all healthcare providers.

The aviation industry classifies human errors into several groups:

Violation	Conscious failure to adhere to procedures and regulations
Procedural	Followed procedures with wrong execution
Communications	Missing or wrong information exchange or misinterpretation
Proficiency	Error due to lack of knowledge or skill
Decision	Decision that unnecessarily increases risk

Impact of complications

When a complication is managed well the outcome for the patient may be favourable. When the outcome of a complication is not favourable this can lead to physical and psychological injury and can be a source of litigation. Data from the UK NHS Litigation Authority for the period 1995 to 2007 indicates that there were 841 claims related directly to anaesthesia, which is 2.5% of all claims with a value of £121 million. The major sources of these claims are detailed in Table 2.1.

Table 2.1 NHS Litigation Authority anaesthesia-related complications resulting in litigation by category from 1995 to 2007. Note that claims may relate to more than one category.

Anaesthesia-related complication	Percentage of all anaesthesia-related claims
Regional anaesthesia	44%
Obstetric anaesthesia	29%
Inadequate anaesthesia	20%
Dental damage	11%
Airway-related	8%
Drug-related	7%
Positioning-related	4%
Respiratory-related	3%
Consent-related	3%
Central venous cannulation-related	2%
Peripheral venous cannulation	2%

Timing of complications management

A complication may be considered to involve three time phases: prior to the complication (risk avoidance, preparation, training); during the complication (recognizing and preventing complication evolution, monitoring); after the complication (postoperative clinical management, record keeping, implementing systems to prevent recurrence of complications, management of complaints).

Anticipating complications

Whilst data analysis of complications worldwide and institutionally relating to a particular procedure, as well as experience, are the most important factors in managing complications prior to their occurrence, anticipating complications is the most important preventive measure. Anticipation relates to a healthcare system as well as the individuals involved in carrying out the procedure.

To ensure successful outcome of medical intervention all healthcare systems have implemented series of procedures to prevent negative outcome. A typical example is anticipating pulmonary complications following thoracic surgery. It is known that the incidence of pneumonia after lung resections is 10 to 25%, but the mortality from it is as high as 20%. Therefore most institutions have implemented a system where the patients are carefully prepared for surgery, receive appropriate intra-operative care, and are cared for in specialist designated areas, where appropriate levels of monitoring, pain control and physiotherapy are administered.

Anaesthetists are highly trained to anticipate complications, and this has led to great improvement of unexpected mishaps. An example is the anticipation of bradycardia as a side effect of neostigmine administration to reverse neuromuscular blockade, and therefore administration of glycopyrronium concomitantly.

Recognizing complications

Experienced practitioners not only anticipate a complication but also recognize it promptly and accurately. Indeed, early recognition may be the key to preventing its evolution. For example, an intra-operative pneumothorax if recognized and treated early is likely to cause little in the way of long-term harm. However, an unrecognized simple pneumothorax may develop into a life-threatening tension pneumothorax.

Failure to promptly and accurately recognize a complication can lead to devastating complications as illustrated in Case 2.1.

Case 2.1: Unrecognized oesophageal intubation

An anaesthetic trainee-induced general anaesthesia in a multiparous woman for an emergency caesarean section. Direct laryngoscopy was difficult. A tracheal tube was passed over the bougie. Mechanical ventilation was commenced and chest movements were seen. The capnograph trace remained 'flat'. The trainee felt certain that the endotracheal tube was correctly sited and wrongly concluded that the capnograph must have been malfunctioning. As hypoxia ensued attempts to increase oxygenation by increasing the inspired fraction of oxygen and increasing the minute volume of ventilation were unsuccessful. Several minutes passed before senior consultant help arrived. Laryngoscopy by the consultant revealed an oesophageal intubation. By the time the tracheal tube was correctly re-inserted irreversible hypoxic brain injury had occurred.

Monitoring

Monitoring of vital signs and other physiological parameters has evolved vastly during the last decades. Importantly, the accuracy and simplicity of interpretation have improved too. Many professional organisations, such as the Association of Anaesthetists of Great Britain and Ireland, are now recommending minimum standards for intra-operative monitoring. Additional monitoring may be required according to the needs of the patient and the possible complications that may occur, as shown in Case 2.2.

Case 2.2: Using monitoring to allow for the early management of complications

An anaesthetic registrar and duty consultant were scheduled to anaesthetize an elderly lady with severe aortic stenosis for emergency hip fracture surgery. Recognizing the need for good intra-operative blood pressure control an arterial line was inserted for perioperative invasive blood pressure monitoring. On induction of anaesthesia, despite appropriately reduced anaesthetic doses, the blood pressure fell precipitously. The invasive blood pressure alarms were set to alert the team to a set limit judged the minimum for adequate cardiac and cerebral perfusion. Once alerted to the fall in blood pressure, vasopressors were immediately given and within 30 seconds the blood pressure had been restored to pre-induction values. Further boluses of vasopressors were required throughout surgery but, as a result of using the additional invasive monitoring, no additional complications occurred.

The role of machines, monitors and engineering

Modern safe anaesthesia in the UK relies on the use of electronic and mechanical systems not only to prevent incidents but also to alert the anaesthetist to abnormal states. Examples include the presence of high-pressure airway alarms and capnometry-based apnoea alarms. Monitors measure, observe, check and continuously record patient physiology and capture the conduct of the anaesthetic. Anaesthetic monitors are used in conjunction with other anaesthetic machinery and clinical observations to detect abnormalities and to bring them to the attention of the anaesthetic team. Most systems can be overridden or may be defaulted to states that disregard abnormal measurements. More commonly, the interaction between humans and machines means that warnings may be ignored or misinterpreted. Managing anaesthetic complications successfully therefore relies on knowledge and understanding of the systems that are in place.

The evolving complication

Some complications can evolve and the earliest intervention to preclude further deterioration and improve the patient condition leads to the best clinical outcomes. It is often easy to deal with an anticipated complication for which the team is prepared, but occasionally unanticipated complications occur and are less easy to deal with. Patient-based experiences are very important in learning to manage complications but simulator-based training is increasingly shown to be helpful. This could be invaluable in dealing with life-threatening complications that are rare in routine training practice as shown in Case 2.3.

Case 2.3: A difficult airway

Anaesthesia was induced in an unconscious adolescent pedestrian who had sustained a severe head injury. Despite two attempts at direct laryngoscopy the glottis could not be visualized and blind attempts at passing a bougie were unsuccessful. The patient became hypoxic and passive regurgitation occurred. Maintaining ventilation using a

---

Case 2.3: (*cont.*)

bag-valve-mask and airway adjuncts was unsuccessful. A laryngeal mask airway was inserted but this also failed to allow oxygenation. The team recognized the need for an emergency surgical airway to prevent hypoxic brain injury and a cricothyroidotomy was performed. Maintenance of anaesthesia was established and the patient was transferred to a regional neurosurgical centre. The patient subsequently made a full neurological recovery. The medical team had undergone simulator-based training to rehearse the management of life-threatening complications, and as a result were able to successfully perform the life-saving cricothyroidotomy.

Record keeping

The medico-legal management of anaesthetic complications hinges in part on the accompanying documentation. A detailed pre-operative assessment which includes, for example, the presence of poor dentition accompanied by an explanation of the risk of dental damage can considerably help both the patient and the anaesthetist when faced with such complications. Record keeping, including of events and discussion both before and after an incident, therefore form an important aspect of managing a complication.

Incident reporting

Part of managing a complication involves sharing lessons learned. All UK anaesthetic departments are required to hold regular governance meetings during which such incidents can be discussed. Presentations at regional and national meetings, as well as formal written publications, are another way of doing this. Furthermore, complications that have resulted in harm or a serious 'near-miss' must be reported for risk management purposes to a local and/or national registry. In the UK, the National Patient Safety Agency (NPSA) provides one such registry.

Systems for managing complications

The Australian Patient Safety Foundation published a Crisis Management Manual, one of the first and most comprehensive to be published. This manual recognizes that a predetermined sequence of actions could be used by anaesthetists to respond to unanticipated incidents. It contains a series of algorithms that are designed to reduce the risk of harm that results from a spectrum of possible complications both common and rare. Knowledge of and an ability to put into practice these algorithms can be readily rehearsed and tested by simulation.

Case 2.4: Can't intubate, can't ventilate

A fit and healthy 37-year-old patient was scheduled for sinus surgery, for which a laryngeal mask airway was planned by an experienced anaesthetist. Following induction the lady developed trismus. A further bolus of sedation was administered but hypoxia developed due to two further unsuccessful attempts at laryngeal insertion. A facemask and oral adjuncts were used in an attempt to provide ventilation but this too was unsuccessful. A second consultant anaesthetist arrived to provide additional help but despite this and several attempts at direct laryngoscopy, the consultants were unable to intubate or ventilate. Twenty minutes of profound hypoxia ensued. Eventually an intubating laryngeal mask was inserted, which allowed some ventilation. Oxygenation was restored and the planned procedure was abandoned. The lady was admitted to the recovery room breathing spontaneously. However, she never regained consciousness and died from a hypoxic brain injury 13 days later in the intensive care unit. An investigation into the incident found that during the repeated attempts to provide oxygenation a surgical tracheostomy set had been made available but was not used. An ear nose and throat consultant surgeon was present in the anaesthetic room throughout the events.

In 2005, Elaine Bromiley died as a result of problems that developed during anaesthesia for elective surgery. An investigation found that the management of the anaesthetic complication, namely the inability to either intubate or ventilate, was inappropriate. Among the recommendations from the investigation were suggestions relating to technical skills (including enhancing equipment familiarity) but also those relating to human factors ('*Ensure an atmosphere of good communication in the operating theatre such that any member of staff feels comfortable to make suggestions on treatment*').

Since then, and in part due to the creation of the Clinical Human Factors Group by her husband, an airline pilot, errors have become culturally more accepted as something to be expected and managed.

The anaesthetists involved had both the knowledge and technical skills required to manage the 'can't intubate, can't ventilate' scenario. It was human behaviours that prevented them from applying their knowledge and skills successfully.

Some systems within the UK, for example Scotland's Emergency Medical Retrieval Service or England's Magpas Pre-Hospital Emergency Medical Teams, have developed emergency action checklists for managing anaesthesia-related complications (Figures 2.1 and 2.2). These contain a series of steps to be followed in the event of a life-threatening complication (e.g. persistent hypoxia in an anaesthetized patient) and are based on emergency checklists used in the aviation industry.

There is currently little evidence to suggest that such manuals or checklists are able to significantly reduce the harm that follows a complication, though in line with the use of preoperative surgical checklists in the UK there is mounting evidence that human errors can be reduced by systematic approaches to the complex anaesthesia and surgical environment.

In addition to the availability of such tools and frameworks, the benefits of rehearsing the management of anaesthetic complications is also increasingly clear. Simulation has advanced a great deal in recent years and patient simulators are increasingly available to allow the practice of actions in a safe learning environment. The 2010 Royal College of Anaesthetist's Anaesthesia Curriculum for Basic Level Training outlines the need for over forty 'critical incident' competencies all of which, the curriculum states, are amenable to simulation. Other assessment methods for incident management include, case-based discussion, clinical evaluation exercises and written examination.

Simulation lends itself well to teaching teams about using the environment and colleagues to best manage a complication. Crisis resource management (CRM, sometimes termed crew or team resource management) originates from aviation practice and refers to a team's ability to use the hardware, software and behaviours available to them to avert and manage crises. Having demonstrated the benefits of good CRM within anaesthetic practice an increasing number of CRM courses are now available to anaesthetists.

SpO$_2$ <92% (Ventilated Patient)
EMERGENCY ACTION CHECKLIST

Inform team of problem

Check probe is on patient & apply oximax forehead oximetry now
Check pulse & BP - exclude cardiac arrest / low cardiac output state
Check EtCO$_2$ - exclude oesophageal intubation

Airway

If chest not rising → change to BVM with 100% O$_2$

☐ Check gas supply failure indicator shows white & cylinder full + turned on
☐ Ensure that 100% oxygen being given (see reverse)
☐ Ensure continuous mandotory ventilation selected (see reverse)
☐ Check the integrity of breathing circuit from ET tube to ventilator
☐ Check ETT cuff adequately inflated (listen for leak at mouth with ventilation)
☐ Check there is no leak from sampling port on filter & port on catheter mount
☐ Ensure ET tube length appropriate (20–22cm) – use aide memoir for children

Breathing

☐ Look for and treat pneumothoraces (see reverse)
☐ Check End Tidal CO$_2$
      – if high (>5.5mmHg) then increase respiratory rate and tidal volume
      – if low (>4.0mmHg) exclude oesophageal intubation or hypotension
☐ Pass suction catheter down ET tube to remove blood / secretions
☐ Change filter if heavily blood / fluid soiled
☐ Minimize dead space in circuit in children (e.g. remove Easycap)
☐ Check tidal volume set to 7ml/kg (chest should rise 1–2cm)
☐ Recruit alveoli using BVM
☐ Insert oro/nasogastric tube

Circulation

☐ Recheck blood pressure / peripheral pulses
☐ Exclude arrhythmias – AF / VF / VT / asystole
☐ Control bleeding (traction splint / pressure / CAT / pelvic splint)
☐ Give 250ml fluid bolus to maintain good peripheral pulse / SBP >100
☐ Look for and treat causes of shock (4Hs 4Ts)

Drugs

☐ Give atracurium if >15 mins since last dose

Evaluate

☐ Does the problem persist? Are there any other problems? Can DAD help?

Persistent unexplained hypoxia is most likely the result of respiratory or circulatory failure secondary to injury.
Perform thoracostomies if hypoxia persists in presence of a chest injury.
© Magpas 2010

Figure 2.1 Pre-hospital 'Emergency Action Checklist' for managing hypoxia in a mechanically ventilated patient. (With permission from Magpas.)

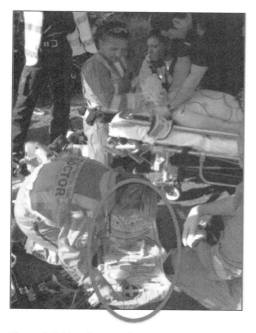 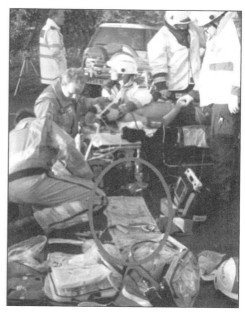

Figure 2.2 Use of a pre-induction anaesthetic checklist in a high-risk pre-hospital environment.

Summary

Complications are common and are to be expected. The way in which the complication is managed, and in particular the anaesthetist's knowledge, skills and behaviours, will have a profound effect on the patient's outcome. A systematic approach at both an individual and organizational level whilst embracing an understanding of human factors can help reduce the risks associated with anaesthetic complications.

List of further reading

Australian Patient Safety Foundation. Anaesthesia Crisis Management Manual. www.apsf.com.au/crisis_management/Crisis_Management_Start.htm (accessed 15 April 2011).

Barach, P. & Small, S. D. Reporting and preventing medical mishaps: lessons from non-medical near miss reporting systems. *BMJ* 2000; **320**: 759–63.

British Journal of Anaesthesia. Postgraduate educational issue: human factors in anaesthesia and critical care. *Br J Anaes* 2010; **105**: 1–90.

Clinical Human Factors Group. www.chfg.org/ (accessed 15 April 2011).

Cook, T. M., Bland, L., Mihai, R. & Scott, S. Litigation related to anaesthesia: an analysis of claims against the NHS in England 1995–2007. *Anaesthesia* 2009; **64**: 706–18.

Hemreich, R. L. On error management: lessons from aviation. *BMJ* 2000; **320**: 781–5.

Chapter

3

Risk management

Mark Dougherty and Stephen T. Webb

Introduction

Risk is the potential for danger, harm, damage or loss. In the context of healthcare, risk is principally applied to patient safety and the possibility of harm that is inherent to the exposure to healthcare services.

Within anaesthesia, critical incident reporting is an established means of gathering information regarding risks and hazards. The critical incident has been defined by the Royal College of Anaesthetists (RCA) as an incident 'that could have led to harm and could have been prevented by a change in process'. When serious failures in the provision of healthcare do happen they have profound effects on patients, their families and healthcare personnel. Risk minimization is the principle that all healthcare providers strive for.

However, many patients are harmed by interaction with healthcare services and this is a growing problem. Risks are inevitable in society and healthcare is not an exception. Runciman has defined risk management as the process of risk reduction to a level deemed acceptable to society.

In the UK, risk management has become an increasingly formalized process within the National Health Service (NHS) over the past ten years. A pilot study performed in 2001 showed an 11% incidence of adverse events for all hospital admissions. This figure correlates with the data from the two landmark trials from the US and Australia. The Harvard study of medical practice performed in 1991 determined an adverse event incidence of 4%, 69% of which were deemed preventable. The study of Australian healthcare quality found a rate of 17%, over half of which were considered preventable. The UK Department of Health (DoH) has used these figures to estimate a frequency of 850,000 adverse events per year, costing a projected additional £2 billion. Litigation settlements declared by the NHS Litigation Authority (NHSLA) rose from £400 million in 1998/99 to £787 million in 2009/10.

The process of risk management involves four processes: identification, assessment, resolution and re-evaluation.

Risk identification

Anaesthesia has been at the forefront in the field of patient safety. In 1978, Cooper first described the process of critical incident analysis to reduce the risk related to anaesthesia using a process modified from the aviation industry. Critical incident analysis forms a cornerstone in determining risks to patients and staff. The mantle for patient safety in

Anaesthetic and Perioperative Complications, ed. Kamen Valchanov, Stephen T. Webb and Jane Sturgess. Published by Cambridge University Press. © Cambridge University Press 2011.

anaesthesia was subsequently progressed in the US by the Anesthetic Patient Safety Forum, and the formation of the closed claim project by the American Society of Anesthesiologists (ASA). The Australian Patient Safety Foundation was formed in 1988 and subsequently coordinated the Australian Incident Monitoring Study, which used critical incident reporting and analysis in order to improve patient safety. Initially the reporting system was specialty-specific, but has evolved to incorporate multiple specialties. In the UK the National Patient Safety Agency (NPSA) was formed in 2001 following the publication of the Department of Health document *An Organization with a Memory*, which raised concerns regarding the ability of the NHS to learn from past mistakes. The NPSA subsequently developed the largest national reporting system for medical critical incidents, the National Reporting and Learning System (NRLS).

Catastrophic incidents within anaesthesia are relatively rare. However, critical incidents and near-miss events are a common occurrence, and may highlight deficiencies in processes that may result in patient harm. Until recently the process for incident analysis remained at a local level. The NRLS provides an excellent opportunity for safety lessons from near-miss events to be disseminated nationally.

Reporting of critical incidents is essential. Having a system that is easily accessible, anonymous and within a culture that encourages reporting should form the basis of an incident reporting system. Analysis of incident reports will only result in meaningful outcomes if the content is comprehensive. During the initial phase of the NRLS, the generic nature of the reporting forms contributed to difficulty in forming meaningful conclusions for action. The result is the development of specialty-specific reporting forms such as the Electronic Anaesthetic Reporting Form, a collaboration between the NPSA and the Safe Anaesthesia Liaison Group (SALG).

Other forms of data collation include closed claims analysis and similar reports from medical defence organisations and the National Health Service Litigation Authority. Root cause analysis, an in-depth investigation of a critical incident, is increasingly used to determine deficiencies in the process of care. Local morbidity and mortality meetings are helpful to identify local risks and permit open discussion. Clinical audit is a useful tool, which permits continual assessment of the efficacy and safety of current practice.

Risk assessment

Errors in patient care will occur and must be expected. However, the events leading to human error are often complex. Many factors involved in healthcare provision may compromise patient safety. The majority of these occur before anaesthesia. Blaming the individual overlooks organizational failures. This approach allows these events to occur again and the risk to continue.

The analysis of the human factor component of medical errors has been well described by Reason (2000) and includes the consideration of active failures and latent failures (Table 3.1). Active failures include cognitive failures (e.g. memory lapses or ignorance) or violations (e.g. deviation from standard safe practice guidelines), and incorporate the factors that may have led to the individual producing the error. Latent factors are those factors that are insidious deficiencies within the environment and organizational system. Latent factors may not produce errors until a certain set of circumstances occur. Vincent *et al.* (1998) describe a framework for the analysis of critical incidents that includes an understanding of both active and latent failures. This system incorporates the analysis of a number

Table 3.1 Active and latent failures.

Failure	Example
Latent	*Organisation failure* – reducing maintenance/updating of equipment to save money *Supervision failure* – inexperienced surgeon and inexperienced anaesthetist attempting an unfamiliar case *Conditions allowing unsafe acts* – fatigued anaesthetist or improper communication
Active	*Unsafe acts* – medical misdiagnosis or incorrect procedure

of domains, including institutional, organisational, environmental, team, individual, task and patient factors. Using this framework a critical incident may be correctly seen in the context of the healthcare system.

Risk resolution

Methods to reduce risk to minimal levels may include physical barriers, e.g. restricting access to concentrated potassium solutions and ensuring gas cylinder yokes are not interchangeable between oxygen and nitrous oxide. Other barriers are less robust, e.g. the reduction of drug administration errors by colour-coded syringe labelling. The *SaferSleep* system, developed in New Zealand and now available in the UK, is a computer system designed to interact with barcode-labelled syringes scanned prior to patient administration.

Some of the most successful methods of improving patient safety come from the development of recommendations and guidelines as a response to critical incident analysis. Examples include the AAGBI minimum monitoring standards for anaesthesia, the AAGBI pre-operative anaesthetic machine checklist and the WHO surgical safety checklist.

Absolute error reduction can be supplemented by training to recognize errors at an early stage and to prevent serious harm. Crisis management training is now established and frequently includes simulation training. Simulation permits experiential learning opportunities with events that are infrequent but serious. Often experience influences the ability of a practitioner to reduce the incidence of adverse events and also to recover from a critical incident before permanent damage ensues.

Increasing emphasis is being placed on improving the non-technical skills of anaesthetists as a method of reducing errors. The Anaesthetists' Non-Technical Skills (ANTS) framework for training and assessment has been developed at the University of Aberdeen. Similar processes exist within aviation and in healthcare crisis management in the US. Non-technical skills incorporate four skill strategies, including: task management (planning and preparation, ability to prioritize, identification of resources); situation awareness (anticipation, the ability to gather information); decision making (the ability to identify options and balance the risks involved); and team working (coordinating activities, interchange of information, assertiveness). Although evidence to conclude that training in ANTS reduces patient harm is currently lacking, the improvement in the ability to remain aware of the environment, improve communication and interact with the dynamic surroundings of theatre can enhance safety.

Most risk reduction strategies are generic and may be applied to all surgical disciplines. Others may require tailoring for risks particular to the discipline. The FOCUS (focused operative cardiovascular unified systems) Project is currently being undertaken by the Society of Cardiovascular Anaesthesiologists (SCA) in the USA. It aims to reduce patient risk in cardiac surgery by first identifying and analyzing potential hazards, then using a holistic approach to work with the theatre team encompassing clinical hazards and non-technical skills. Although this project remains in its infancy it promises to produce a novel and effective means of improving patient safety.

Re-evaluation

Following the institution of methods to reduce risk it is imperative that risk-reduction procedures be reviewed for effectiveness. Robust local and national policies and audit practices with prompt analysis and feedback are essential. Patient safety is more than safe anaesthesia. Anaesthesia has been at the forefront in the nascent field of patient safety. Many ongoing projects pioneered within anaesthesia will continue to push this vital field forward. It is the responsibility of all of us to ensure that we continue to strive for improvements in safe patient care.

List of further reading

Brennan, T. A., Leape, L. L., Laird, N. M. *et al.* Incidence of adverse events and negligence in hospitalized patients. Results of the Harvard Medical Practice Study I. *N Engl J Med* 1991; **324**: 370–6.

Catchpole, K., Bell, M. D. & Johnson, S. Safety in anaesthesia: a study of 12,606 reported incidents from the UK National Reporting and Learning System. *Anaesthesia* 2008; **63**: 340–6.

Cooper, J. B., Newbower, R. S., Long, C. D. *et al.* Preventable anesthesia mishaps: a study of human factors. *Anesthesiology* 1978; **49**: 399–406.

Department of Health Expert Group (Chairman, CMO). *An Organisation with a Memory: Report of an Expert Group on Learning from Adverse Events in the NHS.* London: Department of Health, 2000.

Flin, R., Patey, R., Glavin, R. *et al.* Anaesthetists' non-technical skills. *Br J Anaesth* 2010; **105**: 38–44.

Martinez, E. A., Marsteller, J. A., Thompson, D. A. *et al.* The Society of Cardiovascular Anesthesiologists' FOCUS initiative: Locating Errors through Networked Surveillance (LENS) project vision. *Anesth Analg* 2010; **110**: 307–11.

Merry, A. F. Safety in anaesthesia: reporting incidents and learning from them. *Anaesthesia* 2008; **63**: 337–9.

Reason, J. Human error: models and management. *West J Med* 2000; **172**: 393–6.

Runciman, W. B., Webb, R. K., Lee, R. *et al.* The Australian Incident Monitoring Study. System failure: an analysis of 2000 incident reports. *Anaesth Intensive Care* 1993; **21**: 684–95.

Vincent, C., Taylor-Adams, S. & Stanhope, N. Framework for analyzing risk and safety in clinical medicine. *BMJ* 1998; **316**: 1154–7.

Vincent, C., Neale, G. & Woloshynowych, M. Adverse events in British hospitals: preliminary retrospective record review. *BMJ* 2001; **322**: 517–19.

Webster, C. S., Larsson, L., Frampton, C. M. *et al.* Clinical assessment of a new anaesthetic drug administration system: a prospective, controlled, longitudinal incident monitoring study. *Anaesthesia* 2010; **65**: 490–9.

Chapter

4

Airway complications during anaesthesia

Nick Woodall and Helen Goddard

Introduction

The goal of airway management is to safely maintain ventilation and prevent contamination of the patient's lungs. Following induction of general anaesthesia control of the airway moves from patient to anaesthetist. Airway interventions by the anaesthetist may be responsible for adverse events. Most airway complications are minor and require no treatment but add to the morbidity and discomfort attributed to anaesthesia. Dental damage is the most common cause of anaesthesia-related litigation. Airway trauma, aspiration and prolonged hypoxia can result in severe harm or death. Recent UK figures show complications resulting from airway events account for 20% of the most expensive anaesthesia-related claims settled by the National Health Service Litigation Authority (NHSLA). Aside from the time and expense involved in processing these cases, many of these unfortunate patients, their relatives and anaesthesia providers suffer long-term consequences following serious adverse events.

Approach to airway management

Airway problems may occur at any stage of an anaesthetic. Most (70%) events occur at induction of anaesthesia or during emergence or recovery (15%). These are high-stress periods for anaesthetists as complex pharmacological, physiological and pathological interactions take place. Airway problems often present at a time when the anaesthetist may be distracted by other considerations. When oxygenation is compromised time is limited and prompt action is needed if severe hypoxia and brain injury or death is to be avoided. All anaesthetists should have an airway strategy for managing unexpected problems with mask ventilation and tracheal intubation, including the 'can't ventilate, can't intubate' (CVCI) scenario. The Difficult Airway Society (DAS) have produced guidelines for management of the unanticipated difficult intubation. These guidelines outline the options for maintaining oxygenation and have been widely adopted. An airway strategy (Figure 4.1) should incorporate alternative methods of ventilation, including surgical airway. For the plan to be effective it must be compatible with the skills of the anaesthetist and the equipment available. Airway management plans should emphasize the need to get help, to limit airway trauma by making best use of each intervention, to re-appraise the situation regularly and if feasible to abandon attempts before serious harm results.

Anaesthetic and Perioperative Complications, ed. Kamen Valchanov, Stephen T. Webb and Jane Sturgess.
Published by Cambridge University Press. © Cambridge University Press 2011.

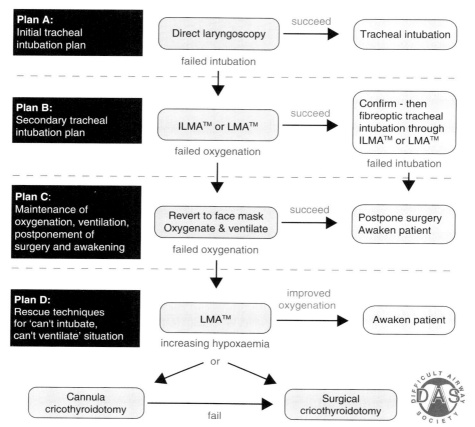

Figure 4.1 Difficult Airway Society failed intubation guidelines. Reproduced with permission from the Difficult Airway Society.

Common symptoms after general anaesthesia

Symptoms suggestive of airway trauma are common (Table 4.1) after general anaesthesia and do not necessarily indicate a problem unless they are very severe or prolonged. Anticholinergic drugs, particularly glycopyrrolate, commonly cause a dry throat. Minor injury and irritation of the pharynx, larynx and trachea can occur after airway insertion or instrumentation. Mucosal erythema, oedema, bruising and haematoma may be observed. The severity of symptoms increase with movement of a device within the airway, use of larger airways or tubes, prolonged duration of use and with higher cuff inflation pressures. Dysphagia is more common following laryngeal mask airway (LMA) use than after tracheal intubation. Recent trends towards tracheal intubation without recourse to neuromuscular blocking drugs are associated with increased incidence of postoperative sore throat.

Aetiology of airway complications

General anaesthesia reduces airway muscle tone and obtunds airway protective reflexes, leaving the airway vulnerable to obstruction or contamination. Airway obstruction impairs gas exchange and oxygenation. Uptake of anaesthetic gases may be delayed leading to

Table 4.1 Incidence of minor morbidity following LMA and tracheal tube use.

Complaint	ETT	LMA
Sore throat	14–50%	5.8–34%
Hoarseness	50%	25%
Dysphagia	12%	24%
Cough	18–28%	<18%
Dry throat	70%	<70%

inadequate anaesthesia and awareness. Contamination of the respiratory tract usually results from gastrointestinal contents or blood. Airway complications result from obstruction, and contamination, or from the methods used to prevent them. The timing of airway events in relation to the stages of anaesthesia is shown in Table 4.2. A problem with the airway can precipitate a whole series of further complications, like a line of falling dominoes. Reviewing each problem in isolation unfortunately creates a gross oversimplification of what may present a very difficult and challenging clinical problem.

Table 4.2 Timing of perioperative airway problems.

At induction

– Airway obstruction

– Misplaced airway device

– Aspiration

– Awareness/inadequate anaesthesia

– Airway trauma

During airway management under local anaesthetic

– As above, plus possible local anaesthetic toxicity

Perioperative problems

– Aspiration

– Displaced airway device

– Leaks

  • equipment failure

  • surgical interference

– Airway fires

Postoperative problems

– Aspiration

– Airway obstruction

  • laryngospasm

  • laryngeal oedema

  • throat pack

  • blood clot

  • neck haematoma

Airway obstruction

Airway obstruction is very common under general anaesthesia due to loss of tone within the musculature supporting the airway. Basic airway management manoeuvres such as jaw thrust, head extension or the insertion of an artificial airway usually remedy the problem. Uncorrected airway obstruction leads to inadequate ventilation, hypoxaemia, brain damage, cardiac arrest or death. Possible sites of airway obstruction are shown in Table 4.3.

The clinical features of airway obstruction vary depending on whether the patient is breathing spontaneously or if breathing is controlled. Conscious patients may exhibit distress, anxiety or restlessness with paradoxical movement of the abdomen and chest. Inspiratory stridor indicates severe narrowing of the extra thoracic airway. Intra thoracic lesions tend to produce expiratory stridor as the airway is compressed during exhalation. Manual lung inflation of apnoeic patients may be impossible.

Table 4.3 Causes of airway obstruction by site.

Within the lumen of the airway
Occluded or misplaced airway device
Gastric contents
Tumour
Foreign body
Blood clot
By the wall
Loss of airway muscle tone or tracheomalacia
Laryngospasm
Tumour
Oedema
External compression
Goitre
Tumour
Neck haematoma causes laryngeal oedema not compression

Anticipated airway obstruction

Airway obstruction should be anticipated in patients with pre-operative airway obstruction and in those with a recognized anatomical problem. There may be a clear anatomical barrier such as limitation of mouth opening, neck problems or known complications during previous anaesthesia.

Anticipated airway obstruction following pre-operative airway obstruction

Obstructive lesions within the airway are not uncommon and may present with severe respiratory distress and stridor. They may require urgent tracheal intubation or an

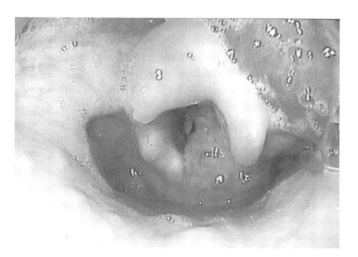

Figure 4.2 Laryngeal hemangioma: distorted laryngeal anatomy may impair ventilation and intubation attempts.

emergency surgical airway. This group represents the most common reason for CVCI during anaesthesia. Causes include laryngeal tumours (Figure 4.2), epiglottitis, laryngeal oedema, or foreign body within the airway. If direct laryngoscopy is attempted the anatomy may be unrecognizable and tracheal intubation difficult or impossible.

Difficult airway management should be expected in patients with advanced airway obstruction. Airway imaging and nasendoscopy findings should be reviewed if available. Total airway obstruction may occur at any time and the need for a surgical airway must be anticipated. Good communication is required between all theatre staff. The anticipated problems and the planned solutions should be made clear to all. A tracheostomy performed under local anaesthesia may be the primary plan. Where tracheal intubation is the preferred airway management option this should still take place in an operating theatre. An experienced surgeon should be scrubbed and ready to proceed to a surgical airway if either mask ventilation or tracheal intubation is impossible. The aim is to achieve maximal oxygenation, therefore 100% oxygen should be used. Inhalational general anaesthesia is slow and difficult in these patients. Spontaneous ventilation may improve during induction with application of CPAP but coughing or premature instrumentation of the airway may precipitate total airway obstruction. Preoxygenation, IV induction and muscle relaxant provides optimal conditions for laryngoscopy, tracheal intubation or an emergency surgical airway if required. This imposes a strict time limit. If mask ventilation is found to be impossible an early surgical airway is needed. Where mask ventilation is possible and laryngoscopy suggests tracheal intubation may be difficult or traumatic it may be safer to avoid tracheal intubation altogether and proceed directly to tracheostomy.

Large or fine bore cricothyroidotomy and surgical cricothyroidotomy are alternatives to emergency tracheostomy. Cricothyroidotomy is usually the quickest route to restore ventilation and oxygenation in an acute emergency. The theatre team must be familiar with the equipment and have had the opportunity to practise the technique. Intrathoracic lesions of trachea represent a particular challenge. They cannot be bypassed with an emergency surgical airway; instead a small tracheal tube (TT), or rigid bronchoscope, should be passed alongside the lesion.

Anticipated airway obstruction due to an anatomical problem

Anatomical abnormalities such as extreme neck flexion or reduced mouth opening indicate that facemask ventilation or direct laryngoscopy will be difficult or impossible. Documented problems with mask ventilation and tracheal intubation during previous operations are likely to recur during subsequent anaesthetics. When difficulty is anticipated, fibreoptic intubation under local anaesthetic is accepted as a safe form of airway management. Spontaneous breathing is maintained, oxygenation is preserved and if awake intubation fails other options remain available. Patient cooperation is required for awake intubation. This may be a problem with some adults and children.

Airway complications during awake intubation

The ASA closed claims studies show serious and fatal complications have been reported during attempted awake fibreoptic intubation. Complete airway obstruction may follow the administration of sedation or the application of local anaesthetic to the airway in patients with severe upper airway obstruction. Sedation must be administered cautiously and monitored closely. Short-acting drugs with an available antagonist are ideal. Over-sedation leads to loss of airway control. The British Thoracic Society recommends doses of up to 8.4 mg/kg lidocaine for diagnostic bronchoscopy. Lidocaine toxicity is unlikely to be a problem if the dose of topical lidocaine remains within this limit. Generous use of local anaesthetic is preferable to over-sedation. However, caution with local anaesthetic dosage should be exercised in patients with severe liver disease as first pass metabolism may be inpaired, leading to higher blood lidocaine levels.

Unanticipated difficulty with ventilation

Problems with ventilation can occur at any stage of anaesthesia. Airway obstruction is not the only cause of impaired ventilation. Possible causes are most logically considered anatomically starting with the delivery system and ending at the chest wall (Figure 4.3). Management of the problem is dictated by the cause. More than one cause may present simultaneously.

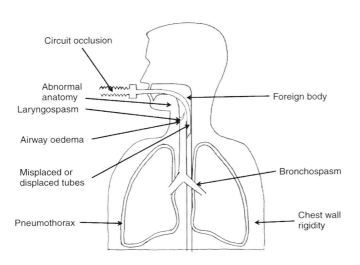

Figure 4.3 Causes of airway obstruction or difficulty with ventilation.

Anatomical factors

Abnormal patient anatomy such as the presence of a lingual tonsil may unexpectedly impede mask ventilation or tracheal intubation. The incidence of difficult facemask ventilation has been quoted as 1.4 to 5%. The incidence of impossible mask ventilation is approximately 0.15% and of those patients who are impossible to ventilate approximately 25% are difficult to intubate. Factors suggesting difficult facemask ventilation are shown in Table 4.4 and those suggesting difficulty with intubation are shown in Table 4.5.

Table 4.4 Factors suggesting difficult facemask ventilation.

1. History of snoring or sleep apnoea
2. Obesity
3. Neck immobility
4. Neck radiation changes
5. The presence of a beard
6. Male sex
7. Mallampati score of >2

Table 4.5 Indicators of a potential difficult intubation.

1. Long upper incisors
2. Receding mandible
3. Class 3 occlusion, unable to advance lower teeth to meet upper teeth
4. Inter-incisor distance <3 cm
5. Mallampati >2
6. High-arched or narrow palate
7. Thyromental distance <5 cm
8. Mandibular space limited, stiff or indurated
9. Short neck
10. Thick neck
11. Reduced neck movement

Routine airway assessment seeks features suggestive of difficulty with mask ventilation. If difficulty occurs insertion of a supraglottic airway (SGA), a tracheal tube (TT) or an emergency surgical airway may be needed. Alternative anaesthetic techniques or intubation under local anaesthesia should be considered.

The Difficult Airway Society created guidelines on *the Management of Unanticipated Difficulty with Tracheal Intubation*. These are based on a series of plans to manage tracheal intubation and oxygenation. The guidelines recommend limited blind instrumentation of the airway in favour of low-skill fibreoptic intubation (through a LMA) and re-appraisal of the situation. If intubation fails, further attempts and anaesthesia are abandoned, when appropriate. Oxygenation techniques include the use of two-person bag-mask-ventilation, supraglottic airway insertion or an emergency surgical airway (Figure 4.4).

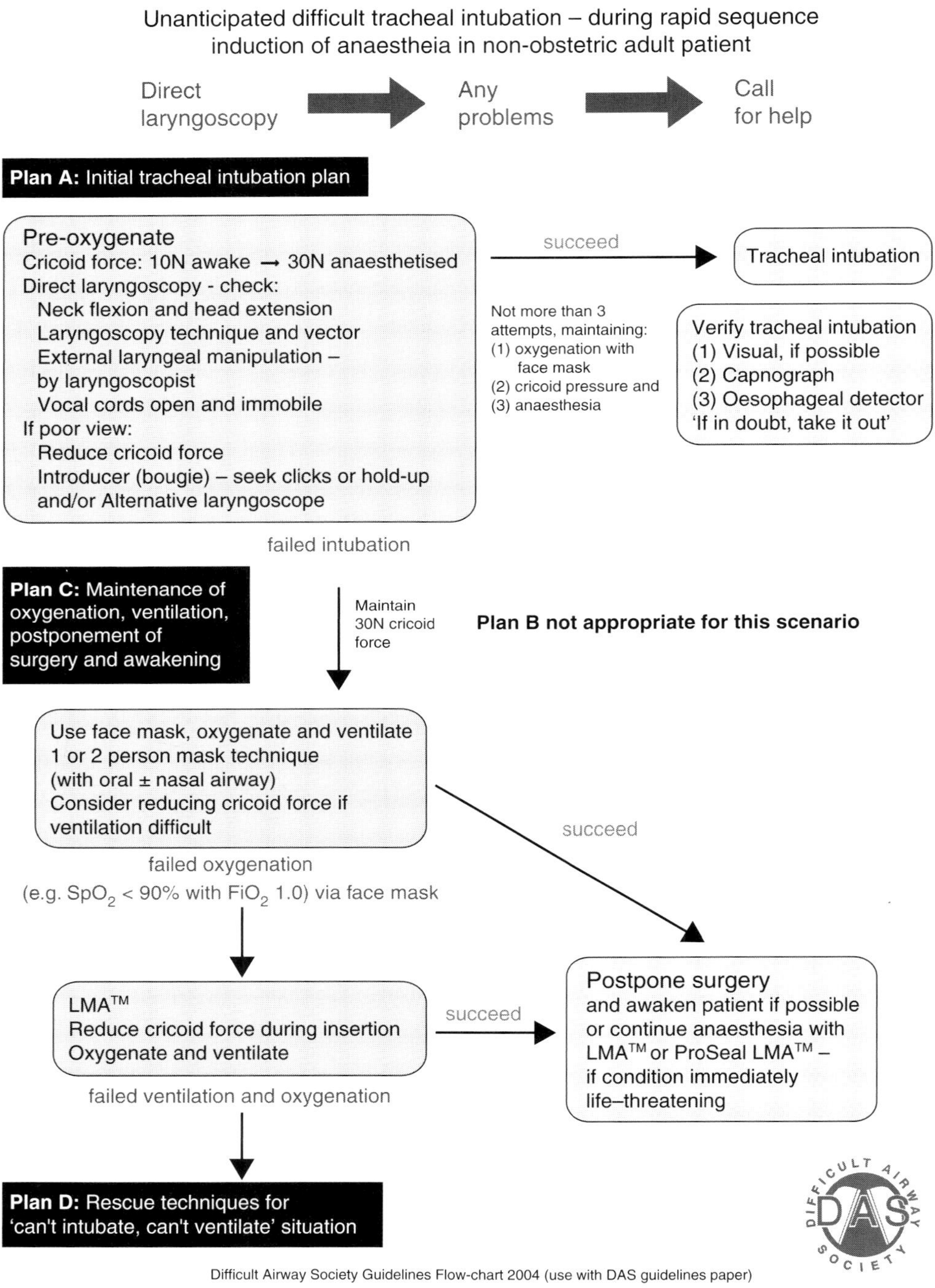

Unanticipated difficult tracheal intubation – during rapid sequence induction of anaestheia in non-obstetric adult patient

Direct laryngoscopy ➡ Any problems ➡ Call for help

Plan A: Initial tracheal intubation plan

Pre-oxygenate
Cricoid force: 10N awake → 30N anaesthetised
Direct laryngoscopy - check:
  Neck flexion and head extension
  Laryngoscopy technique and vector
  External laryngeal manipulation –
  by laryngoscopist
  Vocal cords open and immobile
If poor view:
  Reduce cricoid force
  Introducer (bougie) – seek clicks or hold-up
  and/or Alternative laryngoscope

succeed → Tracheal intubation

Not more than 3 attempts, maintaining:
(1) oxygenation with face mask
(2) cricoid pressure and
(3) anaesthesia

Verify tracheal intubation
(1) Visual, if possible
(2) Capnograph
(3) Oesophageal detector
'If in doubt, take it out'

failed intubation

Plan C: Maintenance of oxygenation, ventilation, postponement of surgery and awakening

Maintain 30N cricoid force

Plan B not appropriate for this scenario

Use face mask, oxygenate and ventilate
1 or 2 person mask technique
(with oral ± nasal airway)
Consider reducing cricoid force if
ventilation difficult

succeed

failed oxygenation
(e.g. $SpO_2 < 90\%$ with FiO_2 1.0) via face mask

LMA™
Reduce cricoid force during insertion
Oxygenate and ventilate

succeed →

Postpone surgery
and awaken patient if possible
or continue anaesthesia with
LMA™ or ProSeal LMA™ –
if condition immediately
life–threatening

failed ventilation and oxygenation

Plan D: Rescue techniques for 'can't intubate, can't ventilate' situation

Difficult Airway Society Guidelines Flow-chart 2004 (use with DAS guidelines paper)

Figure 4.4 Difficult Airway Society unanticipated difficult tracheal intubation during rapid sequence induction. Reproduced with permission from the Difficult Airway Society.

Inadequate anaesthesia or laryngospasm

Laryngospasm may result from stimulation of the upper airway during light levels of anaesthesia. Blood, gastric contents or an artificial airway may be the trigger. Laryngospasm may follow removal of the tracheal tube or supraglottic airway device (SAD). It is also seen with visceral stimulation during surgery, and stimulation of the patient at light levels of anaesthesia should be avoided.

Management should include clearance and opening of the airway with application of 100% oxygen by bag and mask. Continuous positive airway pressure produced by partial closure of the expiratory valve may provide some improvement, as may administration of a sedative dose of induction agent or benzodiazepine. In severe cases administration of suxamethonium will be needed to relieve complete closure of the vocal cords.

Misplaced tracheal tube or airway device

Tracheal tube misplacement or unrecognized oesophageal intubation (OI) has catastrophic consequences and remains an important cause of serious airway morbidity and mortality. Evidence from ASA closed claims studies shows capnography has reduced the frequency of OI in the operating room environment. Oesophageal intubation during emergency airway management outside theatre ranges from 6.7 to 9.7% of intubations.

Oesophageal intubation is more likely if the glottis cannot be seen by direct laryngoscopy and the tracheal tube is placed blindly. Difficult intubation is more likely to occur in inexperienced hands and in isolated locations. Furthermore after difficulty inserting a tracheal tube most practitioners are extremely reluctant to remove it without clear evidence that it is incorrectly placed.

Observation of exhaled CO_2 by capnography after more than three breaths or by endoscopic visualization of the carina with a fibreoptic endoscope are reliable methods of confirming correct placement of the tracheal tube. Where this is not done severe hypoxia and death will continue to occur from oesophageal intubation. Failure to detect exhaled CO_2 in cases of OI has been attributed to cardiac arrest, anaphylaxis or equipment malfunction. Capnography is unavailable on most hospital wards and in some emergency departments and intensive therapy units (ITUs).

Inadvertant OI is not entirely preventable. Even where anaesthetists report that they have seen a TT pass between the vocal cords OI still occurs. Humans are fallible; we sometimes see what we expect to see.

If the tracheal tube has been misplaced the patient requires urgent oxygenation and re-intubation. Where the misplaced TT has been used for ventilation, gastric distension may lead to regurgitation as the tube is removed from the oesophagus.

Displacement of a TT or airway displacement is most likely when the surgeon requires access to the head and neck. Flexion of the head can lead to accidental extubation particularly in children. Extubation is of concern if the patient is apnoeic, or at risk of aspiration, since the lower airway will be unprotected. Effective TT fixation is the solution. Patients with a known difficult airway or in the prone position require greater attention to secure TT fixation.

Foreign body

Perioperative sources of foreign body include misplaced or displaced airway devices, dislodged dentition, gastric contents, retained throat packs and clotted blood. The latter two should be suspected in the presence of airway obstruction after ENT or maxillofacial surgery.

Blood may pool and form a clot in the posterior nasopharynx. Displaced clot can be inhaled or obstruct the airway, 'the coroner's clot'. At the end of surgery the nasopharynx should be cleared and the patient positioned to encourage blood to drain away from the airway.

The use of a throat pack should be justified before placement. Insertion and removal must be documented on the anaesthetic chart and the pack should be included on the theatre swab count. An external indication of the presence of a throat pack, such as a label, should be placed on the patient. Documentation of the presence of a throat pack is a feature of the pre-operative WHO checklist.

Airway oedema

Airway oedema can be a manifestation of an allergic reaction. It may also develop secondary to increased venous pressure produced by haematoma in the neck or following a prolonged period in a head-down position during surgery. Oedema may follow traumatic instrumentation of the airway by a surgeon or anaesthetist leading to complete airway obstruction. This can be problematic at intubation and extubation.

Where possible blind intubation attempts should be avoided. Modern video-laryngoscopes offer a better view of the laryngeal inlet. Alternatively fibreoptic intubation or low-skill fibreoptic intubation through a supraglottic airway are safer alternatives to blind techniques using a bougie. Oxygenation is the priority and may require early recourse to a surgical airway. Intravenous dexamethasone is often used to reduce airway oedema but it may be necessary to delay extubation until swelling subsides.

Circuit occlusion

This is a rare problem but faulty equipment is a very serious cause of airway obstruction and problems with ventilation. Blocked tubes, circuits and catheter mounts may present as total airway obstruction. This has been falsely attributed to asthma or anaphylaxis with fatal consequences. The patency of the whole gas delivery system from the circuit to the alveoli should be considered. A backup system for hand ventilation should be immediately available at all anaesthetic locations. It may be necessary to change the whole circuit to rapidly restore oxygenation whilst the problem is located. If tracheal tube obstruction occurs it should be removed and replaced or mask ventilation performed.

Bronchospasm, pneumothorax and chest-wall rigidity

Bronchospasm, pneumothorax and chest-wall rigidity may all cause difficulty with ventilation. Severe chest-wall rigidity has been attributed to opioids such as remifentanil. However, total airway obstruction has been misdiagnosed as bronchospasm.

Secondary complications and their management

Post-obstructive pulmonary oedema

Post-obstructive pulmonary oedema tends to occur following acute severe airway obstruction in spontaneously breathing, fit, healthy patients recovering from anaesthesia. Laryngospasm or occlusions of a supraglottic airway by the patient's teeth are common causes. It usually presents as persistent hypoxaemia after relief of airway obstruction. Pink frothy sputum of pulmonary oedema may be seen. Clinical and radiological signs support diagnosis. Careful oropharyngeal toilet and the use of a bite block help to prevent this problem. Extreme cases may need diuretics, intubation and a period of intermittent positive pressure ventilation (IPPV).

Hypoxic brain injury

Catastrophic airway problems such as CVCI or unrecognized oesophageal intubation, result in death or hypoxic brain injury (HBI). The ASA closed claims analysis has shown a significant reduction in the number of claims for death and permanent brain damage caused at induction between 1985 to 1992 when compared to 1993 to 1999. Hypoxic brain injury presents as delayed awakening or seizures following a period of profound hypoxia or cardiac arrest. Surgery should only be started when the indication is life-threatening. Postoperative intensive care management should concentrate on ensuring oxygenation, normocapnoea, normoglycaemia and normal cerebral perfusion pressure. Hyperoxaemia and hypocapnoea should be avoided since they worsen neurological outcome. Treatment of seizures is needed to reduce cerebral metabolic rate and reduce the oxygen requirement of the brain. Mild therapeutic hypothermia (cooling to 33 to 34°C for 12 to 24 hours) has been shown to improve neurological outcome after cardiac arrest. Neurological status must be evaluated after rewarming and a period of stability.

Awareness at tracheal intubation

Awareness at intubation results from inadequate anaesthesia and may occur during the management of a difficult airway. Problems with mask ventilation can lead to inadequate alveolar and brain concentrations of inhalational agents to provide anaesthesia for intubation. Furthermore nitrous oxide is often discontinued to provide additional oxygen. Patients tolerant to anaesthetic drugs may also be at greater risk of awareness of intubation in the presence of a normal airway.

Prior to tracheal intubation an assessment should be made of the depth of anaesthesia and if inadequate this should be supplemented by the inhalational or IV route. Total intravenous anaesthesia is unaffected by difficulty with mask ventilation. This may offer some advantage if difficult airway management is anticipated.

If awareness has occurred the patient should be treated sensitively and an explanation of why they experienced recall should be provided. If this resulted from an airway problem the necessary steps to prevent recurrence should be outlined. The patient may benefit from counselling and this should be offered.

Extubation problems

The approach to extubation following an airway complication will be dictated by the primary problem, and requires careful formulation of an extubation and re-intubation plan. Postoperative ventilation may be indicated if a patient is likely to need respiratory support or further surgery. At the end of surgery the airway should be assessed for swelling by confirmation of a leak around the tracheal tube and by laryngoscopy. Fibreoptic laryngoscopy may be required to do this. Removal of the tracheal tube over an airway-exchange catheter may allow adequate inspection. Extubation catheters or an airway-exchange catheter provide a means of re-intubation. These devices are placed through a tracheal tube prior to extubation. The tracheal tube is removed over the device, which is taped in place and retained until re-intubation is considered unlikely. Patients admitted to the ITU following an airway problem are at greater risk if accidental extubation or decannulation of a tracheostomy occurs.

Aspiration

Frequency

Aspiration is reported to occur during 0.01 to 0.06% general anaesthetics. Approximately two-thirds of patients who have evidence of aspiration develop no symptoms or signs within two hours of the event and have an uneventful outcome. Of the remainder just over 50% require mechanical ventilation for more than six hours and 4% of patients who aspirate die. The overall mortality rate attributed to this cause is approximately 1 in 72,000 anaesthetics. Death is more likely in patients with significant co-morbidity.

Cause

Gastric contents are acidic and often contain particulate matter. Their inhalation or passive aspiration may lead to airway obstruction or aspiration pneumonitis, pneumonia and acute respiratory distress syndrome (ARDS). The severity and mortality of the resulting pneumonitis correlates with the volume and acidity of the aspirate. Factors that predispose to regurgitation or aspiration of gastric contents are listed in Table 4.6. Most patients who aspirate have at least one risk factor. The Australian Anaesthetic Incident Monitoring Study (AIMS) identified lack of clinical experience, errors of judgement, faulty technique, poor patient preparation and lack of assistance were commonly associated with cases of aspiration.

Recognition

Aspiration can occur at any time during anaesthesia from induction to the postoperative period. Most of these events occur at induction. Regurgitation may be witnessed, seen at the time of tracheal intubation or during suction of the airway. Coughing or laryngospasm during light anaesthesia may be a manifestation of regurgitation and aspiration. Conscious patients may complain of shortness of breath and chest tightness with wheezing and often require oxygen to maintain peripheral oxygen saturation above 90%. The presence of crackles or wheezes supports the diagnosis particularly if of recent onset. The presence of patchy infiltrates and areas of collapse on a chest radiograph may help to confirm the diagnosis. Approximately 8% of patients with known aspiration have a normal X-ray, but changes may develop at a later stage.

Prevention

The insertion of a cuffed tracheal tube offers the best protection against aspiration under general anaesthesia. The tube should be inserted as soon as the patient loses consciousness as part of a 'rapid sequence induction' (RSI) and it should be retained until protective reflexes return.

Fasting

Pre-operative fasting provides time for the stomach to empty thus reducing the volume of gastric contents. The consensus of the ASA and AAGBI on pre-operative fasting is provided in Table 4.7. However, the studies on which these guidelines are based were performed on healthy adults. Some patient groups have slower gastric emptying times, such as those with diabetes and chronic renal failure.

Table 4.6 Risk factors for aspiration.

Patient factors
Loss of airway reflexes
GCS <8
Bulbar palsy
Stroke
Reduced LOS tone (reduced barrier pressure)
Hiatus hernia
Dyspepsia
Full stomach
Emergency surgery
Pregnancy
Ascites
Obesity
Delayed gastric emptying (increased gastric volume)
Trauma
Opioids
Autonomic dysfunction
Gastric outlet obstruction
Intestinal obstruction
Acute abdomen
Critical illness
Women in labour
Previous upper GI surgery (bariatric surgery)
Surgical factors
Upper abdominal surgery
Laparoscopic surgery
Lithotomy position
Anaesthetic factors
Inadequate anaesthesia
Distension of stomach
IPPV on LMA
Prolonged surgery on LMA

Table 4.7 Fasting guidelines.

6 hours	solid food, infant formula milk
4 hours	breast milk
2 hours	clear, non-particulate, non-carbonated drinks

Table 4.8 Contraindications to nasogastric tube insertion.

Basal skull fracture

Severe midface trauma

Recent nasal surgery

Coagulopathy

Oesophageal varices or stricture

Recent banding or cautery of oesophageal varices

Gastric bypass surgery

Gastric acid reduction

H2 antagonists or proton pump inhibitors can alter the volume and pH of gastric contents. Timing of administration is important, a single dose of ranitidine, lanzoprazole or rabeprazole given a few hours before surgery reduces the volume and acidity of gastric secretions. Omeprazole needs to be given the night prior to and on the morning of operation. There is no evidence to support the routine use of these drugs.

Nasogastric drainage

In the absence of contraindications (Table 4.8) nasogastric drainage should be used to reduce residual gastric volume prior to induction of anaesthesia for patients with bowel obstruction or paralytic ileus. Nasogastric tubes (NGT) reduce lower oesophageal sphincter (LOS) tone and may be associated with gastro-oesophageal reflux around the tube. The presence of an NGT does not appear to reduce the effectiveness of cricoid pressure in cadaver studies.

Rapid sequence induction

In patients at high risk of aspiration, RSI is standard practice. After pre-oxygenation, a predetermined dose of induction agent and muscle relaxant are administered in rapid succession prior to application of cricoid pressure. The cricoid cartilage should be located before induction and a force of 30 N (3 kg) applied when consciousness is lost. The use of cricoid pressure is accepted practice. There is no evidence that cricoid pressure reduces the incidence of aspiration or mortality. When the airway has been secured with a cuffed tracheal tube, the pressure is released. To prevent oesophageal rupture immediate release of cricoid pressure is needed if active vomiting occurs. Excessive or misplaced cricoid pressure can deform the airway causing difficulty with intubation, mask ventilation or SGA insertion. Cautious reduction, removal or relocation of cricoid pressure may be indicated (Figure 4.4). Regular practice is required to provide effective cricoid pressure. Active vomiting, suspected cricotracheal injury and unstable cervical spine injury contraindicate its application.

Airway device

The gold standard for prevention of aspiration is the insertion of a cuffed TT. If used selectively, the risk of aspiration with LMA use has been shown to be similar to that of intubated patients. The LMA reduces LOS and passive reflux occurs in approximately 50% of patients compared to 15 to 22% using facemask ventilation. The LMA produces a low-pressure seal and lifts the larynx away from the oesophagus affording partial protection. Newer supraglottic devices such as the I-gel, Pro-Seal^R LMA and the LMA Supreme^{TM} incorporate gastric drainage ports for regurgitated fluid and gastric tube placement. The Pro-Seal^R LMA and the LMA Supreme^{TM} also have a larger cup and higher sealing pressure thus offering increased levels of protection against aspiration in the event of regurgitation. This may be relevant when selecting a rescue device for use in the event of failed tracheal intubation.

Awake intubation

If difficulty is anticipated with intubation during RSI, tracheal intubation under local anaesthetic is the procedure of choice. After application of local anaesthetic the patient may still aspirate until the airway has been secured. Administration of analgesia and sedation further increase the risk of aspiration therefore sedation, if used, should be cautiously administered and the level closely monitored.

Extubation

The risk of aspiration persists and extubation should be undertaken only after return of muscle tone and protective reflexes in a fully conscious patient. Some anaesthetists choose to extubate high-risk patients in the left-lateral position with slight head-down tilt. This position encourages gastric contents to drain away from the laryngeal inlet and access to the airway with a laryngoscope and sucker is usually good.

Management of aspiration

If the patient is conscious they should be turned to the left-lateral position, the airway cleared and oxygen administered. The unconscious patient should be tipped head down or turned onto their left side. The pharynx should be cleared and oxygen administered prior to insertion of a cuffed TT. Soon after intubation, thorough suctioning of the trachea should take place and bronchoscopy to clear the airway should be considered. Rigid bronchoscopy may be needed to remove particulate matter. Where feasible, it may be better to abandon the operation to allow the patient to recover from the aspiration, rather than to further complicate the recovery with an operation and the need for analgesic drugs.

Many patients aspirate small volumes and do not develop cough, wheeze, significant falls in oxygen saturation or radiological changes. When clinical signs of aspiration are absent the patient may be extubated and observed in the recovery room. Patients who develop symptoms may require admission to a high dependency area and treatment with bronchodilators or CPAP. Gross contamination may lead to severe hypoxaemia and require mechanical ventilation and inotropic support. Routine use of antibiotics is not recommended unless supported by bacteriological evidence.

Airway trauma and complications of airway devices

Airway trauma accounted for one-third of airway-related claims handled by the NHSLA between 1995 and 2007 with 36% of these leading to severe harm and 14% culminating in death. Airway devices may result in patient harm by a number of mechanisms.

Facemasks

Facemask ventilation is a widely used basic airway skill. Injury can be caused by the facemask, or the adjuncts used to aid ventilation. Soft tissue damage of the lips and tongue by the teeth can be avoided by careful attention to mouth closure. Patients with temporo-mandibular joint (TMJ) disease should be identified to avoid further damage to the joint such as subluxation or dislocation. The eyes are at risk from corneal abrasions if the mask is placed incorrectly and pressure on the globe can lead to retinal artery occlusion. Mental nerve injury with lip numbness has been reported following prolonged facemask ventilation.

Table 4.9 Complications of the use of supraglottic airways.

Complication	Incidence (%)
Sore throat	5.8–34
Airway obstruction	1.0
Laryngospasm	0.07–0.9
Pulmonary aspiration	0.02
Nerve palsies	cases reported
Arytenoid dislocation	cases reported

Airway adjuncts

Oropharyngeal airways (OPA) cause damage to teeth and soft tissues. Trauma or obstruction may follow insertion of an incorrectly sized airway. Laryngospasm or vomiting can be induced if an OPA is introduced during light anaesthesia. Nasopharyngeal airways are softer and better tolerated by conscious patients but can damage the delicate nasal mucosa or turbinates.

Supraglottic airways

Supraglottic airways cause less airway morbidity than tracheal tubes. Complications of SGA use are listed in Table 4.9. Airway obstruction can occur due to displacement, laryngospasm or the patient biting on the airway. Some manufacturers incorporate or recommend the use of a bite block to prevent the latter. Malposition may cause obstruction of the glottis with the tip of the SGA or down-folding of the epiglottis or compression of the glottic opening, cuff herniation is also recorded.

Lingular, recurrent laryngeal and hypoglossal nerve palsy have all been reported due to pressure-induced neuropraxia. Symptoms include hoarse voice, dysphagia, sore throat and slurred speech. Care should be taken with patients with bleeding tendency as this increases the risk of bruising to the laryngeal structures and of neuropraxia. High cuff volumes are thought to cause nerve damage and the lowest volume providing an effective seal should be used. Arytenoid dislocation has been recognized after prolonged symptoms. Sore throat is common with SGA use and more likely if blood is present on the device at removal.

Direct laryngoscopy and tracheal intubation

The complications of tracheal intubation are listed in Table 4.10. The incidence of difficult laryngoscopy, defined by the inability to visualize the vocal cords using a conventional laryngoscope, is 1.5 to 8.5%. The incidence of difficult intubation is 1.15 to 3.8% when defined as 'more than two attempts to intubate by an experienced laryngoscopist, or a need to change blade, use an adjunct, or an alternate device or technique'.

The lips, tongue, pharynx and oesophagus can be injured. Minor mucosal injuries are usually superficial and include bruising, mucosal tears and lacerations; these have minimal sequelae but lacerations and haematomas can become infected. Serious mucosal injuries occur where the intubation is rated as difficult and attempts at intubation are blind. Perforation of the pharynx and oesophagus has been reported. Unrecognized perforations can lead to retropharyngeal abscess, mediastinitis and death. Signs are only present in 51% of cases. These include neck pain, difficulty swallowing, subcutaneous emphysema and

Table 4.10 Complications of tracheal intubation.

Complications	Incidence (%)
Difficult intubation	1.15–3.8
Failed intubation	0.13–0.3
Sore throat	14–50
Dental damage	0.02
Trauma:	
mucosal injury	
perforation	
TMJ joint injury	
arytenoid cartilage injury	
vocal cords injury	
vocal cords granuloma	
laryngeal/tracheal stenosis	

pneumothorax. Early recognition and aggressive treatment within 12 to 24 hours with anti-biotics and drainage is required to minimize mortality.

Adjuncts to aid intubation also cause trauma. The use of gum elastic bougies has been associated with perforation of the airway and laryngeal oedema. The device may become fractured or avulsed within the airway. This requires airway instrumentation for their removal. Over-inflation or use of high gas flow via airway-exchange catheters may cause pneumothorax, and death has been reported.

Dental trauma occurs approximately once in 4,500 anaesthetics. Most commonly the upper incisors are involved. Risk factors include poor dentition, and difficult direct laryngoscopy. Of the anaesthesia-related claims to the NHSLA between 1995 and 2007, 11% were for dental damage. It is important to warn patients who are at high risk of dental damage. Mouth guards can be used but have not been shown to reduce the risk. If a tooth is damaged any fragments must be located and removed. Request an urgent dental review if a tooth is avulsed, subluxated or dentine or pulp is exposed.

Temporo-mandibular joint injuries accounted for 10% of airway trauma claims recorded in the ASA closed claims database between 1961 and 1996. All cases were associated with routine intubation. Most claims were by women under the age of 60 years and 30% of the claimants had pre-existing TMJ disease. Immediate reduction should be performed. Soft diet is recommended for two weeks. If symptoms continue referral should be made to an oral surgeon for consideration of treatment with an occlusion appliance.

Arytenoid cartilage damage is most likely if visualization of the vocal cords was poor. The incidence of arytenoid dislocation is approximately 0.1%. Risk factors include chronic renal failure, Crohn's disease, acromegaly and elderly patients with systemic joint disease such as rheumatoid arthritis. Prolonged hoarseness is the cardinal sign, along with breathy voice, weak cough and sometimes aspiration. To prevent dislocation care must be taken with susceptible patients and selection of a smaller TT will reduce the risk. Diagnosis and management include CT or MRI imaging, and prompt reduction. Late diagnosis reduces likelihood of success due to ankylosis of the joint.

Vocal cord injury can lead to prolonged hoarseness. Causes include vocal cord oedema, erosions and vocal cord paralysis. Paralysis is more likely following long-term intubation. Cuff pressure on the recurrent laryngeal nerve is thought to be the cause. Spontaneous resolution is common but intervention may be required to improve glottic closure.

Cervical spine fractures have been reported in patients with ankylosing spondylitis during direct laryngoscopy. Patients with spinal abnormalities such as fractures or rheumatoid disease may be susceptible to spinal cord trauma. If time allows, awake fibreoptic intubation should be considered. In emergencies manual inline stabilization should be maintained during intubation.

Haemodynamic complications of intubation can occur at induction or extubation. Hypertension, tachycardia and dysrhythmias are well documented and are more frequent in patients with pre-existing hypertension or ischaemic heart disease.

Damage to the airway device or tubing may result in large leaks, which mimic tracheal tube displacement. Tracheal tubes may be perforated or cut by surgeons operating around the airway. Manual ventilation will aid recognition of the problem. Some airway devices have inadvertently been sutured in place making removal difficult or dangerous.

Prolonged tracheal intubation can lead to chronic laryngeal problems. Ulcerated vocal cords may form granulomas. Management includes maintaining a clear airway and a period of observation. Laser excision is required for larger lesions. Laryngo tracheal stenosis is associated with increased duration of intubation and carries high morbidity. A stenosis may be glottic, sub-glottic or tracheal and usually presents with reduced exercise tolerance or progressive stridor. Emergency tracheostomy may be required for severe obstruction. Laser or dilatational endoscopy can be used in selected patients. Definitive management is surgical resection. During long-term ventilation fluid collects above the tracheal tube and can track down into the lungs through longitudinal folds in the cuff leading to aspiration pneumonitis.

Nasotracheal intubation

Nasal intubation often leads to bruising of the nasal mucosa (50%) and mild epistaxis (47%). Trauma to the turbinates is common and these may be avulsed, as may nasal polyps or tumours with subsequent intra-luminal obstruction. Laceration to the posterior pharyngeal wall occurs in about 2% of cases and can lead to bleeding or infection. Nasotracheal tubes may pass into the sub-mucosal plane where bleeding produces a retropharyngeal haematoma or an abscess. Uncomplicated nasal intubation produces a bacteraemia in 12% of cases. The majority will be asymptomatic.

Pressure injury to the nostrils can lead to skin necrosis if care is not taken with positioning the tube. Injuries to the septum can be reduced by using small tubes, lubrication, decongestant and by using care when advancing the tube. Contraindications to nasotracheal intubation include basal skull fracture and bleeding diathesis, caution is needed with patients on anti-platelet drugs.

Double lumen tubes and bronchial blockers

Double lumen tubes (DLT) are designed to isolate parts of the respiratory tract or provide single lung ventilation. To enable effective ventilation and aspiration of secretions large tubes are usually selected, these are associated with increased trauma during insertion. Sore throat affects 60% of patients post-operatively. Minor bronchial injuries such as erythema, oedema and haematoma occur in 25% of cases. Tracheal rupture is a rare but serious complication with 20% mortality. Increasing patient age, emergency intubation and delayed diagnosis increase mortality. Conservative treatment produces a better outcome than surgery. The incidence of hoarseness and vocal cord injuries are greater with DLT compared to bronchial blockers (44% vs. 17% respectively).

Fibreoptic intubation

Fibreoptic intubation is indicated where direct laryngoscopy is not possible. The pressor response to fibreoptic intubation is similar to that of direct laryngoscopy. Nasendoscopy produces nasal trauma but probably less than a nasotracheal intubation. Surgical emphysema due to perforation of pharyngeal mucosa and gastric rupture due to massive gastric distension has been reported when oxygen has been administered via the working channel during endoscopy. It is recommended that this practice be avoided.

Rescue techniques

Cricothyroidotomy is used predominantly in emergency situations, such as the CVCI scenario, or in patients with impending airway loss due to trauma. It has a high complication rate. Four techniques are described: fine-bore cricothroidotomy with low-pressure oxygen source, or with high-pressure oxygen source, large-bore cannulae devices and surgical cricothyroidotomy. Fine-bore cricothyroidotomy with a low-pressure oxygen source is ineffective and will not re-oxygenate an adult. Complications during insertion include haemorrhage, damage to surrounding structures including the posterior tracheal wall. These are more common during surgical insertion. Problems with ventilation, such as hypercarbia, surgical emphysema and pneumothorax are more common with fine-bore cricothyroidotomy devices. Reported complication rates appear to be lower for surgical techniques (10 to 48%) compared to small-bore cannula techniques (65%). Cadaver studies show wire-guided methods were more reliable and had fewer complications compared to direct-puncture techniques (13% vs. 75%) but the latter were faster to perform. These procedures should be rehearsed on models at regular intervals in order to maintain skills.

Percutaneous tracheostomy has been used as an emergency airway rescue technique. The acute complications include major and minor haemorrhage, pneumothorax, accidental decannulation, surgical emphysema, wound infection, difficult insertion, false passage, hypoxia, posterior tracheal wall injury, loss of airway and death. Chronic complications include formation of granulation tissue, tracheal stenosis, tracheomalacia, tracheo-innominate-artery fistula, tracheoesophageal fistula and aspiration.

Airway fires

Surgical fires are rare; reports suggest 33% occur in the airway. A fire requires fuel, oxygen and a heat source. Plastic tubes, drapes and cleaning solutions act as a fuel source. Oxygen and nitrous oxide both support combustion, ignition is provided by either diathermy or a laser. Tracheal tube fires can occur during tracheostomy formation or during laser airway surgery. Laser-resistant tubes help prevent airway fires although these will burn and are not totally resistant to diathermy ignition. Saline should be used to inflate cuffs, high concentrations of oxygen and the use of nitrous oxide should be avoided.

In the event of an airway fire, the patient should be disconnected from the anaesthetic machine. Remove the TT and any remaining burning parts in the airway. Consider flushing the area with saline to extinguish flames. Re-establish the airway and ventilate with room air until certain all burning has stopped. Examine the airway to determine extent of damage and transfer to ITU for further management. The patient may suffer airway burns with oedema or develop an inhalational injury caused by heat and smoke. This complication carries a high mortality and morbidity.

Patient management after airway complications

The patient should receive a full explanation of the event and be informed of its significance, including the options available in the future. A written account should be supplied to the patient and their general practitioner. This should include details of the problem and the action taken, with recommendations for future management. Patients should take this information with them to future surgical and anaesthetic consultations. In addition to detailed recording of the event a warning should be placed in the medical records. A medic alert bracelet should be considered.

Finally it is important to complete local critical incident forms and the national anaesthesia critical incident reporting e-form in order to learn from incidents and identify common themes. Presentation of complications at local governance meetings is important to ensure the department is adequately prepared to manage similar events.

Key points

- All anaesthetists should have an airway management plan compatible with the patient, their skills and the equipment available. It will require modification for some patients.
- Airway trauma is common and can lead to severe harm.
- CVCI most commonly follows anticipated difficulty in airway management.
- In a crisis seek help early and regularly re-appraise the situation.
- Capnography and fibreoptic endoscopic visualization of the carina are reliable means of confirming tracheal tube placement.
- In an intubated patient the absence of exhaled CO_2 always indicates tracheal tube misplacement or total occlusion even in the presence of a cardiac arrest.
- Oesophageal intubation, occluded circuits and inhaled foreign bodies, such as blood clots and throat packs, may be misdiagnosed as asthma.

Acknowledgement

The authors would like to thank Mr. Paul Montgomery for the image of the larynx and the Difficult Airway Society for the flow charts.

List of further reading

Cook, T. M., Scott, S. & Mihai, R. Litigation related to airway and respiratory complications of anaesthesia: an analysis of claims against the NHS in England 1995–2007. *Anaesthesia* 2010; **65**: 556–63.

Cook, T., Woodall, N. & Frerk, C. Major complications of airway management in UK; results of the Fourth National Audit Project of the Royal College of Anaesthetists and the Difficult Airway Society. Part I. *Anaesthesia* 2011; **106**: 617–31.

Henderson, J. J., Popat, M. T., Latto, I. P. & Pearce, A. C. Management of unanticipated difficult intubation guidelines. *Anaesthesia* 2004; **59**: 675–94.

Ng, A. & Smith, G. Gastroesophageal reflux and aspiration of gastric contents in anesthetic practice. *Anesth Analg* 2001; **93**: 494–513.

Peterson, G. N., Karen, B., Domino, K.B. *et al.* Management of the difficult airway: a closed claims analysis. *Anesthesiology* 2005; **103**: 33–9.

Chapter 5

Respiratory complications

Andrew Roscoe and Hamish Thomson

Introduction

Pulmonary complications contribute significantly to perioperative morbidity. Respiratory complications run the gamut from the benign self-limiting (basal atelectasis), the acute life-threatening (tension pneumothorax), through to major chronic illness (acute respiratory distress syndrome, ARDS). Table 5.1 lists the more common complications. Postoperative respiratory morbidity has been shown to increase hospital length of stay and resource utilization.

Atelectasis

The term atelectasis is derived from the Greek words *ateles* (incomplete) and *ektasis* (extension). It is defined as the lack of gas exchange within alveoli due to alveolar collapse.

The reported incidence of intra- and postoperative atelectasis ranges from 3 to 60%, depending on the exact definition and type of surgery. Computed tomography scanning has shown that healthy individuals under general anaesthesia in the supine position frequently develop atelectasis in dependent areas of the lungs. The severity varies from a minor, easily reversible condition to complete lobar or even unilateral lung collapse, precipitating critical hypoxaemia.

The closing capacity (CC) is the lung volume at which the airways begin to collapse, leading to shunting of blood through unventilated alveoli and impaired gas exchange. The CC comprises the residual volume (RV) and the closing volume (CV). Physiologically, significant atelectasis occurs when the closing capacity encroaches on the functional residual capacity (FRC), resulting in alveolar collapse during normal tidal volume ventilation (Figure 5.1).

The aetiology of atelectasis may be divided into obstructive and non-obstructive causes.

Obstructive atelectasis

It is typically due to mucous plugging. An increase in the volume and viscosity of bronchial secretions, combined with a reduced ability to cough, results in airway occlusion. Unventilated lung parenchyma distal to this obstruction gradually collapses, creating a V/Q mismatch and shunt. Risk factors include thoracic surgery, upper abdominal operations, vertical laparotomy incision, prolonged operation time, poor postoperative analgesia, cigarette smoking, pre-operative malnutrition and obesity. Less common causes for developing obstructive atelectasis include inhaled foreign body or endobronchial tumour.

Anaesthetic and Perioperative Complications, ed. Kamen Valchanov, Stephen T. Webb and Jane Sturgess.
Published by Cambridge University Press. © Cambridge University Press 2011.

Table 5.1 Common perioperative respiratory complications.

	Incidence
Atelectasis	3–60%
Pneumonia	3–30%
Bronchospasm	up to 10%
Pneumothorax	<1%

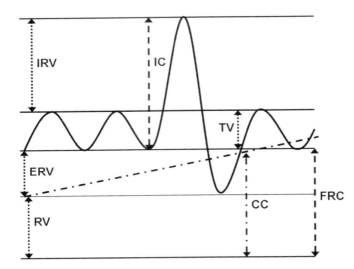

Figure 5.1 Lung spirometry showing the effect of increasing closing capacity. CC: closing capacity; ERV: expiratory reserve volume; FRC: functional residual capacity; IC: inspiratory capacity; IRV: inspiratory reserve volume; RV: residual volume; TV: tidal volume.

Non-obstructive atelectasis

Non-obstructive atelectasis may be classified into compressive, adhesive, infiltrative and absorptive.

External compression of alveoli may be due to a collection in the pleural cavity (effusion or pneumothorax) or by enlarged peribronchial lymph nodes. The lower and middle lobes are more affected by fluid collections, whilst the upper lobes are more prone to collapse in the case of a pneumothorax.

Adhesive atelectasis is caused by a deficiency of alveolar surfactant. The resultant increased surface tension counteracts alveoli expansion, reducing compliance and culminating in lung collapse. This is seen in conditions such as ARDS, oxygen toxicity and radiation pneumonitis.

Infiltrative atelectasis is most commonly due to scarring of lung tissue secondary to a necrotizing infection or granulomatous disease, which leads to loss of lung volume.

When breathing an oxygen–air mixture the alveolus is splinted open by nitrogen. When the fraction of inspired oxygen (FiO_2) is increased to 1.0, such as during pre-oxygenation, alveolar volume diminishes due to the absorption of oxygen into the bloodstream. Ventilating patients with FiO_2 of 1.0 has been shown to cause more rapid progression of atelectasis, compared to oxygen–air or oxygen–nitrous oxide mixtures.

Right middle lobe syndrome is a disease process involving atelectasis of the right middle lobe or lingula segment of the left upper lobe. It is more common in children with a history

Table 5.2 Risk factors for developing postoperative pneumonia.

Thoracic or upper abdominal surgery

Chronic obstructive pulmonary disease

Age >70 years old

Diabetes mellitus

Cigarette smoking

Malnutrition

Immunocompromised

Renal dysfunction

Prolonged intubation/ventilation

Poor postoperative analgesia

Use of nasogastric tube

Recent previous antibiotic usage

of atopy and may be linked to inflammation or bronchial oedema. It has been linked with Sjögren's syndrome.

Prevention of atelectasis is difficult. The use of pre-operative chest physiotherapy has not been shown to be beneficial in the majority of patients. Modifiable risk factors, such as smoking and malnutrition, can be addressed. Attention to quality postoperative analgesia is essential. Perhaps the simplest preventative measures are to avoid administering FiO_2 of 1.0 for any longer than necessary, the addition of positive end-expiratory pressure (PEEP) when providing positive pressure ventilation and the application of frequent recruitment manoeuvres.

The diagnosis of atelectasis is generally made in the first 48 hours post-operatively. It commonly presents with tachypnoea, reduced air entry on auscultation, mild pyrexia, elevated white cell count (WCC) and areas of poor lung expansion on chest X-ray (CXR).

Management begins with providing adequate analgesia and chest physiotherapy. In obstructive atelectasis, nebulized bronchodilators and mucolytics may loosen secretions and assist in expectoration. When lobar collapse has occurred, bronchoscopy may provide the best treatment option.

Pneumonia

The reported incidence of postoperative pneumonia ranges from 3 to 30%, depending on the precise definition used. The mortality from postoperative lower respiratory tract infection can be as high as 40%. It usually presents four to seven days after surgery.

The risk factors for developing postoperative pneumonia are listed in Table 5.2. Of these, thoracic or upper abdominal surgery and chronic obstructive pulmonary disease (COPD) provide the greatest hazard, carrying a four-fold increase in relative risk.

Prevention

Prevention involves identifying and addressing modifiable risk factors, the provision of high-quality postoperative analgesia and prophylactic interventions. Cigarette smoking should cease a minimum of six weeks prior to surgery to allow some recovery of mucociliary function. Good diabetic control and adequate nutrition are important aspects of perioperative care. Provision of excellent postoperative analgesia allows for coughing and clearance of bronchial secretions. Early extubation, where possible, avoidance of unnecessary nasogastric tubes and the use of incentive spirometry combined with aggressive chest physiotherapy may help to reduce the risk.

Diagnosis

The diagnosis of pneumonia is based on clinical, laboratory, radiological and microbiological features. Patients may present with a productive cough, dyspnoea, tachycardia, pyrexia and typical signs on chest auscultation. There is usually elevation of the WCC, c-reactive protein (CRP) and procalcitonin (PCT) levels. Areas of consolidation or infiltration are seen on CXR or CT scan. Isolation of an organism from a sputum sample or bronchoalveolar lavage (BAL) directs further antimicrobial therapy.

Management

The mainstay of management is antimicrobial therapy, complemented by physiotherapy and, in severe cases, intubation of the airway and bronchoscopic toilet. The initial choice of antimicrobial therapy is empirical, based on the most common pathogens, but can be targeted after culture and sensitivities are determined.

Ventilator-associated pneumonia (VAP)

Ventilator-associated pneumonia is a type of hospital-acquired pneumonia in patients who have been mechanically ventilated for more than 48 hours. It can occur in up to 30% of ventilated patients in intensive care units, with a mortality of 20 to 50%.

The presence of an endotracheal or tracheostomy tube provides a route for bacteria to bypass upper airway host defence mechanisms and gain direct access to the lower respiratory tree. Risk factors for acquiring VAP include immunosuppression, COPD, ARDS, lying supine, reduced level of consciousness, presence of a nasogastric tube and use of poor aseptic techniques when handling airway devices. Strategies to reduce risk include adherence to strict protocols for hand washing and patient airway handling, oral antiseptic decontamination, positioning the patient 30 degrees head-up, maintaining adequate airway cuff pressures and minimizing the use of sedative agents.

Purulent tracheobronchial secretions, pyrexia, elevated WCC and new infiltrates on CXR all suggest a diagnosis of VAP. However, the sensitivity of the clinical criteria for VAP may be less than 50%, especially in patients with ARDS, other pre-existing pulmonary disease and systemic sepsis. Scoring systems have been developed to aid in the rapid diagnosis of this serious condition.

Initial empirical antimicrobial therapy is directed at the potential organism. Multi-drug-resistant (MDR) organisms are more common in patients with a history of recent antibiotic use, current hospitalization of more than five days, immunosuppression, chronic dialysis treatment or residence in a long-term care facility. In the absence of the above risk factors, therapy is aimed at *Streptococcus pneumoniae* and *Haemophilus influenzae*. When MDR organisms are suspected, empirical therapy is broadened to cover *Pseudomonas aeruginosa*, *Klebsiella*, *Stenotrophomonas*, methicillin-resistant *Staphylococcus aureus* (MRSA) and *Acinetobacter*.

Bronchospasm

Intra-operative bronchospasm may arise in patients with underlying reactive airways disease or may be precipitated in previously healthy individuals. In asthmatics, the incidence of intra-operative bronchospasm is up to 10% when an endotracheal tube is inserted in combination with general anaesthesia. This incidence is reduced to less than 1% if tracheal intubation is avoided. In non-asthmatics the incidence is very low, but may still be life-threatening. Bronchospasm may be the initial presentation of anaphylaxis.

In patients with reactive airways disease, exaggerated bronchoconstriction and airway oedema develop secondary to a trigger, such as laryngoscopy, insertion of an endotracheal device, drugs or drug preservatives.

The use of prophylactic bronchodilator therapy has been shown to reduce the incidence of intra-operative bronchospasm in susceptible individuals. Potential trigger agents should be identified and avoided if possible.

The diagnosis is made based on a combination of increased airway pressures, wheeze or diminished breath sounds, desaturation, gas-trapping and a high index of suspicion. Manual bag ventilation will elicit compliance. In critical bronchospasm the bag will not re-fill during exhalation.

The immediate management of severe intra-operative bronchospasm is to administer FiO_2 of 1.0 and remove any suspected triggering agent. Hand ventilation is recommended to assess lung compliance and prevent excessive inspiratory airways pressures. Bronchodilation may be achieved by increasing the concentration of inhalational anaesthetic agent, β_2-agonists, magnesium sulphate, aminophylline and adrenaline. Other agents worth considering include corticosteroids, atropine and ketamine.

Treatment of anaphylaxis is directed at the systemic process.

Pneumothorax

Pneumothorax occurring under anaesthesia is a rare but potentially life-threatening event. Identification may be difficult and is often hampered by limited access to the patient during surgery. Due to the mechanics of positive pressure ventilation the risk of tension pneumothorax and severe haemodynamic compromise is of particular concern.

The causes of pneumothorax during anaesthesia are numerous but can be broken down into spontaneous, traumatic and iatrogenic.

Spontaneous

Spontaneous pneumothoraces may occur at any time during anaesthesia or recovery and are classified as primary or secondary. Primary pneumothoraces occur in the absence of lung disease or trauma and are most common in young adults. Other risk factors for spontaneous pneumothorax include smoking, male sex and low body mass index (BMI). Secondary pneumothoraces occur in the context of underlying lung disease particularly COPD. Other causes include asthma, ARDS and congenital cystic pulmonary disease. Secondary spontaneous pneumothoraces carry an increased mortality, which is quoted as 1 to 17% for COPD patients.

Traumatic

Traumatic pneumothorax occurs following major chest trauma. Initiation of positive pressure ventilation may either cause an air leak from injured lung tissue or unmask a subclinical pneumothorax. Patients with significant chest trauma undergoing anaesthesia should be managed with a very high index of suspicion for pneumothorax, and many authors would advocate prophylactic chest drain insertion if intermittent positive pressure ventilation (IPPV) is used. The presence of a chest drain will not completely remove the risk of pneumothorax as drains may become blocked or misplaced.

Iatrogenic

Iatrogenic pneumothoraces can be sub-classified as those occurring due to inadvertent pleural puncture and those due to barotrauma.

Inadvertent pleural puncture

Causes of inadvertent pleural puncture include:

- Subclavian and internal jugular venous cannulation. Subclavian line insertion is associated with 0.5 to 2% risk of pneumothorax while the risk for internal jugular lines is somewhat lower at 0.2 to 0.5%. Risk of pleural injury is increased by high BMI and multiple needle passes.
- Brachial plexus, intercostal and paravertebral blocks carry a risk of pneumothorax. The risk is highest with intercostal blocks and has been quoted to be as high as 19%. The risk for brachial plexus block is dependent on approach but is highest for the supraclavicular approach (0.5 to 6%).

  Surgery around the neck or thorax is also associated with pneumothorax.

  Instrumentation of the airway and fiberoptic bronchoscopy carry a small risk of bronchial trauma and pneumothorax.

Barotrauma

Barotrauma may occur due to user or equipment error. Several case reports exist of accidental barotrauma resulting in pneumothorax due to ventilator malfunction or damage. Inappropriate setting of the ventilator may result in excessive tidal volumes and serious barotrauma. This is a particular problem in children. In some instances normal tidal volume ventilation may result in significant barotrauma, such as in one-lung ventilation or in low-compliance lungs (ARDS). Occasionally partial occlusion of an endotracheal tube may cause a ball-cock effect and hyperinflate the lungs.

Prevention is by far the best treatment. Use of spontaneous ventilation or regional techniques in high-risk patients should be considered. Ultrasound guidance when inserting central venous catheters or undertaking brachial plexus blockade will reduce the risk of pleural injury. Close observation of airway pressure and tidal volumes may help to prevent barotrauma. Nitrous oxide should be avoided in high-risk cases as it will defuse into the pneumothorax and enlarge it.

The identification of pneumothorax requires a high index of suspicion in patients who are at risk and a logical approach, as the signs may be produced by other anaesthetic emergencies. The classic signs are:

- difficulty ventilating
- desaturation
- unilateral air entry
- tracheal deviation

- neck vein distension
- haemodynamic collapse
- widened rib spaces.

Chest X-ray (CXR) confirmation is usually impractical and results in dangerous delays to management in compromised patients. Bedside ultrasound (US), if immediately available, may help to exclude pneumothorax by looking for 'pleural sliding' and 'comet tail artefacts'.

If pneumothorax is suspected the FiO_2 should be increased to 1.0. If the patient is haemo-dynamically compromised then a large-bore cannula should be inserted into the second rib space in the midclavicular line and the pneumothorax decompressed. Definitive chest drainage should then be undertaken in the fifth interspace, just anterior to the midaxillary line.

Acute lung injury/acute respiratory distress syndrome

Acute lung injury (ALI) and acute respiratory distress syndrome (ARDS) are part of the same spectrum of disease. Acute respiratory distress syndrome is defined as acute non-cardiac pulmonary oedema or more precisely as a combination of bilateral pulmonary infiltrates with a PaO_2/FiO_2 ratio of less than 200 mmHg (or 27 kPa) and a pulmonary capillary wedge pressure ≤ 18 mmHg (or clinically normal left atrial pressure). Acute lung injury represents the milder spectrum of the disease with a PaO_2/FiO_2 <300 mmHg (or 40 kPa).

The population incidence of ARDS is often quoted as 1.5 to 8.3 per 100,000 people per year, although more recent studies suggest the incidence may be ten times higher. The exact incidence of ARDS following anaesthesia is not known.

The mortality rate from ARDS is quoted as 30 to 50%. Long-term follow-up of patients with ARDS show significantly reduced quality of life measurements despite the fact that pulmonary function tends to improve after the acute illness. Some patients may be left with long-term respiratory failure.

Both ALI and ARDS are caused by the leakage of protein-rich fluid into the alveoli from the pulmonary capillaries. The factors precipitating capillary leak are numerous and are closely associated with the systemic inflammatory response syndrome (SIRS) or with other causes of lung injury. While anaesthesia itself does not directly cause ARDS, multiple events associated with anaesthesia and surgery may precipitate ALI or ARDS. Volutrauma and barotrauma from over-vigorous mechanical ventilation can produce inflammatory changes in the lung, which may contribute to the development of ARDS and worsen the outcome in patients with existing lung injury. The causes of ALI/ARDS are listed in Table 5.3.

ALI/ARDS should be anticipated in patients with the associated conditions. Diagnosis is confirmed by respiratory distress and hypoxaemia, conforming to the above definition, and with the characteristic CXR findings of bilateral defuse pulmonary infiltrates. Further imaging, such as high-resolution computed tomography (CT) may help if the diagnosis is uncertain and will usually show consolidation of dependent zones. If cardiogenic pulmonary oedema is suspected then echocardiography may help to confirm the diagnosis.

The management of ALI/ARDS is mainly supportive. Increased inspired oxygen concentration and non-invasive ventilation may be sufficient in some cases, but many patients will require full mechanical ventilation to maintain adequate oxygenation. The main principle of treating a patient with ARDS is to correct the underlying condition and to limit further lung injury from mechanical ventilation.

The ARDSNET trial demonstrated that mortality was significantly reduced by adopting a 6 ml/kg (ideal body weight) tidal volume, opposed to a 12 ml/kg tidal volume, in

Table 5.3 Causes of acute respiratory distress syndrome.

Pulmonary causes
Pneumonia
Aspiration of gastric contents
Fat emboli
Inhalation injury
Pulmonary contusion
Reperfusion injury
Non-pulmonary causes
Sepsis
Trauma (and major surgery)
Shock
Transfusion of blood and blood products
Pancreatitis
Cardiopulmonary bypass
Drug overdose

mechanically ventilated patients with ARDS. It is postulated that high tidal volumes, particularly in the context of a patient with significant amounts of unventilated consolidated lung tissue, causes cytokine release due to sheer stresses, which increases lung injury.

Conservative fluid strategies, as compared with liberal fluid approaches, may improve pulmonary function and reduce length of ventilation in patients with ARDS, whilst not worsening other organ functions.

Other treatment strategies include corticosteroids, prone ventilation and inhaled nitric oxide therapy, but the evidence showing survival benefit is still not established.

Pleural cavity collections

Haemothorax

Haemothorax (blood in the pleural space) is a rare, but potentially lethal, complication of anaesthesia. In the period 1990 to 2002 the American Society of Anesthesiologists (ASA) claims database recorded only five haemothoraces, of which three proved fatal.

The aetiology is invariably vascular injury during central venous catheterization, especially of the subclavian vein, or from vascular puncture during nerve blockade in the upper body. Inadvertent arterial puncture would appear to be a significant risk factor. Haemothorax has been reported following paravertebral, intercostal and brachial plexus blocks. Disorders of haemostasis will put the patient at additional risk.

Ultrasound guidance of central venous cannulation and brachial nerve blockade should reduce the incidence of iatrogenic vascular injury and haemothorax. In patients with coagulopathy a risk–benefit assessment should be undertaken beforehand. In such cases, a compressible site (internal jugular or femoral vein) for venous cannulation is preferred.

Patients with haemothorax may develop signs and symptoms of hypovolaemia, shock or respiratory compromise due to compression of the lung. Reduced air entry on the affected side is to be expected. Diagnosis of pleural fluid can be confirmed on CXR or chest US, but the presence of blood will only be confirmed on aspiration and drainage.

Initial treatment should be commenced on an ABC approach with restoration of circulating volume. Drainage should be undertaken with full resuscitation facilities and with large-bore vascular access, as decompression may release tamponade and precipitate new bleeding. Drainage is best performed with a large-bore chest tube inserted just posterior to the midaxillary line in the fifth intercostal space. As with trauma, large volume haemothoraces (>1,500 ml) are associated with significant vascular injury. Such patients should be referred urgently to a cardiothoracic surgical assessment.

Chylothorax

Chylothorax is the accumulation of lipid-rich lymph fluid in the pleural cavity. It is a very rare complication of anaesthesia. The most common cause following anaesthesia is from direct trauma to the thoracic duct during attempted cannulation of the left subclavian or left internal jugular veins. Attempted left brachial plexus blocks also carry a risk. Extensive venous thrombosis from central lines may cause chylothorax by increasing back pressure.

Many chylothoraces are found incidentally on postoperative CXRs. Diagnosis is confirmed by the aspiration of milky pleural fluid with a high triglyceride level on laboratory analysis. The most important differential is that of empyema.

Treatment may be conservative or surgical. Conservative management is effective in approximately half of all cases and is based on intercostal drainage of the effusion and measures to reduce chyle flow (parenteral nutrition and low-fat diet) to allow closure. Surgical options include ligation of the thoracic duct or insertion of a pleuro-peritoneal shunt.

Pulmonary vascular conditions

Pulmonary embolism

By far the most common pulmonary vascular complication following anaesthesia and surgery is pulmonary embolism (PE). The majority of these are secondary to deep vein thrombosis (DVT). The incidence of fatal PE in hip surgery without thromboprophylaxis is 0.4%. Mortality for treated pulmonary embolism is quoted at 2%, accounting for 15% of postoperative deaths, and results in significant morbidity combined with the need for long-term anticoagulation with its attendant risks. Rarely PE may originate from other sites, such as clots on central venous catheters, from the surgery, such as marrow embolism, or embolism following bone cementing.

Multiple patient factors increase the risk of PE in the perioperative period. These include age >60 years, obesity, pregnancy, smoking, COPD, heart disease, thrombophilia, hormone replacement therapy, oral contraceptive medication and malignancy. The factors that contribute to the development of DVT/PE during anaesthesia are listed below:

- Surgical and pre-surgical trauma leading to activation of the clotting cascade.
- Venous stasis during anaesthesia due to immobility, reduced cardiac output and venous pooling, or secondary to tourniquet use. Lower limb venous stasis may occur due to physical obstruction of the veins during pelvic or abdominal surgery.

- Injury to the pelvic or lower limb veins during surgery.
- Dehydration.

Prophylaxis of DVT and PE involves both physical and pharmacological approaches. Compression stockings and early mobilization help to reduce stasis, but patients at higher risk may require prophylactic anticoagulation with low molecular weight heparins (LMWH).

Acute PE may be asymptomatic, but most commonly presents with dyspnea, pleuritic chest pain, cough and haemoptysis. Clinical findings are often non-specific with tachycardia and tachypnoea. Cardiovascular collapse can occur with large PE. Plain CXR is often normal and the investigation of choice is the CT pulmonary angiography (CTPA).

Immediate management of acute PE comprises providing adequate oxygenation and haemodynamic support. Anticoagulation is commenced if the patient is stable. If there is significant cardiovascular compromise thrombolysis should be considered, but may result in life-threatening haemorrhage in the immediate postoperative period. Surgical embolectomy via sternotomy is usually reserved for extreme cases.

Pulmonary haemorrhage

Pulmonary haemorrhage is very rare, but it may be rapidly fatal. Several factors may cause pulmonary haemorrhage during anaesthesia:

- Direct trauma to the airway from instrumentation (e.g. bougie).
- Sheer stresses to abnormal lung tissue from IPPV (cystic fibrosis).
- Negative pressure pulmonary oedema due to upper airway obstruction.
- Lung trauma from attempted neuroaxial blockade (paravertebral block).
- Massive PE.

Prevention is by avoiding precipitants, such as using spontaneous ventilation in cystic fibrosis with recent pulmonary haemorrhage.

The main aims of treatment are to maintain oxygenation and circulating volume. Positive pressure ventilation with PEEP may help to limit bleeding in some cases and help with oxygenation. Isolation of the haemorrhage, with either endobronchial intubation with a double lumen tube or placement of an endobronchial blocker, is required to protect the unaffected lung. Correction of hypovolaemia and coagulopathies should be undertaken. Pro-thrombotics such as tranexamic acid have been used. Radiological embolization may be considered when the patient is stable.

List of further reading

Acute Respiratory Distress Syndrome Network. Ventilation with lower tidal volumes as compared with traditional tidal volumes for acute lung injury and the acute respiratory distress syndrome. *New Engl J Med* 2000; **342**: 1301–8.

Brooks-Brunn, J. A. Postoperative atelectasis and pneumonia: risk factors. *Am J Crit Care* 1995; **4**: 340–9.

Guimaraes, M. M., El Dib, R., Smith, A.F. & Matos, D. Incentive spirometry for prevention of postoperative pulmonary complications in upper abdominal surgery. *Cochrane Database Syst Rev* 2009: CD006058.

Joyce, C. J. & Williams, A. B. Kinetics of absorption atelectasis during anesthesia: a mathematical model. *J Appl Physiol* 1999; **86**: 1116–25.

Koenig, S. M. & Truwit, J. D. Ventilator-associated pneumonia: diagnosis, treatment and prevention. *Clin Microbiol Rev* 2006; **19**: 637–57.

Lawrence, V. A., Cornell, J. E., Smetana, G. W. *et al.* Strategies to reduce postoperative pulmonary complications after noncardiothoracic surgery: systematic review for the American College of Physicians. *Ann Intern Med* 2006; **144**: 596–608.

Schein, M. Postoperative pneumonia. *Curr Surg* 2002; **59**: 540–8.

Thompson, J. S., Baxter, B. T., Allison, J. G. *et al.* Temporal patterns of postoperative complications. *Arch Surg* 2003; **138**: 596–602.

West, J. B. (ed). *Respiratory Physiology*, 6th edn. Philadelphia: Lippincott, Williams & Wilkins, 2000.

Woods, B. D. & Sladen, R. N. Perioperative considerations for the patient with asthma and bronchospasm. *Br J Anaesth* 2009; **103** (Suppl 1): i57–65.

Cardiovascular complications

Victoria Howell and Joseph E. Arrowsmith

Introduction

Acute, life-threatening cardiovascular events during the course of anaesthesia – and, by impli-
cation, surgery – are fortunately uncommon. Intra-operative deaths from catastrophic haemorrhage, cardiac tamponade, tension pneumothorax and severe immune-mediated phenomena
(e.g. anaphylaxis, incompatible transfusion and overwhelming sepsis) are rare. By contrast,
postoperative major adverse cardiovascular events (MACE) occurring after emergence from
anaesthesia are common. It is now widely accepted that, for some patients, the 'window of cardiovascular risk' persists long into the postoperative period and that seemingly trivial haemodynamic perturbations and non-lethal complications may have long-term implications. The
healthcare burden of cardiovascular disease in this setting is significant; as many as 10% of
patients undergoing non-cardiac surgery have, or are at risk of having, cardiovascular disease.

Anaesthesia and surgery have a wide range of short and intermediate-term effects on the
cardiovascular system (Table 6.1). In order to meet that additional metabolic oxygen (O_2)
demand imposed by the neurohumoral ('stress') response to surgery an increase in tissue O_2
delivery is required. The magnitude and duration of the stress response is largely dictated by
both the magnitude of surgery and the occurrence of complications such as haemorrhage
and sepsis. Failure to meet increased O_2 demand increases the likelihood of perioperative
complications.

With a few exceptions, all anaesthetic drugs are cardiovascular system depressants – acting via a range of direct (myocardial depression, vasodilatation) and indirect (central nervous
system) mechanisms. The resulting fall in cardiac output and tissue perfusion directly obtunds
the normal physiological response to surgery. For this reason, even healthy patients undergoing
minor surgery may be subject to significant cardiovascular depression as a direct consequence
of anaesthetic agents and procedures. In patients with pre-existing cardiovascular disease, the
impact of cardiodepression and vasodilatation may be more pronounced. The signs and symptoms of these surgical stresses to the cardiovascular system are often masked by anaesthesia.

Hypotension

Importance

Perioperative hypotension can be defined as a mean arterial pressure (MAP) 25% below the
patient's normal pre-operative value. While many vital organ systems autoregulate blood flow

Anaesthetic and Perioperative Complications, ed. Kamen Valchanov, Stephen T. Webb and Jane Sturgess.
Published by Cambridge University Press. © Cambridge University Press 2011.

Table 6.1 Cardiovascular responses to anaesthesia and surgery.

Drugs	
Vasodilatation	Hypotension
Myocardial depression	Reduced cardiac output
Positive pressure ventilation	Reduced venous return, reduced cardiac output
	Hypotension, antidiuresis
Posture	
Reverse Trendelenberg	Increased venous return may lead to excessive preload
Trendelenberg	Reduced venous return, reduced cardiac output
Pneumoperitoneum	Reduced venous return, hypercapnia
Hypothermia	Impaired peripheral circulation, coagulopathy
	Postoperative shivering
Surgical stimulation	Increased O_2 consumption
Haemorrhage	Reduced venous return, reduced cardiac output, vasoconstriction

Table 6.2 Mechanisms of hypotension.

Heart rate	Vagal reflexes
	Drugs – β-blockers, neostigmine
	Dysrhythmias – heart block
Stroke volume	Preload
	Hypovolaemia – inadequate resuscitation, gastrointestinal fluid loss, haemorrhage
	Intrathoracic pressure – positive pressure ventilation
	Cardiac filling – pneumothorax, pericardial effusion, tamponade, aortocaval compression
	Afterload
	Aortic stenosis, left ventricular outflow tract obstruction, pulmonary embolism
	Contractility
	Hypoxia, hypercapnia, acidosis, hypothermia, drugs, ischaemic heart disease, myocardial ischaemia, cardiomyopathy, cardiac failure
SVR	Drugs – vasodilators, anaesthetic agents
	Hypersensitivity reactions
	Central neuraxial blockade
	Sepsis

over a wide range of perfusion pressures, hypotension may lead to permanent ischaemic damage. Although myocardial and cerebral metabolic rates are reduced by anaesthesia, profound and prolonged hypotension may cause myocardial ischaemia or infarction, renal failure and stroke.

Causative factors

MAP is the product of cardiac output (CO) and systemic vascular resistance (SVR), and CO the product of heart rate (HR) and stroke volume (SV). It follows, therefore, that a reduction in SVR, SV or HR may produce hypotension (Table 6.2).

Prevention

Patients with existing arterial hypertension are more likely to develop intra-operative hypotension than normotensive individuals. This is especially true for those patients treated with angiotensin converting enzyme (ACE) inhibitors or angiotensin II antagonists, where 'refractory' hypotension may in part be related to decreased intravascular volume. Withholding ACE inhibitors or angiotensin II antagonists for at least ten hours prior to anaesthesia is associated with a reduced risk of post-induction hypotension.

Recognition

Hypotension should be anticipated during induction of anaesthesia, particularly in patients with valvular stenosis or concealed hypovolaemia, and in those dependent on increased sympathetic nervous system (SNS) activity (e.g. heart failure, hypovolaemia). Errors or inaccuracies in blood pressure monitoring may lead to an inappropriate diagnosis. Non-invasive monitoring systems tend to be unreliable at low blood pressures and in the presence of some tachyarrhythmias (e.g. atrial fibrillation). Movement artefacts and the use of an inappropriately sized cuff may give spurious readings. While invasive blood pressure monitoring provides a continuous measure of arterial pressure throughout the cardiac cycle, damping, resonance, zero-drift and incorrect calibration may result in erroneous readings. Additional information (i.e. ECG, end-tidal CO_2, central venous pressure, cardiac output and arterial blood gas analysis) may assist diagnosis.

Management

The treatment of hypotension is largely dictated by its severity and consequences. The goals are identification of the underlying cause and restoration of adequate organ perfusion and oxygenation, rather than achieving a specific blood pressure. Preload should be optimized using posture (Trendelenburg position) and repeated fluid challenges as initial steps. Reducing the inhaled concentration or infusion rates of anaesthetic agents may improve hypotension, but care should be taken to avoid awareness. Intropes (e.g. ephedrine, adrenaline, calcium salts) and vasopressors (e.g. metaraminol, phenylephrine) are commonly used. Failure to respond to initial therapy should prompt additional invasive monitoring (e.g. pulmonary artery catheter) or echocardiography.

Arterial hypertension

Importance

Intra-operative hypertension is defined as arterial pressure (systolic, mean or diastolic) greater than 25% above the pre-operative value. Increased afterload and left ventricular wall tension increases myocardial work and the risk of ischaemia and infarction. Moreover, hypertension may increase surgical bleeding. The risk of myocardial ischaemia is compounded by tachycardia, which typically accompanies SNS-mediated hypertension and reduces diastolic coronary perfusion.

Causative factors

Undiagnosed or poorly controlled pre-existing arterial hypertension may present in the perioperative period, and the abrupt withdrawal of antihypertensive medications may cause elevated blood pressure. Increased SNS tone may be secondary to laryngoscopy, inadequate anaesthesia or analgesia, hypercapnia, hypoxia or tracheal extubation. Raised intracranial pressure secondary to cerebral ischaemia or haemorrhage may cause hypertension and bradycardia (Cushing reflex). Drugs including vasopressors and inotropes, but also ketamine, will raise blood pressure. Other causes of intra-operative hypertension include malignant hyperpyrexia, phaeochromocytoma, thyroid crisis, carcinoid syndrome and aortic cross-clamping. Hypertension in the postoperative period may be caused by uncontrolled pain or anxiety, residual neuromuscular blockade or urinary retention. Hypertension is more common after vascular, head and neck, and neurosurgical procedures.

Recognition

As with hypotension, accurate blood pressure measurement is fundamentally important before the commencement of treatment.

Treatment

Pre-operative hypertension should be treated and, wherever possible, elective surgery delayed until the blood pressure is below 180/110 mmHg. It is thought that below this level patients are not at increased risk of perioperative cardiac complications. For this reason, the withdrawal of antihypertensive medication pre-operatively should be avoided as rebound hypertension may occur. Sedative premedication may help to reduce endogenous catecholamine levels. Having excluded and treated inadequate anaesthesia, antihypertensive drugs such as esmolol, labetolol, hydralazine, nifedipine, sodium nitroprusside and glyceryl trinitrate may be used to control hypertension. These should be carefully titrated as anaesthetic agents can potentiate their effects.

A hypertensive crisis may occur as a feature of hypertensive disease, pregnancy, phaeochromocytoma or following cardiac or vascular surgery. Untreated, the initial symptoms (confusion, headaches, visual disturbances) may progress to encephalopathy, seizures and coma. Associated phenomena may include retinal haemorrhages, papilloedema, renal dysfunction, cardiac failure and stroke. Oral therapy is usually advocated as intravenous antihypertensives may cause a precipitous fall in blood pressure, which in itself may result in renal impairment, stroke or myocardial ischaemia.

Haemorrhage

Importance

Bleeding, which is a normal consequence of virtually every surgical procedure, is considered significant when >15% of the circulating volume has been lost and red blood cells are required to maintain the oxygen-carrying capacity. Pre-existing anaemia worsens the physiological impact of blood loss. Haemorrhage leading to massive transfusion can be defined as loss of the entire blood volume within 24 hours, loss of 50% blood volume within three hours or a blood loss of >150 ml/min. Acute blood loss can be classified according to the percentage of total blood volume lost and the degree of hypovolaemic shock produced with its associated symptoms and signs: class I <15%; class II 15 to 30%; class III 30 to 40%; class IV >40%.

Causative factors

Surgical bleeding may be compounded by congenital or acquired coagulopathy. Inherited disorders of coagulation include haemophilia A and B (deficiencies of factors VIII and IX respectively) and von Willebrand's disease. Thrombocytopenia may be drug-induced, immune-mediated or a consequence of sepsis, chronic disease or disseminated intravascular coagulopathy (DIC). Platelet dysfunction may be drug-induced (non-steroidal anti-inflammatory drugs, aspirin, clopidogrel, prasygrel, abciximab and tirofiban), the result of uraemia or the use of extracorporeal circulation. Hepatic disease sufficient to impair production of vitamin K dependent clotting factors (II, VII, IX, X) may be associated with portal hypertension and oesophageal varices.

Prevention

Pre-operative optimization of a patient's haemoglobin will not prevent haemorrhage, but may reduce perioperative transfusion requirements. Anaemia due to iron or vitamin B_{12} deficiency should be treated, although the pre-operative use of erythropoietin is controversial. Surgical steps to prevent excessive haemorrhage include the use of minimally invasive techniques, tourniquets, adrenaline-containing local anaesthetics and topical haemostatic agents. Anaesthetic techniques used to minimize blood loss include avoidance of hypercapnia, hypothermia, high intrathoracic pressures and venous congestion. Hypotensive anaesthesia is associated with reduced blood loss, but risks the possibility of cerebral and coronary ischaemia. Epidural and spinal anaesthesia may reduce blood loss due to the reduction in both arterial and venous pressures. Acute normovolaemic haemodilution and cell salvage may be used to reduce blood transfusion requirements. Pre-operative autologous blood donation is used less commonly.

Recognition

Blood loss should be estimated from the volume of blood in suction bottles and the weight of swabs. This may be difficult when haemorrhage is concealed or occurs during operations where large volumes of irrigation fluid are used, such as transurethral prostatectomy. Indicative clinical signs such as tachycardia and hypotension often occur late. In massive haemorrhage the subsequent fall in cardiac output may be seen as a fall in peripheral oxygen saturation or end-tidal carbon dioxide. The haemoglobin concentration can be checked intra-operatively with point-of-care testing devices. Laboratory investigations should include full blood count as well as a coagulation screen.

Management

Bleeding should be stopped with the appropriate surgical, obstetric or radiological intervention. Although intravascular volume may be maintained initially with intravenous fluids, ongoing haemorrhage will inevitably mandate the transfusion of red blood cells. Although there is no absolute transfusion trigger most guidelines recommend that patients with a haemoglobin concentration <7 g/dl should receive blood. In patients with cardiac or respiratory co-morbidities who tolerate anaemia poorly this level may be higher. A blood warmer should be used where possible and a rapid infuser may be advantageous where there is significant haemorrhage. Fresh frozen plasma and clotting factors will be required when large volumes of blood have been replaced. Recombinant factors VIIa, XIIIa and fibrinogen are used for haemorrhage unresponsive to blood product therapy. Cell salvage may help reduce the amount of packed red cells required and its use may extend into the postoperative period following orthopaedic or cardiac surgery.

Myocardial ischaemia

Importance

Perioperative myocardial ischaemia (PMI) and infarction (MI) are significant events associated with a hospital mortality of up to 25%. Furthermore, a non-fatal perioperative MI is a significant risk factor for death or repeat MI within six months. In most cases PMI and MI are preventable. The peak incidence of PMI occurs within three days of surgery. Patients with a history of coronary artery disease are at highest risk but other risk factors include postoperative anaemia, hypothermia and pain.

Causative factors

The pathogenesis and clinical features of perioperative MI appear to differ from those of MI in the non-operative setting. In addition to coronary plaque rupture and subsequent platelet aggregation and thrombosis, perioperative MI may occur as the result of an imbalance between myocardial O_2 supply and demand, and imbalance between thrombotic and thrombolytic mechanisms.

Induction and emergence from anaesthesia are thought to be periods of vulnerability for developing PMI. Emergence is typically associated with increased HR, blood pressure, SNS tone and procoagulant activity. Increased SNS tone increases myocardial O_2 demand and coronary vascular shear stress.

Recognition

The triad of typical ischaemic chest pain, typical ECG changes and increased serum concentration of creatine kinase (CK)-MB isoenzyme is often absent. The diagnosis of PMI is thus difficult to make and requires both vigilance and a high index of suspicion. Unexplained hypotension, dysrhythmia or non-specific ECG changes during surgery may be the only clinical manifestations. While continuous, multi-lead ECG monitoring using a five-lead ECG system has high sensitivity for the detection of myocardial ischaemia, echocardiographic evidence of a new regional ventricular wall motion abnormality provides earlier detection of ischaemia.

In more than 80% of cases, PMI and MI are clinically 'silent' and there are no standard diagnostic criteria. Symptoms such as dyspnoea and nausea, and physical signs such as hypotension and tachycardia, are so common in the postoperative period that they may be attributed to non-cardiac causes such as bleeding, atelectasis, pneumonia or drug side effects. The ECG is also uncharacteristic; ST segment depression, rather than ST segment elevation or Q-waves, are more commonly seen in perioperative MIs. The duration of ST segment depression (the so-called 'ischaemic burden') appears to be of prognostic significance.

Biochemical markers of myocardial injury may be difficult to interpret in the postoperative period. Creatine kinase levels are invariably elevated in surgical patients, leading to false positive results. However, particularly high CK levels, which result in a low CK-MB : CK

Table 6.3 The Lee Revised Cardiac Risk Index (RCRI). Original outcome data from 4,315 patients >50 years old (2,893 derivation, 1,422 validation). *Circulation* 1999; 100: 1043–9. The score calculated from the left-hand table is used in the second column of the right-hand table to calculate risk.

Factor	Score
High-risk surgery	1
History of ischaemic heart disease	1
History of congestive cardiac failure	1
History of cerebrovascular disease	1
Pre-operative insulin therapy	1
Pre-operative creatinine >177 µmol/l (2 mg/day)	1

Class	Score	Mortality
I	0	0.4–0.5%
II	1	0.9–1.3%
III	2	4–7%
IV	>2	9–11%

ratio, may prompt a false negative result. Assays for cardiac troponins T (cTnT) and I (cTnI) are highly sensitive and specific for myocardial injury. Appropriate cut-off concentrations for defining a clinically significant cardiac event remain the subject of debate. It should be borne in mind that non-cardiac conditions, such as pulmonary embolism and renal failure, may be associated with elevation of cTnT and cTnI. In the setting of acute coronary syndrome, however, a small increase in serum troponin concentrations is an independent predictor for mortality and major cardiac events.

Prevention

Prevention of perioperative myocardial ischaemia requires the assessment and modification of cardiac risk. Risk modification strategies can be considered in two groups; myocardial revascularization and drug therapy. The Lee Revised Cardiac Risk Index (Table 6.3) is widely used to identify patients at increased cardiovascular risk by virtue of their medical history, functional status and the type of surgery proposed. Existing practice guidelines suggest that high-risk patients and *some* intermediate-risk patients benefit from additional investigation (e.g. stress echocardiography, myocardial viability studies) and, if necessary, coronary revascularization. The initial enthusiasm for pre-operative coronary revascularization was soon tempered by the observation that as many as 20% of patients undergoing surgery after percutaneous intervention (PCI) died. At present, pre-operative coronary revascularization is reserved for patients with symptomatic or unstable ischaemic heart disease. Pharmacological risk modification or cardioprotection is summarized in Table 6.4.

A number of perioperative anaesthetic strategies are advocated for reducing the risk of PMI in susceptible patients. Of these, the prevention of inadvertent hypothermia and secondary SNS activation appears to be of benefit. Contrary to conventional wisdom, choice of anaesthetic technique (i.e. regional vs. general) appears to have no impact on cardiovascular outcome.

Management

There is no good evidence to guide the management of PMI. It seems prudent to identify and treat correctable causes such as hypoxia or anaemia. Thrombolytic, antiplatelet and anticoagulant therapies have different risk–benefit ratios in the perioperative setting. Secondary

Table 6.4 Perioperative pharmacological cardioprotection.

Drug	Comments
Beta-blockers	Improve myocardial oxygenation by reducing HR and myocardial contractility.
	Promote coronary plaque stability by reducing mechanical and shear stresses.
	Reduced risk of non-fatal MI and myocardial ischaemia, but at the expense of increased risk of non-fatal stroke, and possibly all-cause mortality.
	In studies where β-blocker dose was titrated to HR there appears to be no increased stroke rate. Heart rate <70 bpm was associated with the best outcome.
Statins	The 3-hydroxy-3-methylglutanyl (HMG) coenzyme A reductase inhibitors exert pleiotropic effects to stabilize vulnerable atherosclerotic plaques as well as reducing inflammatory activity. Their perioperative use is associated with a significant reduction in cardiovascular morbidity and mortality. Current evidence suggests that statin therapy should be restarted as soon as possible after surgery.
Calcium antagonists	Calcium channel blockers dilate coronary arteries, but there is no good evidence to support their perioperative use.
α_2-agonists	Suppress release of catecholamines and they have been shown to reduce postoperative MI and mortality, but only in select groups of patients.
	May be a suitable alternative in patients with contraindications to β-blockers.
Opioids	Ischaemic pre-conditioning.
Volatile anaesthetic agents	Ischaemic pre-conditioning. Ischaemic post-conditioning.

prevention and long-term management with aspirin, ACE inhibitors, beta-blockers and statins may not have the same benefits in this cohort of patients.

Pulmonary oedema

Importance

Pulmonary oedema is a major perioperative event associated with increased length of ICU and hospital stay, and significant mortality. The postoperative risk may be as high as 7.6%, with a peak incidence within 36 hours of surgery.

Causative factors

Four Starling pressures (P_c, capillary hydrostatic pressure; P_i, interstitial fluid pressure; π_p, plasma colloid osmotic pressure; and π_i, peri-capillary interstitial fluid colloid osmotic pressure) determine the equilibrium of extracellular fluid across pulmonary capillary membranes (Table 6.5). Any disruption of this equilibrium or changes in membrane permeability may cause pulmonary oedema.

Transmembrane flow $\alpha \, [(P_c - P_i) - (\pi_p - \pi_i)]$.

Table 6.5 Classification and causes of pulmonary oedema.

Cardiogenic	Chronic congestive cardiac failure, myocardial infarction, arrhythmias, mitral valve disease, left ventricular outflow tract obstruction	
Non-cardiogenic	Acute lung injury	Sepsis, inflammation, aspiration, pulmonary reperfusion, pulmonary re-expansion, blood transfusion reactions
	Fluid maldistribution	Hypotonic fluid – TURP syndrome Isotonic fluid – amniotic fluid embolism Hypoalbuminaemia
	Negative pressure	Laryngospasm, obstructive sleep apnoea, bronchial obstruction, airway trauma
	Neurogenic	Subarachnoid haemorrhage, intraparenchymal bleed, brain or spinal cord trauma, encephalitis, meningitis, hypoglycaemia
	Drugs	Naloxone, opioid poisoning, tocolytics
	Anaphylaxis	–

Recognition

Pulmonary oedema is a relatively rare during surgery as both intermittent positive pressure ventilation and reduced SVR reduce capillary hydrostatic pressures and cardiac afterload. Signs that may be seen in anaesthetized patients include tachycardia, arterial desaturation, increased respiratory efforts, reduced pulmonary compliance and copious pink frothy secretions in the endotracheal tube. Fine inspiratory crackles may be heard on auscultation together with cardiac murmurs and a third heart sound. ECG changes may be seen with arrhythmias and evidence of ischaemia or right heart strain. The erect chest radiograph characteristically shows upper lobe venous diversion, 'bat wings' appearance, Kerley B lines, interlobar fluid lines, effusions and cardiac enlargement. An echocardiogram may be required for confirmation of the cause.

Management

Management is directed to the underlying cause and avoidance of lethal hypoxaemia. In spontaneously breathing patients, the sitting position and oxygen administration are initial measures. Continuous positive airway pressure (CPAP) may be required. In mechanically ventilated patients the application of positive end-expiratory pressure (PEEP) may be helpful. Morphine helps to reduce respiratory distress as well as causing venodilatation. Diuretics may be indicated especially if there is an element of fluid overload, with furosemide causing venodilatation as well as a diuresis. It is important to control arrhythmias. In cases of severe myocardial dysfunction inodilators may be required.

Dysrhythmias

Importance

Cardiac dysrhythmias affect up to 29% of patients having non-cardiac surgery and are a significant cause of morbidity and mortality in the perioperative period. Although dysrhythmias

Table 6.6 Causes of perioperative dysrhythmias.

Reversible problems	Pre-existing cardiac conditions	Drug effects	Rarer causes
Hypoxia	Ischaemic heart disease	Halothane	Phaeochromocytoma
Hypercarbia	Congenital heart disease	Local anaesthetic toxicity	Thyrotoxicosis
Hypotension	Cardiomyopathy	Inotropes	Carcinoid syndrome
Hypertension	Wolff–Parkinson–White syndrome	Digoxin toxicity	Malignant hyperthermia
Hypothermia	Long QT syndrome	Prolonged QT – ondansetron, droperidol, sevoflurane, class III antiarrhythmic agents, some fluroquinolone and macrolide antibiotics, antipsychotic and antidepressant drugs	Subarachnoid haemorrhage
Metabolic and electrolyte abnormalities			Drug or solvent abuse
Mechanical irritation – CVC insertion, PA catheter, chest drains			

may be the manifestation of an underlying cardiac disorder, they are an independent risk factor for future cardiac events. The incidence of dysrhythmias is greater following cardiac surgery. Postoperative atrial fibrillation (AF) is associated with a 2.3-fold increase in the risk of stroke, as well as an increased incidence of ventricular dysrhythmias, myocardial infarction, congestive cardiac failure and renal failure.

Causative factors

The majority of cardiac dysrhythmias occur in patients with pre-existing heart disease who have sustained an additional insult in the perioperative period. Cardiac, thoracic and laparoscopic surgeries are the commonest settings for perioperative dysrhythmias, with more than 15% of thoracic patients having an arrhythmia. Other causes of dysrhythmias are summarized in Table 6.6.

Long QT syndrome, whether congenital or acquired, is significant as it predisposes to the development of polymorphic ventricular tachycardia torsade de pointes, which can degenerate to ventricular fibrillation and sudden death. Patients with cardiomyopathy are at a significantly increased risk of PMI or sudden death during non-cardiac surgery.

Prevention

In order to prevent dysrhythmias reversible causes such as hypoxia, hypotension, acidosis and electrolyte abnormalities should be avoided, particularly in those at high risk. Beta-blockers have been shown to reduce the incidence of perioperative AF by up to 61%. However, the addition of prophylactic magnesium to β-blockers therapy is supported by limited evidence.

As increased intravascular volume is a common contributing factor to the development of dysrhythmias, fluid overload should be avoided.

Recognition

ECG monitoring is standard during anaesthesia but a 12-lead ECG may be required postoperatively to confirm the diagnosis. Evaluation of the ECG should include heart rate and regularity, the presence of p-waves and the configuration of the QRS complex. It is also important to note the existence of myocardial ischaemia, which may be a cause or consequence of the dysrhythmia. Assessment of the degree of cardiovascular compromise caused by the dysrhythmia is also crucial.

Sinus arrhythmias (tachycardia and bradycardia) are the most frequently encountered intra-operative dysrhythmias. Bradycardia may follow activation of vagal reflexes such as the oculocardiac reflex during ophthalmic surgery, or the Brewer–Luckhardt reflex during anal or cervical stretching. Hypoxia, high-sympathetic block, acute myocardial infarction or drugs may all lead to bradycardia. Sinus tachycardia may be due to pain, light anaesthesia, sepsis, hypoxia, hypovolaemia, hypercapnia or drugs.

Conduction abnormalities may cause complete heart block, which may require temporary or permanent pacing. However, it is rare for patients with intraventricular conduction delays even in the presence of left- or right-bundle branch block to progress to complete heart block intra-operatively.

Management

The urgency of dysrhythmia management is determined by the degree of cardiovascular compromise. When associated with profound hypotension, synchronous DC cardioversion may be appropriate. Any reversible cause should be corrected prior to consideration of antidysrhythmic medication. In patients with new onset AF, the clinical picture will determine whether rhythm or rate control is most appropriate. Amiodarone, digoxin, β-blockers and rate-limiting calcium channel blockers all have a place in the management of tachyarrhythmias. Atropine, glycopyrrolate or temporary pacing may be appropriate in bradyarrhythmias or heart block.

Venous thromboembolism

Importance

Venous thromboembolism (VTE) encompasses a spectrum of conditions ranging from asymptomatic leg vein thrombosis to fatal pulmonary embolism (PE). It is the third most common cause of death in hospitalized patients. Chronic venous insufficiency secondary to venous thrombosis is associated with significant long-term morbidity. Non-fatal PE is associated with significant short- and long-term morbidity and represents a considerable healthcare burden. In a significant number of patients repeated episodes of asymptomatic PE may eventually lead to chronic thromboembolic pulmonary hypertension.

Causative factors

Surgical patients are considered to be at increased risk of VTE if they meet one or more of the criteria shown in Table 6.7.

Prevention

Published by the National Institute for Health and Clinical Excellence (NICE) in 2010, *Clinical Guideline 92* provides a framework for VTE risk reduction in hospitalized adults. General measures to reduce the risk of VTE include avoiding dehydration if possible, encouraging early mobilization and considering cessation of oestrogen-containing oral contraceptive pills or hormone replacement therapy. The benefits of regional over general anaesthesia, with its reduced risk of VTE should be contemplated.

Table 6.7 Risk factors for venous thromboembolism.

Patient factors	Surgical factors	Disease processes
Age >60 years	Any surgery >90 minutes duration	Active cancer/cancer treatment
Obesity (BMI >30 kg m^{-2})		
Existing varicose veins with phlebitis	Pelvic surgery >60 minutes	Thrombophilia – PS, PC, APS
	Lower limb surgery >60 minutes	
Dehydration	Acute intra-abdominal condition	Heart disease
Personal family history of VTE		Metabolic/endocrine conditions
Pregnancy and puerperium	Significant immobility expected	
Hormone replacement therapy	Critical care unit admission	Acute infectious disease
Oestrogen-based contraceptives		Inflammatory conditions

BMI, body mass index; VTE, venous thromboembolism; PS, protein S deficiency; PC, protein C deficiency; APS, antiphospholipid syndrome.

Perioperative VTE prophylaxis comprises both pharmacological and non-pharmacological measures. Pharmacological measures include low molecular weight heparin (LMWH), unfractionated heparin (UFH), fondaparinux sodium, dabigatran etexilate and rivaroxaban. Non-pharmacological or mechanical methods comprise anti-embolism (graduated compression) stockings, intermittent pneumatic leg compression devices and foot impulse devices. Temporary inferior vena cava (IVC) filters may be considered for patients at very high risk when pharmacological and mechanical prophylaxis is contraindicated.

Recognition

The clinical features of a deep vein thrombosis (DVT) occur due to the obstruction of venous drainage and include pain, tenderness, unilateral leg swelling, warmth, erythema and dilation of surface leg veins. However, up to 50% may be asymptomatic. Clinical prediction rules such as the Well's score are used to predict the likelihood of DVT or PE and are used to guide further investigations. D-dimers are highly sensitive (97%) for VTE but have low specificity, particularly in the postoperative period. Venous duplex ultrasound is usually the investigation of choice as it is non-invasive and has both high sensitivity (97%) and specificity (94%).

Pulmonary embolization often presents with non-specific signs such as progressive dyspnoea, but if peripheral occlusion of a pulmonary artery causing parenchymal infarction occurs, pleuritic chest pain, cough and haemoptysis may occur and a pleural rub or wheeze heard on auscultation. In massive PE there is cardiovascular collapse with hypotension, tachycardia, dyspnoea and acute pulmonary hypertension. The arterial blood gas will typically show hypoxaemia, hypocapnia and a respiratory alkalosis. A chest radiograph, often done to exclude other causes of dyspnoea, is usually initially normal although wedge-shaped infarcts may be seen. The classical ECG right-sided strain pattern of S_1-Q_3-T_3 only occurs in 20% of patients with proven PE but an echocardiogram is often diagnostic in massive PE. A CT pulmonary angiogram is the recommended initial lung-imaging modality. Isotope lung scanning may be considered if CT is unavailable, provided there is no underlying cardiopulmonary disease and the chest radiograph is normal. Conventional pulmonary angiography is rarely performed.

Management

Anticoagulation is the mainstay of management in VTE and should be initiated as soon as a DVT or PE is suspected. This is usually with LMWH, although unfractionated heparin may be used in patients with renal dysfunction. Oral anticoagulation is then commenced once VTE has been confirmed. Warfarin is typically used in the long-term aiming for an international normalized ratio (INR) of 2 to 3. The duration of therapy varies and depends on the aetiology and individual patient risk factors. Three months is usually recommended for a first episode related to a transient reversible risk factor, although indefinite therapy may be required for those with recurrent episodes or with irreversible risk factors.

Thrombolysis is the first-line treatment for massive PE and cardiovascular support may also be required in these patients. An inferior vena cava (IVC) filter may be required in patients with a contraindication to anticoagulation therapy, those who have recurrent VTE despite being anticoagulated or those who survive a massive PE but in whom recurrent embolism may prove fatal.

Pulmonary hypertension

Importance

Pulmonary hypertension is defined as a persistent mean pulmonary artery (PA) pressure greater than 25 mmHg, with a wedge pressure less than 15 mmHg. Elevation of PA pressure on exercise is no longer considered to be a diagnostic criterion. It is associated with increased perioperative morbidity, with respiratory failure, cardiac arrhythmias and congestive cardiac failure being the most common complications. Due to these complications, patients have an increased risk of dying in the early postoperative period with mortality rates of up to 25%.

Causative factors

Hypoxic pulmonary vasoconstriction is the physiological mechanism that causes shunting of blood to well oxygenated (ventilated) areas of the lungs, thus improving ventilation and perfusion matching. Transient hypoxic pulmonary vasoconstriction is therefore useful; however, persistent hypoxaemia and pulmonary vasoconstriction may result in sustained raised PA pressures and pulmonary hypertension may develop. Chronic pulmonary hypertension leads to right ventricular dilatation, hypertrophy and failure.

In the perioperative setting the commonest causes of acute pulmonary hypertension include VTE and amniotic fluid embolism (AFE). Amniotic fluid embolism is a rare but potentially fatal complication of the peripartum period, whose aetiology is not clear but is related to the exposure of maternal blood vessels to fetal tissue. Hypoxia associated with hepatic dysfunction and intrapulmonary shunts may lead to portopulmonary hypertension in patients with end-stage liver disease. Pulmonary hypertension may also develop post-cardiopulmonary bypass due to various perioperative factors. The ischaemia-reperfusion injury causes an imbalance of vasoconstrictors and vasodilators at the pulmonary vascular bed, and this, combined with intra-operative hypoxia, acidosis, hypothermia and micro-embolism, may exacerbate pulmonary hypertension. Protamine used for heparin reversal is also associated with the development of pulmonary hypertension.

Prevention

Exacerbating factors should be avoided in patients with pulmonary hypertension. These include hypoxia, hypotension, hypervolaemia, acidosis, hypothermia and raised intrathoracic pressures as pulmonary vascular resistance is lowest at functional residual capacity. Anaesthetic drugs also have an effect on pulmonary vasculature, although the results of various studies are contradictory. Standard teaching states that inhalational, but not intravenous, agents blunt hypoxic pulmonary vasoconstriction and ketamine is known to cause pulmonary vasodilatation.

Recognition

Symptoms suggestive of pulmonary hypertension include dyspnoea, fatigue, syncope and chest pain secondary to right ventricular ischaemia. With the progression to right heart failure a raised jugular venous pressure is seen with giant cv-waves and peripheral oedema, hepatomegaly and ascites may develop. A loud second heart sound (P2) is suggestive of a raised PA pressure, and pulmonary regurgitation due to the dilatation of the pulmonary valve annulus can occur.

Cardiac catheterization is the gold standard investigation to measure pulmonary artery pressures, but other less invasive investigations may be of use. The ECG may demonstrate right ventricular hypertrophy, which has high specificity but low sensitivity for pulmonary hypertension. A chest radiograph may demonstrate right atrial and ventricular enlargement as well as a large pulmonary artery. An echocardiogram can assess PA pressures and a CT scan may detect evidence of thromboembolic disease.

Management

Oxygen is indicated if the patient is hypoxic and anticoagulation is required. In anaesthetized patients, sodium nitroprusside or glyceryl trinitrate were traditionally used, acting as nitric oxide donors to reduce pulmonary vascular resistance. However, both these drugs also reduce SVR, which may further impair right ventricular perfusion. Nitric oxide is an inhaled selective pulmonary vasodilator increasing blood flow to ventilated areas of the lungs. This reduces pulmonary vascular resistance, but also improves oxygenation by improving ventilation perfusion matching. Sildenafil, a phosphodiesterase-5 inhibitor, produces pulmonary vasodilatation and also enhances the effects of nitric oxide. Inhaled prostaglandins are also used for perioperative pulmonary hypertension. The endothelin inhibitor Bosentan is also used for pulmonary hypertension control in outpatient settings. Prostacyclin can be given via a nebulizer or intravenously as epoprostenol. Iloprost is a prostacyclin analogue that can be inhaled by non-intubated patients. Calcium channel blockers may be used but are effective in only 15 to 25% of patients.

Air embolism

Importance

Air embolism is due to the inadvertent administration or entrainment of air into blood vessels. This typically occurs in the venous system where air enters the right side of the heart. The air often becomes localized initially at the junction of the SVC and RA before passing through to the right ventricle. Small emboli may be eliminated into the pulmonary arteries; however, larger volumes cause right ventricular outflow tract obstruction with the subsequent fall in cardiac output. The true incidence of air embolism will probably never be established, as it is dependent on the method of detection, as much subclinical air embolism may go undetected and thus unreported.

Causative factors

Venous air embolism can occur when there is a communication between a vein and a source of air and a pressure gradient down which the air can enter the circulation.

Patients positioned in the head-up position during head and neck surgery are at risk of air embolism when large veins are opened. However, those in the sitting position for posterior fossa surgery are at even higher risk as the dural sinuses do not collapse and an incidence of air embolism of up to 58% has been reported. Other surgical procedures of increased risk are open-heart surgery, hepatic resection, hip arthroplasty and caesarean section where air may enter the uterine sinuses in up to 40% of patients. The use of gas-cooled laser probes can lead to gas emboli, and laser surgery to bronchial carcinoma has been associated with the formation of fistula between bronchi and the pulmonary veins. The inadvertent insufflation of gas into a vessel or organ during laparoscopic surgery also causes gas embolism.

Entrainment of air also occurs through intravenous cannulae. The incidence of air embolism associated with central venous catheters is reported to be 1:47 to 1:3,000. Common causes include faulty connections, incorrect use of taps, failure to prime tubing and the administration of fluids under pressure. Other causes of air embolism include epidural insertion with a loss of resistance to air technique and chest trauma.

Recognition

The clinical features of gas emboli are dependent on the volume of gas in the circulation as well as the rate of accumulation. A rate of 0.5 ml/kg/min can produce symptoms and a total air volume of 200 to 300 ml (3 to 5 ml/kg) has been described as a fatal dose. The use of nitrous oxide also influences the clinical picture as administration of 50% N_2O can increase the size of the bubble by 200% and 75% N_2O by 400%.

Cardiovascular complications including dysrhythmias, most commonly sinus tachycardia but also ventricular ectopics or fibrillation, can occur. The ECG may show evidence of right heart strain with non-specific ST changes. Tinkling sounds may be heard on precordial auscultation but the classical 'mill-wheel' murmur only occurs as a late sign with large volumes of air in the circulation. A loss of the end-tidal CO_2 trace is seen due to decreased dead space caused by the emboli and reduced cardiac output. The CVP is often raised and the jugular veins distended. Circulatory collapse is common with larger emboli although there may be a brief preceding period of hypertension. Dyspnoea, hypoxia, cyanosis, increased pulmonary artery pressures, bronchospasm and pulmonary oedema may all be seen.

Around 20 to 35% of the population have a patent foramen ovale and if right atrial pressure exceeds left atrial pressure there is a possibility that venous air may enter the systemic circulation. These paradoxical air emboli can cause seizures, loss of consciousness and transient or permanent focal deficits.

A transoesophageal echocardiogram is the most accurate way of diagnosing venous air embolism, although it may over-diagnose the problem identifying as little as 0.02 ml/kg of air. Precordial Doppler is the most sensitive non-invasive method, detecting 0.05 ml/kg of air. The chest radiograph is often normal, but may show gas in the pulmonary arteries, focal oligaemia or pulmonary oedema. Computerized tomography may also aid diagnosis, demonstrating air in the central veins, right ventricle or pulmonary veins.

Prevention

As the majority of air emboli are iatrogenic, this condition can be prevented. The sitting position is now less commonly used for posterior fossa surgery, and Trendelenburg positioning can raise venous pressure during hepatic resection. The Trendelenburg position is also recommended during central venous cannulation, and the supine position during active exhalation for catheter removal. During procedures where there is a high risk of air embolism the avoidance of nitrous oxide is recommended, although the routine use of PEEP is controversial.

Management

The aims of management are to identify the source of entry in order to prevent further air entrainment, reduce the volume of air if possible and give haemodynamic support. The site of entry should be covered or flooded with fluid. If possible open veins in the surgical field should be ligated, cauterized, packed or surgical bone wax applied. Mechanisms to increase venous pressure such as intravenous fluid administration and jugular venous compression may help. If cardiac output is seriously compromised cardiopulmonary resuscitation may be required although a left-sided, head-down tilt in order to relocate the air to the right atrium and reduce pulmonary outflow tract obstruction is of questionable benefit. Specialized wide-bore, multi-orifice catheters are available to aspirate air from the right atrium, although the therapeutic benefit of this is doubtful. Hyperbaric oxygen has also been used where facilities exist to reduce the size of the embolus and improve oxygenation.

List of further reading

Daumerie, G. & Fleisher, L. A. Perioperative beta-blocker and statin therapy. *Curr Opin Anaesthesiol* 2008; **21**(1): 60–5.

Devereaux, P. J., Yang, H., Yusuf, S. *et al.* Effects of extended-release metoprolol succinate in patients undergoing non-cardiac surgery (POISE trial): a randomised controlled trial. *Lancet* 2008; **371**(9627): 1839–47.

Fleisher, L. A., Beckman, J. A., Brown, K. A. *et al.* ACC/AHA 2007 guidelines on perioperative cardiovascular evaluation and care for noncardiac surgery: a report of the American College of Cardiology/American Heart Association Task Force on Practice Guidelines. *Circulation* 2007; **116**(17): e418–99.

Kneterpal, S., O'Reilly, M., Englesbe, M. *et al.* Preoperative and interoperative predictors of cardiac adverse events after general, vascular and urological surgery. *Anaesthesiology* 2009; **110**(1): 58–66.

MacKnight, B., Martinez, E. A. & Simon, B. A. Anesthetic management of patients with pulmonary hypertension. *Semin Cardiothorac Vasc Anesth* 2008; **12**(2): 91–6.

National Institute for Health and Clinical Excellence. Venous thromboembolism: reducing the risk. *NICE Clinical Guideline 92*, 2010.

Poldermans, D., Bax, J. J., Schouten, O. *et al.* Should major vascular surgery be delayed because of preoperative cardiac testing in intermediate-risk patients receiving beta-blocker therapy with tight heart rate control? *JACC* 2006; **48**(5): 964–9.

Priebe, H-J. Perioperative myocardial infarction: aetiology and prevention. *Br J Anaesth* 2005; **95**(1): 3–19.

Subramaniam, K. & Yared, J. P. Management of pulmonary hypertension in the operating room. *Semin Cardiothorac Vasc Anesth* 2007; **11**(2): 119–36.

Webb, S. & Arrowsmith, J. Perioperative cardioprotection. In Hunter, J., Cook, T., Priebe, H-J. & Struys, M. (eds). *The Year in Anaesthesia and Critical Pain*, Volume 2. Oxford: Clinical Publishing, 2008, pp. 71–99.

Wijeysundera, D. N., Beattie, W. S., Austin, P. C., Hux, J. E. & Laupacis, A. Non-invasive cardiac stress testing before elective major non-cardiac surgery: population based cohort study. *BMJ* 2010; **340**: b5526.

Complications of blood products and fluid infusions

Dafydd Thomas and Tom Holmes

Introduction

There are potential complications involved in the administration of any intravenous (IV) fluid. These can arise from a patient reaction to the fluid, which could be at the site of infusion, or a systemic effect, which may be immediate or delayed. Complications may also be related to inappropriate or poor administration procedures. This chapter will cover the complications of blood, colloid and crystalloid administration.

Blood

Approximately 30% of all blood issued by the blood services is given to surgical patients during the perioperative period. Therefore it is crucial that the anaesthetist has a clear knowledge of potential complications related to fluid administration.

The benefit of blood transfusion in saving life has been recognized for some time. In 1818, a British obstetrician, Dr James Blundell, successfully transfused a woman with her husband's blood to treat post-partum haemorrhage. However, the dangers of blood transfusion have been known for even longer. It was banned for the previous 150 years following catastrophic events. The first series of documented blood transfusions in England and France resulted in a number of fatalities.

At the turn of the twentieth century, ABO blood grouping and its significance in acute haemolytic reactions was realized by Landsteiner. Between the two World Wars (WW) it became evident that anticoagulation could enable the storage of blood. This led to the organization of blood services providing a stored supply of blood for injured patients. Clearly the soldiers during the Second World War benefited from improved resuscitation as a result of blood component availability. Hepatitis was a major hazard when those soldiers who had been transfused returned home. Over the ensuing 40 years it became apparent that many diseases could be transmitted by blood transfusion. In fact it took 30 years to identify hepatitis B (then known as hepatitis virus) and then develop a test, but today we have seen near eradication of its transmission via blood transfusion.

Today, the leading causes of allogeneic blood transfusion (ABT)-related mortality in both the USA and UK are transfusion-related acute lung injury (TRALI), ABO and non-ABO haemolytic transfusion reactions (HTRs) and transfusion-associated sepsis (TAS).

Anaesthetic and Perioperative Complications, ed. Kamen Valchanov, Stephen T. Webb and Jane Sturgess. Published by Cambridge University Press. © Cambridge University Press 2011.

Table 7.1 Strategies to reduce risk from blood transfusion.

Strategy	Risks minimized by strategy
Minimize exposure to transfused blood: • transfusion guidelines • avoid pooled products • cell salvage	Reduction in all adverse reactions
Identification systems	Acute and delayed HTR
Fresh frozen plasma and single-donor platelets from males or females without a history of pregnancy	TRALI PTP TAS
Leukoreduced blood	Possible reduced TTI, TAS, TRALI, TRIM and PTP

Data show that the most frequent reported root cause of HTRs is incorrect or inappropriate transfusion of a blood product. The error can arise anywhere within the system, from donor choice, laboratory and administrative errors, to unnecessary transfusion.

The realization that there can be many adverse events resulting from blood component administration has led to the formation and development of a haemovigilant culture. Reporting of complications from transfusion is now undertaken in many countries including the UK (Serious Adverse Bloods Reactions and Events – SABRE). The Serious Hazards of Transfusion (SHOT) initiative was created as a hub for reporting and responding to transfusion-related incidents. Over the first 11 years of reporting (1996 to 2007) in the UK, transfusion was considered to have a causal or contributory role in 115 deaths reported. The lowest transfusion-related mortality rate, since SHOT began in 1996, was recorded in 2007 when there was no death definitely attributable to ABT. A well developed haemovigilance programme monitors the risk of ABT-related adverse events and from the data develops strategies to overcome the risks. Table 7.1 shows some examples of strategies that can be used and Figure 7.1 shows the cumulative cases reviewed by SHOT from 1996 to 2009.

Immune transfusion reactions

Febrile non-haemolytic transfusion reaction

The most common transfusion reaction is a febrile non-haemolytic transfusion reaction (FNHTR). Fever occurs within six hours of the transfusion starting and is sometimes accompanied by mild dyspnoea and rigors. Febrile non-haemolytic transfusion reactions are benign and have no lasting sequelae. Only 15% of patients who have an FNHTR will have a second reaction on subsequent transfusion.

A number of studies have shown that the degree of leukocyte contamination and the presence of cytokines (such as interleukin (IL)-1, IL-6, IL-8 and tumor necrosis factor-alpha) within the blood product are associated with FNHTR. Evidence for these theories would seem to be backed up by the observations that leukoreduction and decreased storage time (i.e. less time for cytokine generation and accumulation) are both associated with lower incidence of FNHTR.

The importance of early recognition is that initial symptoms and signs of serious (acute haemolytic) and benign (FNHTR) immune reactions are similar. Initial management of FNHTRs therefore most importantly consists of stopping the transfusion, administration of antipyretics

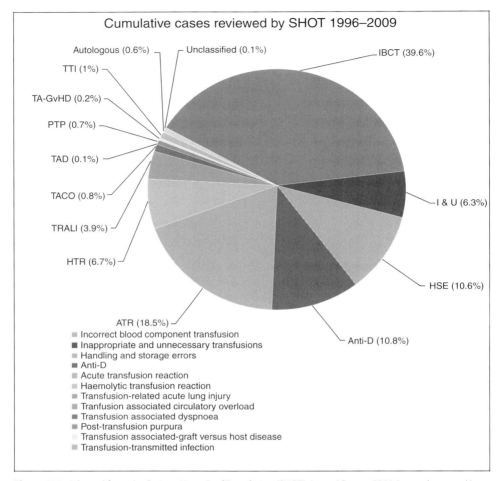

Figure 7.1 Adapted from the Serious Hazards of Transfusion (SHOT) Annual Report 2009 (www.shot.org.uk).

and ruling out acute haemolytic reaction. This is more complicated in unconscious or anaesthetized patients. Recognition of signs rather than symptoms becomes important. Relevant clinical signs, such as a raised temperature or skin rashes, help diagnosis and treatment.

Acute haemolytic transfusion reaction

An acute haemolytic transfusion reaction (AHTR) is a medical emergency that results from the rapid destruction of donor erythrocytes by pre-formed recipient antibodies, e.g. ABO incompatibility. Most fatalities from haemolytic transfusion reactions have been associated with RBC transfusions of 200 ml or more, and mortality is approximately 44% for transfusions exceeding 1,000 ml.

Between 1996 and 2007 there were 213 ABO-incompatible RBC transfusions reported to SHOT. This included 24 deaths. Only three AHTRs were reported in 2007. It is thought that development of improved procedures and systems for checking the identity of units and

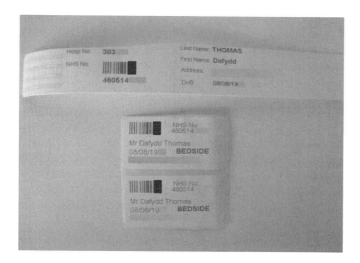

Figure 7.2 Bar-coded identification wrist band with bar-coded labels.

patients has led to the very low error rate. Evolving technologies e.g. barrier systems, bar codes and patient identification systems (Figure 7.2), have been associated with low rates of sample collection errors – too low to estimate.

When an AHTR occurs, the classic presentation is a triad of fever, flank pain and red-brown urine (i.e. haemoglobinuria). This is not often seen. As mentioned, fever may be the only initial manifestation. In patients under anaesthesia, delayed recognition may mean DIC is the presenting manifestation.

Management includes confirming the diagnosis with the direct antiglobulin (Coombs) test, informing the blood bank and aggressive supportive care. Cardiovascular collapse, renal failure and DIC can occur.

Delayed haemolytic transfusion reactions

Delayed haemolytic transfusion reactions (DHTRs) are due to an anamnestic antibody response following alloimmunization to a foreign red cell antigen during a prior transfusion, transplantation or pregnancy. The antibody, often of the Kidd or Rhesus systems, is undetect-able on pre-transfusion testing but increases rapidly in titre following the transfusion.

These delayed reactions are usually seen within two to ten days after transfusion. Haemolysis is mainly extravascular, gradual and less severe than with acute reactions. Rapid haemolysis can occur. A falling haematocrit, slight fever, mild increase in serum unconju-gated bilirubin and spherocytosis on the blood smear may be seen. The diagnosis is often made by the blood bank when a new positive direct antiglobulin test and a new positive antibody screen are found when more blood is ordered.

No treatment is required in the absence of brisk haemolysis. However, future transfu-sions containing the implicated red cell antigen need to be avoided. It is therefore important to make the diagnosis and maintain hospital and blood bank records.

Transfusion-related acute lung injury (TRALI)

The National Heart, Lung and Blood Institute Working Group and Canadian Consensus Conference have defined TRALI as a new acute lung injury (ALI) occurring within six hours after a blood product transfusion. This ALI can present anywhere on a spectrum, with ARDS at one extreme. Most patients recover fully within 96 hours.

Transfusion-related acute lung injury has been reported as occurring following all types of blood components; however, fresh frozen plasma (FFP) has been the most frequently implicated component. In 65 to 90% of TRALI cases, WBC antibodies have been identified in the plasma of the implicated donors and most implicated donors have been multiparous women. These antibodies are thought to be due to alloimmunization during previous pregnancies. Transfusion-related acute lung injury has been reported in all age ranges and equally between gender, and mortality is estimated at between 5 to 10%.

In 2003, the UK started using FFP primarily from male donors, discarding plasma from female donors. The SHOT data showed no death definitely attributed to TRALI after 2004, and the group concluded that the reduction in TRALI observed in 2006 and 2007 was 'likely' to be due to the UK's decision to change to preferential use of male plasma. Transfusion-related acute lung injury will continue to occur despite this measure due to the remaining plasma found in platelet and red cell components.

Transfusion-related acute lung injury is also more common following transfusion of stored components and the '2-hit' model proposed by Silliman *et al.* may explain this phenomenon. In this model, the initial insult to the vascular endothelium (due to infection, surgery, trauma or massive transfusion) attracts and primes neutrophils that adhere to the endothelium. In the second 'hit', biological response modifiers contained in transfused plasma (e.g. lipid-priming molecules, cytokines, CD40 ligand or leukocyte antibodies) activate the sequestered neutrophils. The activated neutrophils release oxidases and proteases that damage the endothelium producing capillary leak and acute lung injury. This model would support the transfusion of fresher RBC and platelet components to prevent TRALI.

Management of the patient with TRALI is supportive, with the expectation that clinical improvement will occur spontaneously as the lung injury resolves.

Transfusion-related graft versus host disease (TR-GVHD)

Transfusion-related graft versus host disease is a rare and almost invariably fatal complication of transfusion. It is mediated by the presence of viable donor lymphocytes that, once transfused, go on to proliferate and damage the recipient's organs – in particular bone marrow, skin, liver and GI tract. The clinical syndrome comprises fever, skin rash, pancytopenia, abnormal liver function and diarrhoea. The usual onset is eight to ten days post transfusion. It occurs in two clinical settings. The first occurs when the recipient is immunodeficient and the second, more common situation, is when there is a specific type of partial HLA matching between the donor and recipient. The technique of choice to prevent TR-GVHD is irradiation of blood products.

Anaphylactic transfusion reactions

Severe anaphylactic reactions have a reported incidence of 1:20,000 to 1:50,000. One well characterized mechanism for this reaction is the presence of class-specific IgG, anti-IgA antibodies in patients who are IgA deficient. Selective IgA deficiency is not uncommon, occurring in about 1:300 to 1:500 people. Fortunately, few IgA-deficient patients develop antibodies. Prevention consists of establishing the diagnosis and using IgA-deficient blood products.

Urticarial transfusion reactions (UTRs)

Urticarial transfusion reaction occurs when donor plasma proteins react with pre-existing IgE antibodies in the recipient. This causes mast cells and basophils to release histamine, leading to urticaria.

Post-transfusion purpura (PTP)

Post-transfusion purpura is rare. It occurs primarily in women sensitized by pregnancy but can occur in males who develop antibodies to a human platelet antigen (HPA) during a previous transfusion. Thrombocytopenia, lasting days to weeks, develops about five to ten days following transfusion of a platelet-containing product. Post-transfusion purpura is an immune thrombocytopenia and may be confused with drug-induced or idiopathic thrombocytopenic purpura, since the blood and bone marrow smears are essentially the same. In the UK the current recorded incidence is 1:700,000.

Diagnosis is confirmed by detecting the presence of circulating alloantibodies to a common platelet antigen, most often against HPA-1a, and that the patient's own platelets lack this antigen. The donor has always been a female with a history of pregnancy. Implicated donors should be deferred from subsequent donations. Current recommended therapy is intravenous immune globulin in high doses and usually takes about four days for the platelet count to exceed $100,000/\mu l$.

Transfusion-related immunomodulation (TRIM)

The immunosuppressive activity of allogenic blood has been known since the studies on renal allograft survival were published in the 1970s. Recent interest has looked at the impact of the immunosuppressive effect of allogenic blood (particularly the leukocyte component) on postoperative infection, tumor recurrence and nosocomial infection in critically ill patients. The evidence that postoperative infection is increased in patients receiving allogenic blood during surgery is compelling, though not absolute, as are the data implicating transfused leukocytes as the cause.

Transfusion-transmitted infection

Transmitted infections can be bacterial, viral, prion or parasitic.

Bacterial contamination

Since 1996, there have been 34 cases of transfusion-associated sepsis (TAS) reported, of which eight recipients died due to the transfusion. The majority of these cases (28) relate to platelet units (10 apheresis, 18 pool). Most bacterial contamination occurs either at the time of venepuncture or during component preparation and less frequently because the donor has a silent bacteraemia at the time of donation.

The most common organisms of clinical relevance are Gram negative, endotoxin-secreting bacteria that can survive cold storage, e.g. *Yersinia enterocolitica*, some *Pseudomonas* and *Enterobacter* species. Studies have shown that leukoreduction performed 2 to 12 hours after collection ('pre-storage' leukoreduction) can significantly reduce bacterial proliferation of *Y. enterocolitica*. The benefit may be mediated by the removal of bacteria ingested by leukocytes, filtration of bacteria and/or prevention of release and subsequent proliferation of viable bacteria from disintegrating leukocytes.

Platelets are responsible for 70% of the fatalities and RBCs for 30%. Moreover, platelets are most often given to patients who have an impaired immune system and are also often neutropenic. Many episodes of TAS in this group are not reported as transfusion transmitted. Before the introduction of routine testing for bacteria and use of apheresis (single-donor) platelets in March 2004, TAS occurred with a frequency of approximately 1 per 25,000 platelet transfusions. Since this date deaths from TAS have approximately halved.

Viral contamination

Between 2006 and 2007 SHOT reported no cases of transfusion-transmitted viral infection, largely due to the success of systems in place from donor selection through to transfusion. In 2007 the UK Health Protection Agency published the following estimated rates of transmission due to transfusion:

- Hepatitis B – 1 in 850,000
- HIV – 1 in 5 million
- Hepatitis C – 1 in 51 million
- HTLV – 1 in 11 million.

Better pre-donation screening criteria and a decrease in the incidence of these infections in the general population has meant the incidence of hepatitis B virus (HBV), hepatitis C virus (HCV) and human immunodeficiency virus (HIV) infections has fallen dramatically.

Data obtained in 1985 prior to the availability of HIV testing showed that approximately 90% of transfused recipients acquired HIV infection when given an HIV seropositive blood component. Transmission rates of HIV are equal with red cells, platelets or plasma. In 1999/2000, HIV minipool nucleic acid testing (MP-NAT) was introduced into routine blood-donor screening. This assay detects HIV RNA, which appears earlier than the p24 viral protein or HIV antibody. Due to the increased sensitivity of HIV MP-NAT for detecting early window period infection, the risk of HIV infection from transfusion has further decreased.

In 2002, the US mosquito-borne West Nile virus (WNV) epidemic resulted in 23 confirmed cases of transfusion-transmitted infection and seven subsequent deaths. West Nile virus nucleic-acid amplification testing was introduced in the US in 2003; however, WNV transmissions and deaths have still occurred since the introduction.

Dengue fever virus (DFV) is transmitted by mosquitoes, has a median viraemia of five days and causes asymptomatic infection in most cases. At least two cases of transfusion transmission of DFV have been documented. Concern exists regarding repeat of the WNV 2002 experience.

Variant CJD cases worldwide have just exceeded 200. Of these, 167 have occurred in the UK and the incidence appears to be falling. Four probable cases of transfusion transmission of vCJD have been reported from the UK in patients who had received blood products from asymptomatic donors who later developed vCJD. The transmissible spongiform encephalopathies (such as vCJD) may, however, have an incubation period of up to 50 years. Measures to protect the blood supply from vCJD are being evaluated in the UK. Possible measures include the filtration of blood components through prion-retention filters and testing of donor blood for the abnormally conformed prion protein.

Transfusion associated circulatory overload

Pulmonary oedema secondary to congestive failure can occur following blood transfusion. This is called transfusion associated circulatory overload (TACO). It occurs mainly in elderly patients, small children and/or those with compromised cardiac function.

In order to reduce the risk of TACO in those at risk, the rate should be minimized (approximately 1 ml/kg per hour) and number of units transfused in a 24-hour period limited. In very high-risk patients where transfusion time would exceed the four-hour limit products should be out of storage, the blood bank may be able to provide smaller 'split' units. Alternatively small doses of a diuretic can be administered between transfusions or isovolemic exchange can be performed. While TACO should not be mistaken for transfusion-related lung injury (TRALI), it may be difficult to distinguish one from the other. The distinction between hydrostatic/cardiogenic (TACO) and permeability/non-cardiogenic (TRALI) pulmonary oedema after transfusion is difficult, in part because the two conditions may coexist.

Management is the same as for any other presentation of cardiogenic pulmonary oedema secondary to heart failure.

Hyperkalaemia

Stored red cells leak potassium proportionately throughout their storage life. Irradiation of red cells (to prevent graft versus host disease) increases the rate of potassium leakage. Clinically significant hyperkalaemia can occur after rapid transfusion. Newborn infants are particularly at risk. Blood that is less than seven days old is generally used in this age group.

Iron overload

Transfusion iron overload can occur in chronically transfused patients. When the storage sites are saturated, iron is deposited in organs, e.g. the heart and liver, leading to damage and eventually organ dysfunction.

Massive blood transfusion

Massive blood transfusion has a number of definitions, one of which is the replacement of the patient's total blood volume within 24 hours. All of the above complications are increased after massive transfusion and the following complications are also seen.

Citrate toxicity

Citrate binds to ionized calcium and therefore prevents activation of clotting factors of donated blood. Each unit of blood contains approximately 3 g of citrate and a healthy human liver can metabolize 3 g every five minutes. Impaired liver function or transfusion rates exceeding this will cause hypocalcaemia (and hypomagnesaemia) and consequent cardiovascular compromise. Citrate is also rapidly metabolized to bicarbonate, which then 'drives' potassium into the cells. Therefore hypokalaemia and alkalosis are possible after massive transfusion.

Hypothermia

Hypothermia has many effects including reduced metabolism of citrate, lactate and impairment of other enzyme systems including clotting factors. This is the triad of hypothermia, acidosis and coagulopathy.

Fluid infusion

Crystalloids versus colloids

Debate over the relative merits of crystalloids versus colloids has been ongoing for over 50 years. Theory suggests colloids would have benefits due to their greater colloid osmotic pressure. Because of this they remain within the intravascular space longer and also reduce the potential for oedema. Colloids also have various non-oncotic properties that may influence vascular integrity, inflammation and pharmacokinetics, although the clinical relevance of these properties is not yet known. Despite these theoretical benefits, randomized controlled trials and systematic meta-analyses have failed to demonstrate improved patient outcome when colloids are compared to crystalloids.

In 2004 the SAFE (Saline versus Albumin Fluid Evaluation) study randomized a heterogeneous group of 6,997 critically ill patients requiring fluid resuscitation to receive either colloid (4% albumin) or crystalloid (0.9% saline). All-cause mortality at 28 days (the primary end point of the study) was not statistically different between the groups. Secondary end points (multi-organ failure, the duration of hospital stay, days of mechanical ventilation and days of renal replacement) were also similar in both groups.

Local adverse effects

Unless excessively warm or cold, isotonic solutions do not adversely affect the vessel wall. Solutions with a grossly abnormal osmolality, e.g. glucose solutions over 10% concentration, are associated with painful thrombophlebitis secondary to an inflammatory response.

Oedema

Highly compliant tissues such as skin and connective tissue tend to accumulate the most fluid; however, vital organs such as lungs, kidney and gut are also at risk.

In 2003, Brandstrup *et al.* conducted a randomized controlled trial of colorectal surgical patients, which showed a significantly higher mortality in groups given more fluid intra-operatively. Benefits were also shown in a later study in which patients undergoing intra-abdominal operations who received a restrictive regime of 4 ml/kg/h Ringers had fewer complications, shorter hospital stay and earlier passage of flatus.

A study by Singer *et al.* of patients undergoing elective pneumonectomy recommended an intra-operative fluid balance of not more than 2 l and not more than 3 l in the first 24 hours post-operatively as more than this was associated with increased complications (respiratory failure and pneumonia) as well as increased in patient mortality.

The Fluids and Catheters Treatment Trial (FACTT) compared outcomes of patients with ALI who were managed with defined 'liberal' and 'conservative' fluid regimes. Although it did not show a difference in the mortality between the groups it did show a reduction in mechanical ventilation by approximately 2.5 days and subsequent shorter ITU and hospital stay.

Hyponatraemia

This is the most frequent electrolyte abnormality post-operatively and has potentially catastrophic neurological consequences. The most common cause post-operatively is the administration of hypotonic fluid, in the presence of increased antidiuretic hormone (so the capacity to excrete free water is impaired). Oestrogens seem to impair the brain's ability

(Na-K ATPase system) to adapt to hyponatraemia and therefore women (especially menstruant women) are at more risk.

All children are at particular risk of cerebral oedema. This is in part due to the difference in cranial capacity to brain size, relatively smaller CSF volume and brain intracellular Na approximately 27% higher than in adults. Initial brain response to hyponatraemia is to transport intracellular sodium to the extracellular space via the Na-K ATPase pump. In pre-pubertal animal models this enzyme mechanism is reduced. Lack of timely treatment has also been blamed for poor outcome in children as symptoms may not be recognized. For these reasons many centres have abandoned the 'traditional' perioperative use of hypotonic fluids for isotonic fluid therapy.

Hyperchloraemic acidosis

There is controversy as to whether the hyperchloraemic acidosis caused by fluid therapy has clinical relevance. Although evidence is conflicting, it has been shown that this acidosis is associated with impaired urine output and abdominal discomfort when patients are given 0.9% saline compared to Ringers. Evidence for its impact on mortality is controversial.

Specific risks of colloids

Colloids can be either non-synthetically produced, such as albumin, or synthetically produced. This second group are made up of three groups; hydroxyethyl starch (HES), dextrans and gelatin.

Many of the differences demonstrated have been between albumin and HES, possibly because these two colloids have been most extensively investigated. Compared to crystalloids, colloids have more risks. Newer colloid preparations are being produced that may offer a lower incidence of side effects.

Anaphylactoid reactions

Reactions to colloids make up about 4% of all perioperative anaphylactic reactions. A French prospective multicentre study published in 1994 observed an overall frequency of 0.2% among 19,593 patients treated with albumin (0.1%), gelatin (0.3%), dextrans (0.3%) or HES (0.05%). Multivariate analysis revealed four independent risk factors for anaphylactoid reactions; gelatin infusion (odds ratio, OR, 4.81), dextran infusion (OR 3.83), history of drug allergy (OR 3.16) and male gender (OR 1.98).

Pruritus

Pruritis is almost exclusively restricted to HES solutions. A study of intensive care patients showed that 44% of patients who experienced pruritis following HES developed a severe, persistent form that was resistant to treatment.

Coagulopathy

All colloids affect the coagulation system, with dextran and starch solutions having the most potent antithrombotic effects. The effects of HES on coagulation are dependent on its molecular weight and elimination. Coagulation is most effected by dextrans and high molecular weight (>200 Da) highly substituted starches.

In vivo and in vitro studies have shown that crystalloids cause a perhaps counter-intuitive hypercoagulable state. The theory of this phenomenon is an induced imbalance in the anti-coagulant (antithrombin III in particular) and procoagulants. This may have consequences particularly in vascular patients.

Renal dysfunction

All synthetic colloids are mainly eliminated via the kidney. Impaired renal function may contribute to colloid accumulation. The proposed mechanism for colloid-induced renal failure is due to increased renal tubular viscocity, decreased urine flow and uptake of molecules into proximal tubule cells via pinocytosis causing cell swelling. The incidence of renal dysfunction is highest following dextrans. The initial studies to demonstrate this were conducted in the 1960s and used large fluid volumes in dehydrated patients. Compared with dextrans, HES solutions are less likely to cause renal dysfunction. Before 1991 no case had been reported. Gelatins are generally regarded as the safest of the synthetic colloids in terms of renal impairment.

Future

Avoiding blood transfusion altogether is the only way of eradicating blood transfusion related complications. Potential future technologies in this field include 'red blood cell substitutes'; haemoglobin-based oxygen carriers and enzymes that potentially enable blood from groups A, B and AB to be converted into group O.

Monitoring tools to guide fluid therapy are being developed, and research into the way these tools should be applied is ongoing. For example, we cannot objectively quantify blood volume, fluid overload or tissue perfusion at the bedside. A method to give us this information is likely to help refine fluid therapy and therefore minimize complications. Ultimately we need an approach to fluid therapy that is rational, monitored and goal directed. Future developments in these areas will undoubtedly improve future practice of fluid therapy.

List of further reading

Finfer, S., Bellomo, R., Boyce, N. et al. The Saline versus Albumin Fluid Evaluation (SAFE) Study investigators. A comparison of albumin and saline for fluid resuscitation in the intensive care unit. N Engl J Med 2004; 350: 2247–56.

Hahn, R. G., Prough, D. S. & Svensen, C. H. Perioperative Fluid Therapy. Informa Healthcare, 2006.

Klein, H., Mollison, P. & Anstee, D. Mollison's Blood Transfusion in Clinical Medicine. Wiley-Blackwell, 2005.

Serious Hazards of Transfusion (SHOT). Annual reports. www.shotuk.org/ (accessed 15 April 2011).

Vamvakas, E. C. & Blajchman, M. A. Transfusion-related mortality: the ongoing risks of allogeneic blood transfusion and the strategies for their prevention. Blood 2009; 113: 3406.

Chapter

8

Complications during obstetric anaesthesia

Felicity Plaat and Matt Wilkner

Introduction

Obstetric anaesthesia promotes the highest standards of anaesthetic practice in the care of mother and baby. Anaesthetists are becoming involved in more and more cases. This is a positive evolution but there are a number of complications that occur in obstetric anaesthetic practice. Many are minor and improve with time. Some are serious and lead to disability and death. Importantly, obstetric anaesthesia is the leading cause of litigation against anaesthetists. In this chapter we will discuss the management of the commonest problems in obstetric anaesthesia.

Inadequate regional analgesia for labour

The size of the problem

One of the commonest problems in labour is inadequate analgesia (0.2 to 24%). Maternal satisfaction is multifactorial and complex to measure. However, poor pain relief, especially in the context of high expectations, gives rise to dissatisfaction.

The need to replace an epidural catheter is an unequivocal indication that the preceding analgesia has been or has become inadequate. Catheter re-site rates between 4.7 and 5.6% have been reported. Higher rates may indicate prompt replacement of a poorly functioning catheter and thus be a marker of good care. Following re-sites, 98.8% patients achieved adequate pain relief in one series.

Box 8.1 Factors associated with inadequate analgesia
Obesity
Spinal deformity/pathology
Catheter length in space <2 cm or >8 cm
Failure of initial dose
Duration of labour >6 hours
Malpresentation of fetus
Continuous infusion
Infrequent top ups
Inadequate volume top ups
Inexperienced operator

Anaesthetic and Perioperative Complications, ed. Kamen Valchanov, Stephen T. Webb and Jane Sturgess.
Published by Cambridge University Press. © Cambridge University Press 2011.

Prevention

The addition of an opioid to the local anaesthetic improves the quality of analgesia with either combined spinal and epidural (CSE) anaesthesia or epidural blockade. The combined spinal–epidural technique provides more rapid analgesia. Some studies have shown increased maternal satisfaction and a reduced need for rescue top ups and re-siting compared to epidural alone. If a CSE technique is used, angling the bevel of the spinal needle cephalad improves quality of analgesia and reduces lower limb motor block. In addition epidural volume extension (flushing the epidural catheter with 5 to 10 ml saline immediately after the spinal injection) improves the spread of the spinal dose, and thus analgesia.

In cases where epidural catheterization is performed the sitting-patient position is associated with a higher success rate, but the lateral position has lower incidence of vein cannulation and risk of intravenous local anaesthetic injection. Inserting minimal length of catheter 4 to 6 cm into the epidural space minimizes the risk of displacement as well as the development of a one-sided block. Although there is scanty evidence to date, it seems likely that ultrasound visualization may improve success rates, especially in the presence of obesity and anatomical abnormality.

Withholding pain relief in the second stage does not improve the chance of a normal delivery. The result is simply poor analgesia. When low-dose regimes are used, the level of midwifery care is crucial to maintain analgesia and patient satisfaction. The required one-to-one supervision is rarely achieved in many units.

Patient-controlled epidural analgesia is associated with high levels of user satisfaction but the optimum dose, timing and the use of a background infusion has not been established.

Recognition

Most obstetric units have a written protocol for management of regional analgesia. Regular checks of adequacy of pain relief, level of sensory block, presence of sympathetic block and motor block should be documented. One-sided pain relief and inadequate sacral analgesia are common complaints, and should be dealt with promptly according to local guidelines.

Management

The patient complaining from inadequate labour analgesia should be reassured that the epidural catheter could be re-sited. A one-sided block may be corrected by withdrawing the catheter, although recent publications have shed doubt on this. Giving a high-volume, low-concentration top up with patient lying on the painful side may be effective. If block density is the problem (such as with sacral discomfort), adding additional opioid medication may overcome the problem.

Inadequate regional anaesthesia for caesarean section

Severity and frequency

Pain during caesarean is disturbing for the patient and her partner, and can interfere with the mother's ability to care for her baby as a result of post-traumatic stress disorder. Not surprisingly this is a major source of litigation in the field.

The true incidence of failed regional anaesthesia for caesarian section is difficult to accurately assess. The easiest definition of failure to measure is conversion to general anaesthesia, but may not reflect the unpleasant experiences of patients who require supplemental pain relief or those who refuse general anaesthesia, despite pain. The Royal College of Anaesthetists in the UK has proposed the following standards: <1% conversion of regional anaesthesia to general anaesthesia in elective caesarean section; <3% conversion from regional anaesthesia to general anaesthesia in emergency caesarean section.

Epidural anaesthesia (topping up indwelling epidural catheters) is associated with highest failure rates (2 to 13%) and CSE the lowest (0.5 to 1.2%), with intermediate rates associated with single-shot spinal anaesthesia.

Box 8.2 Factors associated with inadequate anaesthesia during caesarean section

As for labour analgesia (Box 8.1) plus:
- epidural opposed to intrathecal block
- inadequate dose
- time pressure (inedaquate anaesthesia is associated with degree of urgency)

Poorly functioning, existing labour epidural:
- extra clinician top ups
- catheter in situ >6 hours
- block below T5 to *light touch* during surgery

Prevention

The most efficient way of avoiding failed regional anaesthesia for caesarian section is to administer an adequate dose of local anaesthetic in the intended space. The following doses have been associated with high rates of success:

- Spinal anaesthesia: ED95 11.2 mg heavy bupivacaine with fentanyl 10 mg or morphine 200 µg as part of CSE technique.
- CSE: lower doses (5 to 7.5 mg heavy bupivacaine) *can be used* as part of a CSE technique. However, epidural supplementation rates are 50% with 5 mg bupivacaine and 8% with 9.5 mg bupivacaine.
- Epidural: 0.5% bupivacaine or 0.75% ropivacaine or 2% lidocaine 15 to 20 ml to give block to T5 to light touch.

Testing the block

Before proceeding with surgery the regional anaesthetic block has to be tested. The original method of assessing the level of the block with either cold or pin-prick sensation has been shown to be inferior to testing light touch. More than 97% women suffering intra-operative pain have a block to touch below T5. The block to cold or pin-prick may be higher in most cases.

Management

The most important aspect of management is to trust the patient when reporting pain. Recommended actions include:

- pause surgery if possible
- offer general anaesthesia and convert
- top up epidural, if in situ
- Entonox via facemask
- intravenous opioids, e.g. alfentanil 250 µg, Fentanyl 25 to 50 µg, repeated to effect.

It has to be remembered that opioids can cross the placenta and cause fetal respiratory depression if used prior to the delivery.

Complications of regional analgesia and anaesthesia post-dural puncture headache (PDPH)

Severity and frequency

Post-dural puncture headache is caused by low cerebrospinal fluid (CSF) volume as a result of leak following a dural puncture. Uncomplicated spinal anaesthesia or CSF can produce this side effect. Post-dural puncture headache is related to the type and gauge of the needle. A cutting tip 27G Quincke is associated with a 2.7% PDPH opposed to the same gauge atraumatic tip Whitacre. This has a rate nearly ten times lower. Similarly there is a ten-fold reduction in the incidence of PDPH between a 22G and 27G needle. Multiple dural punctures have been reported to produce higher incidence of PDPH.

Inadvertent dural puncture with an epidural needle during insertion is the commonest cause of PDPH. This is often easy to recognize but can also remain unnoticed during the procedure. The leak of CSF is usually larger compared to spinal anaesthesia and therefore PDPH likelier. The Royal College of Anaesthetists suggests <1% as an acceptable rate of accidental dural puncture (ADP). The likelihood of PDPH after accidental dural puncture with a 16G Tuohy needle in labour is 50 to 80%.

The symptoms include severe headache, worse in sitting position, visual and auditory disturbances, nausea and vomiting. The headache is often severe and not alleviated by simple analgesics. It reliably improves when lying down. The symptoms may dissipate with time but more frequently are disabling for the new mother and require further treatment.

Alternative diagnoses (meningitis, intracranial haemorrhage, cerebral sinus thrombosis) should be considered, especially if there are atypical symptoms, epidural blood patch (EBP) does not bring relief and the headache recurs after patching.

Management

If accidental dural puncture occurs the conventional recommendations are:

- not to perform prophylactic EBP – there is no proven benefit
- thread the catheter intrathecally – this allows top ups to be given without the risk of epidural doses leaking unintentionally into the intrathecal space
- small studies suggest that leaving an intrathecal catheter in situ for at least 24 hours reduces the PDPH rate to <50%, and provides a route for analgesia and anaesthesia – this carries the risk of infection and dosing error if mistaken for an epidural catheter.

Epidural blood patch is more effective if delayed and reduces PDPH rate at one week from 86 to 16%. Oral analgesics can be given for symptomatic relief for the first 24 to 48 hours. Intrathecal or epidural saline infusions have only a marginal effect.

Nerve damage

Obstetric palsies

Obstetric palsies are surprisingly common; a prospective study of women delivering in a single centre in the United States over a one-year period found a 0.92% incidence of lower limb nerve injury. A UK study supported this with an incidence of 0.58%. These are notoriously difficult to distinguish from neurological deficit resulting from regional anaesthesia for labour.

Box 8.3 Obstetric palsies	
% of cases	
Lateral femoral cutaneous nerve	41%
Femoral nerve	35%
Radiculopathy	9%
Peroneal nerve	5%
Lumbosacral plexus	5%
Other	5%

Nerve injury

Neuraxial procedures are generally safe in labour. However, temporary and permanent nerve damage could complicate these and is a common reason for litigation. A recent national audit suggested the incidence of permanent damage in the obstetric population to be approximately 1:80,000. Temporary damage is estimated to occur between 1:3,000 and 1:6,700 procedures.

Direct needle or catheter trauma

Direct trauma to the spinal cord is infrequent but could cause devastating complications. To minimize the risk of damaging the conus medullaris with spinal or epidural needles, it has been recommended that dural puncture should not be undertaken above the level indicated by Tuffier's line. Recent work suggests this may be overly cautious. Pre-procedure ultrasound visualization improves accuracy of estimation of spinal level.

Arachnoiditis

The preservatives sodium metabisulphite and sodium methyparaben have been shown to be neurotoxic in the past. Only preservative-free preparations of drugs should be used in modern practice. Chlorhexidine and povidone iodine have been shown to be neuro-toxic to adrenergic nerves in rats. The lowest effective concentration should be used: 0.5% chlorhexidine in 70% alcohol, in spray form to reduce the contamination of equipment, is recommended.

Cauda equina syndrome

Cauda equina syndrome is a complex of symptoms resulting from damage of the lowest part of the spinal cord: loss of bladder or bowel control, paraplegia or paraesthesia. Hyperbaric 5% lidocaine injected via intrathecal microcatheters has been implicated in cases of cauda equina syndrome. This practice has now been abandoned. Other hyperbaric local anaesthetic solutions could still cause cauda equina syndrome and should therefore be used in small doses. If cauda equina syndrome is suspected, the cause should be investigated as an emergency. Causes such as spinal canal haematoma are amenable to emergency surgical treatment.

Transient neurological symptoms

Intrathecal lidocaine has a higher incidence of transient neurological symptoms (pain or dysaesthesia in the legs or buttocks) than bupivacaine (11.9% vs. 1.3%). Whilst lidocaine has the advantage of faster spinal block onset than bupivacaine, its use has largely been abandoned in the UK due to the risk of these transient neurological symptoms.

Vertebral canal haematoma

Vertebral canal haematoma is a rare but devastating complication of spinal and epidural anaesthesia. If not promptly surgically decompressed it leads to paraplegia. One meta-analysis reported an incidence of 1:168,000, although no obstetric cases were identified in a recent national, year-long audit in the UK. Spinal haematoma is due to direct or indirect injury to epidural blood vessels. Use of anticoagulants and antiplatelet medication as well as deranged patient clotting are risk factors. The obstetric population may be protected by the low use of anticoagulant and antiplatelet medication and the hypercoagulable state of pregnancy. Current consensus-based guidelines stipulate that there should be a 10- to 12-hour period between a thromboprophylactic dose of low molecular weight heparin and siting or removing a neuraxial block. This should be extended to 24 hours when a therapeutic dose is used. Low molecular weight heparin should not be given within two hours of removal of an epidural catheter. Patients on antiplatelet medication (apart from low-dose aspirin) are at particular risk.

Vertebral canal haematoma presents as rapidly developing focal neurological deficit of lower motor neurons. It is a neurosurgical emergency. If promptly treated it has good prognosis whereas paraplegia is the more likely outcome if a delay of more than 12 hours to surgical decompression occurs.

Vertebral canal abscess

Vertebral canal abscess results from local, systemic or haematogenically spread infection. It presents with neurological deficit, which may be accompanied by symptoms of sepsis. In the UK national audit only one case out of 320,000 was reported. There was a much higher incidence in the general surgical population. The infecting organism is usually *Staphylococcus aureus*. Early surgical treatment is believed to produce good outcome.

Meningitis

Meningitis is an infection of the dura mater. It spreads through the CSF. The infecting organism is usually an oropharyngeal commensal, frequently a streptococcus species. The reported incidence varies with the highest being 1 per 7,000 spinal anaesthetics. Breach in sterility during spinal and epidural injections have been implicated in its development. Systemic sepsis during spinal or epidural injections has also been suspected, although there has been no evidence to support this theory.

Hypotension and nausea and vomiting

Intra-operative nausea and vomiting have been associated with systemic and cerebrospinal hypotension. These occur in approximately 80% of parturients receiving intrathecal anaesthesia as a result of CSF loss and sympathetic block leading to hypotension. The incidence of nausea and vomiting can be reduced to 4% by using rehydration and prophylactic vasopressor infusion. Once the blood pressure is corrected the symptoms of nauseas normally subside.

High regional anaesthesia block

Using a predetermined dose of intrathecal local anaesthetic often produces the desirable level of motor and sensory block. Occasionally the local anaesthetic spreads unexpectedly high rostrally. This produces profound hypotension and can induce phrenic nerve motor block and apnoea. Although the estimated incidence (1:2,500 to 1:13,000) is much lower than failed intubation, the sheer number of regional procedures performed in obstetrics means that the numbers of incidents are similar. The risk of a high block is increased when spinal anaesthesia is used following a failed epidural top up; in this situation, a lower dose CSE technique may be safer. The high regional block presents with hypotension and dyspnoea. Treatment is supportive, and consists of vasopressor support and mechanical ventilation until the block has worn off.

Subdural block

When local anaesthetic is deposited inadvertently between the dura mater and the arachnoid membrane it produces subdural block. It is characterized by late-onset, high-distribution, uneven or poor quality block, sometimes associated with pain on injection. This is thought to occur in up to 1% of epidural insertions and may not give rise to any problems.

Local anaesthetic toxicity

Local anaesthetic toxicity can result from inadvertent intravenous injection or dosing exceeding the safe limits. Death due to wrong route local anaesthetic injection continues to occur. New connectors are being developed to prevent intravenous administration of solutions intended for epidural use. Administering local anaesthetics in doses higher than the safe limits is often by error. The symptoms of neurotoxicity are often followed by cardiotoxicity with arrhythmias and cardiovascular collapse. The use of lipid emulsion has been advocated for all regional anaesthetics but lacks evidence in obstetric practice. The consequences for the fetus of a large lipid load are thus unknown.

The newer amide local anaesthetics (levobupivacaine and ropivacaine) have a lower cardiotoxicity and have superceded racemic bupivacaine in high-dose epidural anaesthesia for caesarean section.

Opioid-related complications

Minor complications associated with opioid use in obstetric practice are common. Pruritus is commonly associated with neuraxial opioids (60 to 100%). This appears to be dose dependent. Intrathecal doses greater than 200 µg of morphine and 300 µg of diamorphine do not add to the analgesic effects, they merely increase pruritus.

As intrathecally and epidurally administered opioids can spread centrally they produce a risk of respiratory depression. Non-lethal respiratory depression has been documented in 0 to 0.9% of parturients when neuraxial morphine is used for caesarean section. However, severe respiratory depression in parturient patients is rare. The onset of respiratory depression is slower (up to 12 hours after injection) for hydrophilic opioids. Lipophilic drugs are less likely to cause delayed effects and are recommended. If respiratory depression is noticed the patient can be transferred to a safe place for monitoring and respiratory support.

Pressure ulceration

This has been reported in labour and is thought to be related to the lack of pain-induced changing of position compounded by motor block. In contrast to other patient populations hypotension does not appear to play a causative role.

Long-term back pain

Back pain complaints are very common after labour. Many of the patients have also received spinal or epidural analgesia. These tend to be patients with more complicated progression of labour who are at high risk of developing labour-related back pain. Prospective and randomized studies have shown no difference in the incidence of long-term backache between women choosing epidural or other forms of analgesia. It is, to date, not possible to suggest that back pain is a direct result from spinal or epidural analgesia during labour.

Effect of regional anaesthesia on labour

Large meta-analyses have shown that neuraxial analgesia lengthens the second stage of labour by approximately 15 minutes. There is a greater requirement for oxytocin augmentation and the risk of instrumental delivery is increased by approximately 10%, although the majority of these are ventouse deliveries. However, the caesarean section rate is not increased irrespective of the stage at which regional analgesia is initiated.

Complications of general anaesthesia for caesarian section

Anaesthetic-related maternal mortality has fallen dramatically in the last five decades. This has in part been due to a decreased use of general anaesthesia. Performing general anaesthesia for caesarian section is challenging as it considers the wellbeing of two patients, airway management is more difficult, and can cause severe haemodynamic disturbances during induction.

Failed intubation

Severity and frequency

In recent years concern has grown that declining experience with general anaesthesia in obstetrics is leading to a rise in cases of difficult and failed intubation.

Recent prospective studies have found that whilst Grade 3 or 4 laryngoscopy views occur in 1:24 obstetric cases, and 'difficult' intubation in 1:30, failed intubation is much rarer 1:238 to 1:274.

Prevention and management

Regional anaesthesia should be employed whenever feasible and pre-operative airway assessment is mandatory in all patients whatever the intended anaesthetic. Failed intubation drills and simulation-based training are recommended for anaesthetists.

When failed intubation occurs the crucial decision is whether to continue surgery. The only absolute indication to continue is a threat to the mother's life. If the airway can be maintained using a supraglottic device, many anaesthetists would allow surgery to continue in the case of fetal distress.

Aspiration of gastric content

Severity and frequency

In one large prospective study, aspiration occurred in 0.1% when rapid sequence induction and cricoid pressure were employed. Regurgitation was more frequent (0.7%). Both occurred more commonly during extubation.

> **Box 8.4 Risk factors for aspiration in obstetrics**
> - Increased incidence of difficult intubation
> - Emergency anaesthesia
> - Reduced lower oesophageal sphincter tone
> - Variable fasting regimes in labour

Prevention

Whilst antacids, rapid sequence induction (RSI) and cricoid pressure have become routine in many parts of the world, there are no robust large-scale studies to show that regurgitation or aspiration of gastric contents are reduced. Recent evidence suggests that gastric emptying is the same in the non-labouring woman at term as her non-pregnant counterpart, and it has been suggested that RSI and cricoid pressure may not be necessary for elective surgery. Metoclopramide increases gastric emptying and reduces gastric volume. H2 antagonists and alkali-based antacids reliably increase gastric pH. There is no difference in aspiration mortality between countries with liberal or strict oral intake policies.

Awareness during caesarian section under general anaesthesia

> **Box 8.5 Risk factors for awareness**
> Increased cardiac output at term:
> - faster redistribution of IV induction agents
> - delayed establishment of volatile agent partial pressures in CNS
> Surgery started before adequate partial pressures established
> Human error due to time pressure (drug/equipment)
> Increased incidence of difficult intubation
> Avoidance of opioids pre-delivery
> Lower concentrations of volatile anaesthetics due to concerns over uterine tone

Awareness is more common in the obstetric population despite a decrease in minimal alveolar concentration (MAC) for volatile anaesthetics during pregnancy of 2 to 40%. Twenty-nine per cent of claims for awareness to the NHS Litigation Authority under general anaesthesia are related to general anaesthesia for caesarian section. It is essential to use adequate doses of anaesthetic agents (e.g. thiopentone 5 to 7 mg/kg). A rapid onset volatile agent reduces risk of awareness at the beginning. Bispectral index (BIS) and entropy monitoring have been recommended.

Anaphylaxis

Severity and frequency

Anaesthesia-related anaphylaxis in the general population occurs between 0.5 and 1 per 10,000 anaesthetics. The incidence in pregnancy is unknown, but there is evidence that women are at higher risk for anaphylaxis to certain drugs than men. Progesterone level changes during pregnancy may increase this risk further.

Management

There is some debate as to whether the general guidelines for management of anaphylaxis under anaesthesia need modifying for the parturient. Although vasopressors may detrimentally affect placental blood flow, early restoration of maternal arterial pressure is probably more important and there is no definite evidence to support the avoidance of adrenaline at present.

Hypertensive response to laryngoscopy and intubation

There were two deaths in the 2003–5 report on maternal mortality in the UK from cerebral haemorrhage in which anaesthesia was judged to have played an indirect part. Both patients had pre-eclampsia. Laryngoscopy and intubation was associated with severe hypertension. Labetalol, hydralazine, GTN, magnesium and alfentanil have all been used to dampen the response in the obstetric population. Remifentanil has been shown to be very effective at a dose of 1 µg/kg. If high-dose opioids are used, neonatal respiratory depression should be anticipated.

Maternal cardiac arrest

Severity and frequency

Cardiac arrest occurs in approximately 1 in 7,000 pregnancies. As parturients become older, more obese with more complex medical problems, cardiac arrest may become more common.

Box 8.6 Causes of cardiac arrest

Massive haemorrhage
Pre-existing cardiac disease
Anaphylaxis
Drug toxicity
Massive pulmonary embolism
Amniotic fluid embolism
Sepsis
Other causes of hypoxia, e.g. pneumonia, pulmonary oedema, failed intubation

---

Prevention

Although a large proportion of obstetric cardiac arrests happen without warning some, such as haemorrhage or severe sepsis, may involve a period of decline and the obstetric early warning score has been developed to identify cases earlier.

Management

Resuscitation skills were judged to be poor in a significant number of cases in the two most recent reports on maternal mortality in the UK. Obstetric cardiac arrest should be managed according to the adult advanced life support algorithm, with a few modifications. Aortocaval compression must be minimized by lateral tilt and left uterine displacement.

Early intubation is required. If there is no return of spontaneous circulation the uterus must be emptied within five minutes to maximize the chances for both mother and child, as the gravid uterus significantly impedes resuscitation.

Pain after caesarean section

Severity and frequency

One prospective study found an incidence of severe pain of 17% at 24 hours post-caesarean section. There is also a significant likelihood of chronic pain and some evidence suggests this is related to the intensity of acute pain in the first few days post-operatively. One retrospective study reported an incidence of 18% at 12 months, although only 1% of patients experienced intense or unbearable pain. Given that this is the most commonly performed operation worldwide, it presents a major health burden.

Box 8.7 Risk factors for postoperative pain following caesarian section

General	Acute pain	Chronic pain
Psychological state	General anaesthesia	Severe acute pain
Pain threshold	Uterine exteriorization	Previous chronic pain
Younger patients	Closure of parietal peritoneum	Back pain
Genetic variability	Epidural anaesthesia > spinal	Chronic disease
	Reluctance to take medication (concerns over breastfeeding)	

Prevention and management

Adequate analgesia during surgery is essential for smooth postoperative recovery. In addition multimodal analgesia should be used. The following are suggested:

- regular paracetamol and NSAID if not contraindicated
- use of regional anaesthesia whenever possible
- long-acting neuraxial opioids
- transversus abdominis plane block and rectus sheath block
- wound infiltration with local anaesthetics and continuous infusion catheters
- rescue opioid medication.

Medico-legal issues in obstetrics

Obstetrics is a high-risk medico-legal area for anaesthetists. Pregnant mothers are generally young and healthy with high expectations and are more likely to litigate if these are not met. Informed consent may be difficult in the context of labour pain and analgesic drugs. Regional anaesthesia per se carries a high medico-legal risk and women are more likely to make a medico-legal claim than men.

Box 8.8 Legal action related to obstetric anaesthesia

Pain during caesarean section
Nerve injury
Delay in anaesthesia for caesarean section
Poor outcomes related to the anaesthetist's 'team role', e.g. post-partum haemorrhage management, pre-eclampsia

Consent

Although pain, exhaustion, anxiety and drugs might be expected to have an effect, their presence has been deemed not to necessarily decrease capacity to consent in legal terms. The majority of women prefer to be given comprehensive information about associated risks, although they are less interested in exact incidences. Such information has little effect on whether they subsequently consent to a procedure.

Delays in anaesthesia

In the United States 22% of obstetric claims for neonatal death or disability include a claim against the anaesthetist. A significant proportion of these were for delays in anaesthesia. A robust system for anaesthesia delivery is pivotal for successful running of all obstetric units.

Prevention and management

A named anaesthetist should be responsible solely for anaesthesia in the labour ward. If the decision is made for caesarean section, the following must be communicated:

- the maximum time until surgical readiness
- when attempts at regional anaesthesia should be abandoned.

Good communication between obstetrician, anaesthetist and midwifery staff (as well as the patient) not only reduces medico-legal action but makes the whole process of providing anaesthesia and analgesia safer overall.

List of further reading

Cooper, G. & McClure, J. Anaesthesia chapter from *Saving Mothers' Lives*: reviewing maternal deaths to make pregnancy safer. *Br J Anaes* 2008; **100**: 17–22.

Davies, J., Posner, K., Lee, L. *et al.* Liability associated with obstetric anesthesia: a closed claims analysis. *Anesthesiol* 2009; **110**: 131–9.

McDonnell, N., Paech, M., Clavisi, O. *et al.* Difficult and failed intubation in obstetric anaesthesia: an observational study of airway management and complications associated with general anaesthesia for caesarean section. *Int J Obstet Anesth* 2009; **17**: 292–7.

Paech, M. J., Godkin, R. & Webster, S. Complications of obstetric epidural analgesia and anaesthesia: a prospective analysis of 10,995 cases. *Int J Obstet Anesth* 1998; **7**: 5–11.

Robins, K. & Lyons, G. Intraoperative awareness during general anesthesia for cesarean delivery. *Anesth Analg* 2009; **109**: 886–90.

Royal College of Anaesthetists. 3rd National Audit Project (NAP3). National audit of major complications of central neuraxial block in the United Kingdom. Report and findings, January 2009. www.rcoa.ac.uk (accessed 15 April 2011).

Sng, B. L., Lim, Y. & Sia, A. T. An observational prospective cohort study of incidence and characteristics of failed spinal anaesthesia for caesarean section. *Int J Obstet Anesth* 2009; **18**: 237–41.

Thew, M. & Paech, M. Management of postdural puncture headache in the obstetric patient. *Curr Opin Anaesthesiol* 2008; **21**: 288–92.

Williamson, R. & Haines, J. Availability of lipid emulsion in obstetric anaesthesia in the UK: a national questionnaire survey. *Anaesthesia* 2008; **63**: 385–8.

Yentis, S. High regional block – the failed intubation of the new millennium? *Int J Obstet Anesth* 2001; **10**: 159–61.

Perioperative neurological complications

Nick Lees and Andrew A. Klein

Introduction

Neurological complications as a direct result of anaesthesia are fortunately rare. From a National Health Service Litigation Authority (NHSLA) claims analysis, regional anaesthesia (obstetric and non-obstetric) was the largest category (44% of all anaesthetic claims), and with most claims related to epidurals. Airway and respiratory complication claims commonly had devastating outcomes, leading to hypoxic brain injury and death, and made up 12% of all anaesthetic claims and 53% of anaesthetic-related deaths. Brain damage carried the highest costs followed by neurological damage from spinal or epidural anaesthetics. Nerve injury as a result of poor positioning was responsible for 4% of all claims. Anaesthetists may encounter other neurological complications during the perioperative period, with a variety of causes. In this chapter we will discuss perioperative seizures, stroke, spinal cord ischaemia not related to regional anaesthesia, cerebral hypoxia/ischemia and neuroprotective strategies, perioperative changes in mental status and neuropathic pain.

Perioperative seizures

A seizure is a paroxysmal event due to abnormal excessive hypersynchronous discharges from an aggregate of central nervous system (CNS) neurons. The lifetime risk of having a seizure is about 5 to 10% and the incidence of epilepsy, i.e. recurrent seizures due to an underlying process, is 0.3 to 0.5%. Consequently, the anaesthetist will encounter patients with seizure disorders frequently. A multicentre prospective study reported an incidence of postoperative seizures of 3.1 per 10,000 patients for all types of surgery and anaesthesia. The incidence of perioperative seizures in epileptic patients is 2 to 3.4%. There are many different causes of seizures, and during the perioperative period the possible aetiologies encountered are listed in Table 9.1. In patients with existing seizure disorders, there are many factors that may reduce the seizure threshold during the perioperative period such as omitted anticonvulsant medication, reduced absorption of medication and electrolyte imbalance. One retrospective review showed that of those patients with seizure disorders who did have a seizure during the perioperative period, it was their usual seizure type and not influenced by anaesthetic or surgery.

Most perioperative seizures occur after surgery, usually within the first 24 hours postoperatively but occasionally after that. The risk associated with epileptogenic drugs may extend up to 72 hours post-operatively.

Anaesthetic and Perioperative Complications, ed. Kamen Valchanov, Stephen T. Webb and Jane Sturgess. Published by Cambridge University Press. © Cambridge University Press 2011.

Table 9.1 Causes of seizures.

Idiopathic

Genetic and developmental disorders

CNS infection

Febrile convulsions

Intracranial mass lesions

Cerebral hypoxia, ischaemia and infarction

Trauma

Degenerative CNS disorders

Alcohol and alcohol withdrawal

Illicit drug use

Metabolic: hypocalcaemia, hypoglycaemia, hypomagnesaemia, hyponatraemia, pyridoxine deficiency, porphyria

Cerebrovascular disease

Uraemia

Hepatic failure

Drug-related, e.g. local anaesthetics, phenothiazines, tricyclics, monoamine oxidase inhibitors, tramadol

Drug withdrawal, e.g. anticonvulsants, benzodiazepines

Many anaesthetic drugs are anticonvulsant and are therefore used in the treatment of status epilepticus. Few anaesthetic agents have been reported to have proconvulsant effects (Table 9.2). This may be epileptiform activity seen on the electroencephalograph (EEG) or less commonly, partial seizures and generalized tonic-clonic seizures. Myoclonus, dystonias or abnormal movements occur more frequently after many anaesthetic drugs including halothane and isoflurane, but are not associated with seizure activity. There is a weak correlation between EEG epileptiform activity and clinical seizures. Epileptiform activity is more likely to be seen in epileptic patients and seizures are usually witnessed at the beginning or end of anaesthesia; however, the proconvulsant effect of a drug may last into the postoperative period. Most proconvulsant drugs exert effects at synapses and affect the interaction of excitatory and inhibitory neurons in the neocortex, leading to excitation and development of an oscillatory seizure state. The drugs with proven seizurogenic activity in epileptics and non-epileptics are enflurane, sevoflurane, etomidate, local anaesthetics and possibly opioids.

Epileptic patients should be carefully managed during the perioperative period to ensure that anticonvulsant medication is not missed and there are no drops in serum levels. Benzodiazepines and thiopentone are γ-amino-butyric acid (GABA)-ergic and reduce the likelihood of seizures. Etomidate and enflurane should probably be avoided in epileptic patients. The use of propofol is controversial. There is no convincing evidence of propofol causing seizures. However, it can cause a variety of abnormal movements that may mimic seizures. If there is doubt about seizure activity, EEG monitoring should be used.

The initial priorities of management of any patient with seizures are attention to airway, breathing and circulation and then treatment of seizures if they resume with anticonvulsant

Table 9.2 Drugs reported to cause seizure activity.

Enflurane	Abnormal movements, tonic-clonic activity, epileptiform activity on EEG reported, potentiated by hypocapnia and increased MAC.
Sevoflurane	Abnormal movements (5%), major seizures potentiated with high MAC and hypocapnia. Mechanism possibly similar to enflurane.
Nitrous oxide	No seizure activity seen on EEG. One case report of convulsions.
Propofol	Excitatory and tonic-clonic movements reported. Predominantly anticonvulsant.
Methohexital	Excitatory and abnormal movements seen. Epileptogenic in psychomotor epilepsy, no effect in generalized convulsive disorders.
Etomidate	Myoclonic movements common. Convulsions reported. Pro- and anticonvulsive effects. Epileptiform activity reported on EEG.
Ketamine	Myoclonus and abnormal movements reported. EEG seizure activity not seen in non-epileptics. Can activate epileptogenc foci in patients with seizure disorders. Anticonvulsant properties.
Diazepam	Anticonvulsant but may cause seizures in a form of secondary generalized epilepsy.
Opioid analgesics	Abnormal movements, myoclonus and grand-mal seizures reported with fentanil and sufentanil. Potent mu agonists can increase epileptiform activity in epileptics and non-epileptics. Tonic-clonic seizures seen after intrathecal and epidural morphine.
Pethidine	Abnormal movements, myoclonus and seizures with epileptiform EEG changes seen due to neurotoxic metabolite norpethidine.
Tramadol	Seizures reported at recommended and high doses with monotherapy but more commonly in conjunction with antidepressant medication.
Local anaesthetics	Well known convulsants after intravenous administration or absorption. Also anticonvulsant membrane-stabilizing properties.

drugs. If the cause of the seizure is uncertain, hypoxia, metabolic derangements, drug toxicity or CNS infection must be recognized and treated accordingly.

Perioperative stroke

A stroke is a sudden-onset focal neurological deficit of vascular origin lasting longer than 24 hours. A transient ischaemic attack (TIA) usually lasts from minutes to 24 hours and implies resolution of cerebral blood flow. A perioperative stroke has a significant impact on the patient and leads to increased length of stay, morbidity and a high mortality (around 26%). Perioperative strokes are usually either ischaemic or embolic in aetiology. Haemorrhagic strokes are rare.

Perioperative strokes usually occur post-operatively. Strokes occurring within the first day post-operatively are usually due to embolism. Surgery may lead to a hypercoagulable state, which increases the likelihood of stroke.

Cerebral hypoperfusion is a common cause of stroke. However, there is no evidence that deliberate hypotensive anaesthesia is associated with an increased risk. On the other hand hypotension in the immediate postoperative period is associated with stroke. Other

Table 9.3 Risk factors for perioperative stroke.

Patient risks	Hypertension
	Advanced age
	Atrial fibrillation
	Peripheral vascular disease
	Symptomatic carotid stenosis >70%
	Diabetes mellitus
	Systolic impairment of the heart
	History of stroke
	Renal impairment
	Discontinuation of antiplatelet or anticoagulant therapy
Intra-operative risks	Cardiac or vascular surgery
	Neck hyperextension
	Long duration of surgery
Postoperative risks	Sustained hypotension
	Hypercoagulability from surgery or dehydration or failure to resume antiplatelet or anticoagulant drugs

rare causes of stroke are air or fat embolism and carotid or vertebral artery disruption or plaque dislodgement during head and neck manipulation as part of anaesthesia or surgery. The incidence of perioperative stroke varies depending on the type of surgery. The lowest risk is associated with non-cardiac surgery and general surgical patients without a previous history of cerebrovascular disease have a risk of 0.2 to 0.7%. The risk is highest with vascular and cardiac surgery and especially combined cardiac procedures (cardiac valve surgery with coronary grafting or more than one valve surgery). The overall risk of stroke in cardiac surgery is 4.6%, and for double- or triple-valve surgery 9.7%. Carotid endarterectomy carries a 30-day rate of stroke of at least 3%. However, symptomatic patients have twice the risk of perioperative death or stroke compared with asymptomatic ones. Risk factors identified are previous TIA or stroke, heart failure and atrial fibrillation. The risk of stroke for any surgical patient increases with age as there are more risk factors for cerebrovascular disease in the elderly such as hypertension, atrial fibrillation and atherosclerosis (Table 9.3).

Prevention of perioperative stroke involves addressing any modifiable risk factors such as treating atrial fibrillation and hypertension and starting statin therapy. There should be consideration to not stopping antiplatelet and anticoagulant drugs during the perioperative period as the risk of significant bleeding is usually low. If these drugs are stopped they should be resumed as soon as possible after surgery. If warfarin is stopped then heparinization should be considered in the early perioperative period. If a patient has risk factors for cerebrovascular disease then sustained intra-operative hypotension should be avoided, as should be hyperglycaemia, which has been shown to increase the extent of neurological injury. Isoflurane and thiopentone have cerebral protective properties but only in doses sufficient to cause burst suppression on the EEG. Post-operatively, hypercoagulability should be avoided through hydration and resumption of antiplatelet and anticoagulant drugs. Any further anaesthesia or surgery should be delayed for four to six weeks because of changes in regional cerebral blood flow, disrupted autoregulation and enhanced thrombin activity.

Perioperative spinal cord injury not associated with regional anaesthesia

Perioperative spinal cord injury (SCI) can result from direct or indirect physiological insult to the spinal cord leading to motor, sensory and/or autonomic impairment. Injury to the spinal cord may be complete or incomplete, and can result in temporary or permanent impairment. Spinal cord injury is a rare but potentially devastating complication of spinal surgery although the incidence is low (<0.1 to 0.5%). In thoraco-abdominal aortic (TAAA) surgery, the spinal cord is also at significant risk of ischemic injury and the incidence of paraplegia or paraparesis is around 4%. After the initial injury, there follows a cascade of events that promotes tissue damage and ischaemia. The mechanisms of this secondary injury include vascular changes, ionic derangements, glutamate accumulation, arachidonic acid and free radical production, oxidative stress, oedema, inflammation and apoptosis.

Pre-operatively SCI may also occur during intubation and patient positioning. Patients at risk include those with spinal stenosis, cervical spondylosis, rheumatoid arthritis and traumatic cervical spine injuries. During surgery the spinal cord may be damaged directly, or indirectly through disruption of its vascular supply, e.g. the artery of Adamkiewicz, and consequent ischemia. Hypotension is another cause of SCI by decreasing cord perfusion and also worsening an existing SCI. Postoperative causes of SCI include epidural haematomas, inadequate decompression and infection.

Neurological injury can be reduced if SCI is recognized and secondary injury reduced. This involves multimodal neurophysiological monitoring during surgery and regular neurological testing post-operatively. The most frequently used modalities for spinal monitoring are somatosensory evoked potentials (SSEPs), motor evoked potentials (MEPs) and electromyographs (EMGs). Motor evoked potential monitoring may also be useful in TAAA repair. If SCI is suspected any precipitating factor, e.g. screw insertion or spinal manipulation, should be reversed if possible. The MAP should be maintained above 80 to 85 mmHg. High-dose methylprednisolone can be given soon after the identification of SCI. It offers potential neuroprotective benefits as exhibited in several randomized controlled trials although these applied only to blunt, closed SCI and not open spinal cord trauma. Relative systemic or local cooling can also be performed to reduce oxygen demand of the spinal cord, reducing the potential ischemic damage. For TAAA repair, cooling the epidural space using cold saline to 25°C has been shown to be effective in minimizing postoperative neurological complications. Cerebrospinal fluid drainage is often used as a method of spinal cord protection following TAAA repair. By decreasing CSF pressure to <10 mmHg, perfusion of the cord is improved and the risk of ischaemic damage reduced. In a randomized control trial with and without CSF drainage following TAAA repair there was an 80% reduction in the relative risk of postoperative deficits with CSF drainage.

Cerebral hypoxia and ischaemia

Cerebral hypoxia or ischaemia can occur in a variety of perioperative circumstances. This may be respiratory or hypoxic, such as airway disasters, or ischemic due to a compromised circulation, such as cardiac arrest. Brain damage may be termed hypoxic-ischaemic encephalopathy and can vary in clinical severity. The brain has a high metabolic demand and is sensitive to reductions in blood and oxygen supply. Regions of the brain requiring higher metabolic rates and vascular border zone areas are particularly vulnerable. A global ischaemic insult causes a reduction in energy substrates such as glucose and ATP, compromising cerebral metabolism and causing neuronal damage and irreversible brain damage within minutes. During cardiac arrest the degree of neuronal injury is proportional to the length of ischaemia with up to 95% of brain tissue damaged after 15 minutes. There are various biochemical changes that lead to neuronal damage and breakdown. These include impaired cell membrane function, ATP depletion, glutamate release, free radical formation and nitric oxide production. Functional changes occur such as mitochondrial dysfunction and lead to cell damage. If resumption of blood flow occurs there is often a period of hyperaemia followed by hypoperfusion due to changes in the cerebral circulation, but cell death can be diminished. 'Reperfusion injury' may still occur as a result of inflammation, oedema and oxidative damage. After a hypoxic arrest the brain injury seen is different and does not tend to be as severe as after cardiac arrest, with functional changes occurring without cell death. Hypoxia and hypercarbia cause an increase in cerebral blood flow so nutrient supply to the brain is not compromised. Hypoxia causes cerebral oedema, which causes encephalopathy. Hypoxia can also lead to delayed demyelination and subsequent neurological symptoms.

Neuroprotection and reducing perioperative neurological injury

There has been a lot of interest in reducing the neurological injury seen as a result of cerebral ischemia. This may be by attenuating the injury before or after an episode of ischemia. The most compelling evidence has come from resuscitation, where trials have shown that mild (32 to 35°C) hypothermia following out-of-hospital ventricular fibrillation (VF) cardiac arrest leads to reduced neurological injury. This has been widely extrapolated to cardiac arrests other than VF and occurring in hospital. Hypothermia is neuroprotective by reducing the cerebral metabolic rate (CMR). Deep hypothermia (18 to 22°C) is used routinely in certain cardiac surgical procedures, e.g. aortic surgery, to allow periods of circulatory arrest of up to 40 minutes with few adverse neurological consequences. Hyperthermia is known to worsen neurological injury and should be avoided. Anaesthetic drugs, particularly the barbiturates, propofol, and volatile anaesthetics reduce neurotransmission and therefore energy requirements and are neuroprotective during an ischaemic period. Hyperglycaemia worsens ischemic injury perhaps by causing intracellular acidosis. Hyperventilation, causing cerebral vasoconstriction, and hyperoxaemia, which may expose the brain to oxygen toxicity, should also be avoided. There is evidence of harm and no evidence of benefit from glucocorticoids (Table 9.4).

Reducing the risk of neurological injury in cardiac surgery

There has been a lot of work in trying to attenuate the neurological injury seen in cardiac surgery. The aetiology of the neurological injury seen is multifactorial and due to cerebral microemboli and hypoperfusion, exacerbated by ischaemia and reperfusion injury. The injury may vary from cognitive dysfunction to stroke and depends on the duration of ischaemia and whether it was regional or global. Strategies to reduce the risk include haemodynamic management, i.e. maintaining an adequate cerebral perfusion pressure (CPP) by avoiding low mean arterial pressures (MAP) and high central venous pressures (CVP) and

Table 9.4 Summary of considerations during perioperative hypoxia and ischemia.

Induced mild-moderate hypothermia if global ischaemia

Avoid hyperthermia

Optimize oxygen delivery

Avoid hyperoxaemia

Maintain normocapnia

Avoid hypocapnia

Avoid hyperglycaemia

Volatile anaesthetic agents

aiming for a higher MAP in high-risk or chronic hypertensive patients who may have altered cerebral autoregulation. Mild to moderate hypothermia reduces the cerebral metabolic rate and excitatory neurotransmitter release. To date pharmacological neuroprotection has had disappointing clinical results. There are a variety of monitors that have been used in the effort to identify and quantify neurological injury during cardiac surgery, such as transcranial Doppler, single- or multi-channel electroencephalography (EEG) and cerebral oximetry. Cerebral oximetry determines the saturation of blood in cerebral tissue (rSO_2) using near-infrared spectroscopy (NIRS). It is non-invasive, has a fast signal–response time, and has been subject to a number of randomized controlled studies. One group studied the use of cerebral oximetry in 200 patients undergoing CABG surgery and used targeted interventions if the rSO_2 dropped any more than 20% from the baseline. Interventions included checking for mechanical problems such as obstruction to venous drainage in the neck and at cannulation sites, increasing $PaCO_2$ in the presence of hypocapnia and increasing FiO_2, MAP and haemoglobin through transfusion of packed red cells. They showed a trend towards stroke reduction and overall improved outcome. Patients that had higher morbidity had more desaturations and lower mean rSO_2 levels and there was a significant inverse correlation between intra-operative rSO_2 and duration of postoperative hospitalization. Another group showed a correlation between prolonged desaturation as seen on cerebral oximetry and increased postoperative cognitive decline and increased length of hospital stay.

The interventions and class of evidence used to reduce the risk of neurological injury in cardiac surgery are:

- heparin-bonded cardiopulmonary bypass circuit
- epi-aortic ultrasound (Class IIb)
- modified aortic cannula
- leukocyte-depleting filter
- cell-saver processing of pericardial aspirate
- CO_2 wound insufflation
- maintaining 'higher' MAP targets (>50 mm Hg) (Class IIb)
- non-pulsatile (versus pulsatile) perfusion (Class IIb)
- alpha-stat versus pH-stat acid–base management (Class IIb)
- minimal haematocrit target during CPB of 27%
- thiopental, propofol, nimodipine, prostacylin, GM1 ganglioside, pegorgotein, clomethiazole (Class III)

- remacemide, lidocaine, aprotinin, pexelizumab
- 'tight' glucose intra-operative control
- hypothermia.

Perioperative changes in mental status

Awareness

Awareness is defined as postoperative, explicit recollection of intra-operative events, at a time when general anaesthesia was intended. Although uncommon, it can lead to significant long-term psychological problems for patients as well as medico-legal consequences. The widely quoted incidence of awareness with explicit recall as demonstrated in large prospective studies is 0.1 to 0.18%, although one review found it to be as low as 0.007%, or 1 in 14,560 patients. In a large review of awareness case reports from 1950 to 2005, patients who experience awareness are more likely to be younger, female and undergoing obstetric or cardiac surgery; however, the principal 'risk factors' are light or insufficient anaesthesia and previous history of awareness. Other associative factors identified from other studies such as age, gender, the use of benzodiazepines and type of anaesthetic have been inconsistent.

Patients who experience awareness report a variety of distressing memories: hearing voices and noises, inability to move, sensation of weakness or paralysis and feelings of helplessness, anxiety and fear. Pain is experienced in 28 to 38% of patients. The commonest complaints are of auditory perception and loss of motor power. Late psychological and psychiatric symptoms are reported in 22 to 33% of patients. These may persist post-operatively for a variable duration and include fear, anxiety, sleep disturbances and post-traumatic stress disorder. There are significant medico-legal and financial implications too. An analysis of all claims made to the NHS Litigation Authority from 1997 to 2007 found that 21% of all anaesthetic claims related to inadequate general anaesthesia and the mean cost for anaesthetic awareness was £32,680 and £24,364 for brief awake paralysis. Most claims led to financial compensation.

Awareness occurs when anaesthesia is insufficient to cause amnesia, analgesia and lack of sensation and recall. This may happen by a number of methods. Firstly, there are patients in which the anaesthetist may choose to give smaller doses of anaesthetic drugs as a result of their low physiological reserve, or when the haemodynamic and depressant side effects of many of these drugs is undesirable. This explains the higher incidence of awareness of up to 1% reported in sicker patients (ASA status III to IV), obstetrics, cardiac surgery and major trauma. Secondly, there are some patients who have an increased anaesthetic dose requirement, the reasons for which are unclear but multifactorial, and include chronic use of alcohol, opioids and sedative drugs, and perhaps in part due to pharmacogenetic differences. Thirdly, the incidence is slightly higher in children (0.8%), maybe due to altered pharmacology and anaesthetic techniques. The most common reason, however, is insufficient anaesthesia due to equipment failure, lack of vigilance and human error. Examples include the vaporizer not being turned on or empty; medication error, such that the muscle relaxant is given to an awake patient; and prolonged difficult intubation without sufficient maintenance of anaesthesia. These cases were characterized by less use of amnesic premedication, induction and maintenance anaesthetics and less opioids compared to control. Patient movement during the operation, hypertension and tachycardia were also common. It is important to note that if a patient has received muscle relaxants then movement after surgical incision, as a sign of light anaesthesia, will not occur and increases the chance of awareness. Equally if a patient has received pre-operative beta-blockade medication then the haemodynamic sympathetic responses will be damped. A significant proportion of awareness cases occur during periods of intense stimulation such as incision or endotracheal intubation.

Prevention and management of awareness

Most cases of awareness are potentially avoidable. Vigilance and experience of the anaesthetist are the best way of reducing the risk. Thorough checking of the anaesthetic machine and equipment, adequate anaesthetic dosage and attention to the patient and monitors throughout the anaesthetic is essential. Amnesic premedication and continuous dosing of anaesthesia may be ways to avoid awareness. One should pay attention to patients with a higher risk of awareness. Other considerations are setting the low alarm of end-tidal volatile anaesthetic concentrations appropriately; administering additional intravenous anaesthetic during a prolonged intubation; ensuring a patent and preferably visible intravenous line when using total intravenous anaesthesia; routinely using a nerve stimulator, and ensuring adequate anaesthesia with muscle relaxation. Syringes should all be labelled and visibly checked before administration. One study found that awareness amongst patients without neuromuscular blockade is less concerning, as long as operating-room conversations are respectful. It may be prudent to mention the risk of awareness during one pre-operative visit of high-risk for awareness patients.

The use of the bispectral index (BIS) monitor (Aspect Medical Systems, Massachusetts, USA) has been advocated to prevent awareness and also allows a reduction in the use of anaesthetic agents. The BIS monitor is marketed as a depth-of-anaesthesia monitor, and works by processing frontal electroencephalogram signals. There are a number of commercially available monitors, but the BIS has the largest body of literature evaluating it. To date there have been two large trials done on BIS and awareness. The B-Aware randomized controlled trial showed a reduction in the risk of awareness of 82% with BIS monitoring compared to routine care in an at-risk group. There were still aware patients in the BIS-guided group (2 out of 1,225 patients), although in these patients the BIS value was at the upper end or over the recommended range of 40 to 60 for sufficient anaesthesia. A subsequent study, the B-Unaware trial, where patients were randomized to BIS-guided care (BIS value 40 to 60) or end-tidal anaesthetic gas analysis (using alarm limits and MAC over 0.7), was unable to reproduce these results but still demonstrated a similar low incidence of awareness. Awareness was no more likely to occur if using the BIS or alarms for limits on volatile anaesthetic concentration. Moreover awareness occurred when BIS and end-tidal values were within the target ranges. This trial, however, has attracted criticism and a meta-analysis supported the use of BIS in preventing awareness. Two large randomized controlled trials are underway to help clarify these conflicting results.

Not all aware patients report spontaneous recall. Provoked recall by direct questioning may be required to elicit the actual incidence of awareness. If a potential case of awareness is identified it should be distinguished from dreaming, which is common (6%). If awareness is thought to have occurred the patient should be visited by an anaesthetist and given reassurance and an explanation. The patient should be reminded to tell future anaesthetists. It would be prudent to offer psychological follow-up.

Postoperative delirium

Delirium is a syndrome described as disturbance of consciousness (i.e. reduced clarity of awareness of the environment) with reduced ability to focus, sustain or shift attention; change

Table 9.5 Postoperative delirium risk factors.

Patient factors	Perioperative factors	Postoperative factors
Female sex	*Anaesthetic factors:*	Hypoxia
Age >70	Anticholinergic, antimuscarinic or benzodiazepine use	Hypocarbia
Pre-existing cognitive impairment	Intra-operative polypharmacy	Acute pain
Depression or anxiety	Long-acting or residual anaesthetics	Anaemia
Previous delirium	Complications: hypotension or hypoxia	Fluid and electrolyte abnormalities
Alcohol or smoking history		Polypharmacy
Visual impairment	*Surgical factors:*	Physical restraints
Polypharmacy	Orthopaedic, ophthalmic, cardiac, vascular surgery	Malnutrition
Benzodiazepine or narcotic use	Long duration of surgery	Sepsis
Severe illness	Increased blood loss or transfusion	Sensory deprivation
Endocrine or metabolic disorders		Sensory overload, e.g. ICU
BUN:Cr[1] >18	Complications: embolism	Sleep deprivation

[1] BUN:Cr – blood urea nitrogen/creatinine ratio.

in cognition (e.g. memory deficit, disorientation, language disturbance and perceptual disturbance) that is not better accounted for by a pre-existing, established or evolving dementia and development over a short period of time (usually hours to days) and the tendency to fluctuate during the course of the day. There should be evidence from the history, physical examination or laboratory findings that the disturbance is caused by the direct physiological consequences of a general medical condition. Delirium is divided into substance intoxication; substance withdrawal; delirium due to multiple aetiologies; and delirium of unclear aetiology.

The mechanisms of delirium are not fully understood, but increased dopaminergic activity and decreased cholinergic and GABA-ergic activity is important. It may involve changes in neurotransmitter activity of acetylcholine, or as a result of the inflammatory response to surgery. Delirium may be seen on emergence from anaesthesia, or in intensive care. Postoperative delirium (POD) is a well recognized condition with significant implications, including increased morbidity, delayed recovery and increased hospital length of stay. The incidence of POD is 5 to 15% although there are certain groups where it is higher, such as cardiac surgery patients (13.5 to 21%) and fractured hip patients (35%). There is a high incidence of POD in the elderly. Postoperative delirium is usually seen between the first and third postoperative days and the typical features are that of an acute confusional state (characterized by fluctuating mental status), inattention and either disorganized thinking or altered level of consciousness. There are a variety of tools used for the assessment of delirium such as the mini mental state exam and confusion assessment method (CAM). The risk factors associated with developing POD are listed in Table 9.5.

The incidence of POD is significantly reduced if geriatricians and anaesthetists implement a specific intervention programme. This can be thought of as a care bundle of pre- and postoperative interventions, including oxygen therapy, early surgery, prevention and treatment of perioperative blood pressure falls and prompt treatment of postoperative complications. An intervention programme using standardized protocols for the management of six risk factors for delirium (cognitive impairment, sleep deprivation, immobility, visual impairment, hearing impairment and dehydration) showed significant reductions in the number and duration of episodes of delirium in hospitalized older patients. A proactive geriatrician review of patients before and after surgery also reduces the incidence of delirium. Prevention of POD should start at pre-assessment when the at-risk patient may be identified. Intra-operatively the anaesthetist should avoid drugs such as atropine and pethidine, hypotension, hypoxia and metabolic derangements. There does not seem to be a difference in POD when regional or general anaesthesia are compared in elective surgery; however, a Cochrane review concluded that with hip fracture surgery, regional anaesthesia is associated with a two-fold reduced risk of acute postoperative confusion. Post-operatively, good nursing care is essential, as is attention to acute pain, cognitive stimulation, allowing adequate sleep at night, mobilization and avoiding certain drugs.

Prevention of POD is more effective than treatment. The treatment of POD involves avoiding precipitating factors, treating any organic causes such as hypoxia or infection and intervention programmes as above. For refractory cases or in situations of hyperactivity, the butyrophenone haloperidol is the drug of choice.

Emergence delirium is classified as substance-induced delirium and occurs on waking in the recovery unit. It differs from POD in that it is not fluctuant. It is short-lived and usually resolves spontaneously or once any identifiable factor has been dealt with such as anxiety and pain. It is characterized by hyperactive behaviour, agitation and restlessness with consequences including self-extubation and removal of indwelling catheters and poses a significant risk of injury and harm to the patient and a burden to staff. The incidence is around 5% and is more common in children (10 to 50%). Risk factors include benzodiazepine premedication; use of etomidate; musculoskeletal, breast and abdominal surgery; age under 40 or over 64 years; and postoperative pain. The presence of an endotracheal tube, urinary catheter and residual neuromuscular block are other suspected factors. The use of antidepressant medication and previous hospitalization appear to be protective factors. Hypoactive emergence is delayed recovery from anaesthesia, and may represent a hypoactive form of emergence delirium or POD. The incidence is around 3% and it carries a risk of increased length of stay in hospital.

ICU delirium is a well known entity with an incidence of around 30% but up to 80% in sicker, ventilated patients. Intensive care unit delirium is an independent predictor of increased length of stay and hospital mortality and may predispose patients to prolonged neuropsychological disturbances after they leave intensive care. There may be hyperactive or hypoactive subtypes and patients often fluctuate between the two. The hyperactive form is well recognized and often the patient is labelled as 'agitated'. Hypoactive delirium may go unnoticed and is associated with a worse outcome. Known risk factors are high APACHE II scores, history of hypertension and alcoholism, and sedative and analgesic drug use. Many drugs used in the ICU can precipitate delirium but in particular benzodiazepines, anticholinergics (crossing the blood–brain barrier) and dopaminergic drugs, and opiate analgesic drugs are implicated.

The Intensive Care Delirium Screening Checklist (ICDSC), the Delirium Detection Score (DDS) and the Confusion Assessment Method for the Intensive Care Unit (CAM-ICU) are screening tools validated for use in the diagnosis of ICU delirium. Prevention is primarily good medical and nursing care, i.e. alleviating anxiety and pain, mobilization, good communication and trying to maintain a normal sleep–wake cycle. Sedation should be used judiciously with sedation-level assessment on a validated scale and regular sedation holds. Organic causes should be identified and treated promptly, such as infection, metabolic and physiological abnormalities such as hypoxaemia, acidosis and ventilator dys-synchrony. Finally, care should be taken to avoid or limit the risk factors such as implicated drugs. Once delirium has been identified, haloperidol should be the first-line pharmacological treatment. The atypical antipsychotic olanzepine may be an appropriate second-line drug or for those patients who cannot tolerate haloperidol.

Postoperative cognitive dysfunction

Postoperative cognitive dysfunction (POCD) is a deterioration of cognition such as memory, learning, attention or perception from pre-operative levels. Postoperative cognitive dysfunction can lead to significant impact on the individual, their safety, relationship with others and environment. It is also associated with an increased morbidity and mortality. It differs from delirium in that it may take days or weeks to manifest, is more persistent in duration and is associated with different risk factors. There is no clear relationship between delirium and POCD and many patients with delirium do not develop POCD and vice versa. The aetiology is unclear, perhaps involving inflammation, release of stress hormones, ischaemia or hypoxaemia, but it is related to major surgery and patients over 60 years. There is no difference in POCD incidence between regional or general anaesthesia. Postoperative cognitive dysfunction usually improves with time but it may persist at six months. For an accurate diagnosis of POCD and objective evidence of cognitive decline, a number of neuropsychiatric tests assessing memory and learning and other aspects of cognitive function should be made pre-operatively and post-operatively, in a standardized manner, and compared. The incidence of POCD is high. A large study of 1,218 patients undergoing non-cardiac major surgery aged over 60 years showed a 26% incidence one week after surgery and 10% at three months. Risk factors identified for early POCD were increasing age, long duration of anaesthesia, a second operation, postoperative infection, respiratory complications and low baseline education level. Increasing age was a risk factor for late POCD and, interestingly, use of benzodiazepines was protective. These results were confirmed in a later prospective study of 1,064 non-cardiac surgery patients where POCD was identified in 37% of young patients aged 18 to 39 years, 30% in middle-aged patients 40 to 59 years and 41% in patients aged 60 and above. At three months the young and middle-aged patients had POCD of around 6% but the elderly group had a significantly higher incidence of 13% than age-matched controls. A subgroup analysis of the older patients showed that the type and severity of cognitive decline varied. At three months after surgery, more elderly adults experienced memory impairment, but only those with executive (ability to process information, concentrate and self-monitor) or combined cognitive decline had functional limitations of daily activities. There are no specific recommendations in the prevention and treatment of POCD, but for elderly patients undergoing major surgery it poses a significant risk and subsequent impact on life and should be considered when seeing a patient and providing information pre-operatively.

Patients undergoing cardiac surgery have the highest incidence of POCD (30 to 80%). A study of 261 patients undergoing coronary artery bypass grafts showed cognitive decline in 53% at discharge, 36% at six weeks, 24% at six months and 42% at five years. Cardiac surgery patients are usually older, with atherosclerosis and cerebrovascular disease, so are already at increased risk before surgery. Cardiac surgery is major surgery and consequently generates a significant inflammatory response, implicated in the development of POCD. Cardiopulmonary bypass (CPB) is often thought to be a factor, with the risk of embolization and generation of an inflammatory response; however, randomized trials comparing CPB with off-pump techniques have not shown a difference in POCD at three months or five years. Cerebral microemboli are the likely cause, and these still occur during off-pump surgery during manipulation of the heart and great vessels.

Neuropathic pain

Neuropathic pain (NP) is defined by the International Association for the Study of Pain as 'pain arising as a direct consequence of a lesion or disease affecting the somatosensory system'. It is characterized by a variety of sensory symptoms and signs such as spontaneous pain, paraesthesia, dysaesthesia, hyperalgesia and allodynia. A lesion of afferent pathways is necessary for the development of NP. The broad classes of aetiology are focal and multifocal lesions of the peripheral nervous system (e.g. post-traumatic neuralgia); generalized polyneuropathies of the peripheral nervous system (e.g. diabetes); lesions in the central nervous system (e.g. spinal cord injury); and complex regional pain syndromes I and II. Surgery may lead to NP via central lesions during spinal surgery and peripheral lesions after thoracotomy, mastectomy or orthopaedic surgery for example. Trauma can also cause NP, e.g. traumatic brain injury and post-traumatic neuralgia.

Management of NP includes assessing the pain and establishing the diagnosis, involving a pain specialist if necessary. Any relevant co-morbidities such as cardiac, renal or hepatic disease, depression and gait instability that might be relieved or exacerbated by NP should be addressed. Any underlying cause such as diabetes or nerve compression should be treated. The management of NP requires an interdisciplinary approach, centred around pharmacological therapy. On the basis of randomized clinical trials, the medications recommended as first-line treatments for neuropathic pain include tricyclic antidepressants, dual reuptake inhibitors of both serotonin and norepinephrine, calcium channel alpha$_2$-delta ligands (gabapentin and pregabalin) and topical lidocaine. Opioid analgesic drugs and tramadol are second-line treatments that can be considered for first-line use in selected clinical circumstances. Other medications that generally would be used as third-line treatments include certain other antidepressant and antiepileptic medications, topical capsaicin, mexiletine and N-methyl-d-aspartate (NMDA) receptor antagonists.

List of further reading

Deiner, S. & Silverstein, J. H. Postoperative delirium and cognitive dysfunction. *Br J Anaesth* 2009; **103** (Suppl 1): i41–6.

Fukuda, S. & Warner, D. S. Cerebral protection. *Br J Anaesth* 2007; **99**: 10–17.

Ghoneim, M. M., Block, R. I., Haffarnan, M. & Mathews, M. J. Awareness during anesthesia: risk factors, causes and sequelae. A review of reported cases in the literature. *Anesth Analg* 2009; **108**: 527–35.

Hogue, C. W., Jr., Palin, C. A. & Arrowsmith, J. E. Cardiopulmonary bypass management and neurologic outcomes: an evidence-based appraisal of current practices. *Anesth Analg* 2006; **103**: 21–37.

Kent, C. D. & Domino, K. B. Depth of anesthesia. *Curr Opin Anaesthesiol* 2009; **22**: 782–7.

Lowenstein, D. H. Seizures and epilepsy. In Braunwald, E., Fauci, A. S., Kasper, D. D. *et al.* (eds) *Harrison's Principles of Internal Medicine.* McGraw Hill, 2001.

Monk, T. G., Weldon, B. C., Garvan, C. W. *et al.* Predictors of cognitive dysfunction after major noncardiac surgery. *Anesthesiology* 2008; **108**: 18–30.

O' Connor, A. B. & Dworkin, R. H. Treatment of neuropathic pain: an overview of recent guidelines. *Am J Med* 2009; **122**: S22–32.

Sekhon, L. H. & Fehlings, M. G. Epidemiology, demographics, and pathophysiology of acute spinal cord injury. *Spine* 2001; **26**: S2–12.

Selim, M. Perioperative stroke. *N Engl J Med* 2007; **356**: 706–13.

Chapter 10

Hepatic, renal and endocrine complications

A. James Varley and Fay J. Gilder

Hepatic complications

Clinically significant derangements of the liver enzymes alanine aminotransferase (ALT) and aspartate aminotransferase (AST) are uncommon after anaesthesia in healthy individuals. Elevations in serum bilirubin are more common, multifactorial in nature, and usually clinically insignificant. De novo acute liver dysfunction as a complication of anaesthesia occurs rarely. However, anaesthesia-induced hepatitis (AIH) is associated with significant mortality. Severe liver dysfunction as a consequence of anaesthesia is not uncommon in patients with pre-existing liver disease. It is important that this high-risk patient group is recognized pre-operatively.

De novo acute liver dysfunction

Perioperative de novo acute liver dysfunction is associated with the use of volatile anaesthetic agents. There are two types:

- **Type I** is a mild subclinical hepatotoxicity reported after halothane and enflurane anaesthesia only. It is characterized by clinically insignificant rises in serum transaminases or glutathione-S-transferase, which resolve within 48 hours. The mechanism is thought to be a hepatotoxic effect of the anaerobic metabolites of halothane and enflurane.
- **Type II** is also known as anaesthesia-induced hepatitis (AIH). It is a rare form of liver injury associated with volatile anaesthetic agents. The incidence varies according to the causative agent.

Anaesthesia-induced hepatitis

Anaesthesia-induced hepatitis (AIH) has been associated most commonly with halothane. The incidence is between 1 in 3,500 to 1 in 35,000. There have been only a handful of case reports in the literature implicating enflurane (incidence 2 in 1,000,000), isoflurane and desflurane as causes for AIH. Oxidized reactive metabolites can bind to the liver forming trifluoroacetylated macromolecules. In susceptible individuals these altered liver proteins are seen by the immune system as foreign antigens. Massive liver necrosis follows as a result of immune activation. The variation in incidence is related to the percentage of the agent oxidized by the liver cytochrome P450 2E1 – halothane (20%), enflurane (2%), isoflurane (0.2%) and desflurane (0.02%).

Anaesthetic and Perioperative Complications, ed. Kamen Valchanov, Stephen T. Webb and Jane Sturgess.
Published by Cambridge University Press. © Cambridge University Press 2011.

Although sevoflurane metabolites are not reactive there have been case reports implicating this agent as the cause of hepatic dysfunction. The mechanism of injury is unknown.

Anaesthesia-induced hepatitis occurs in healthy individuals. It can occur after a brief anaesthetic and minor surgery. The signs and symptoms appear three to six days post-operatively and comprise fever, anorexia, nausea, chills, myalgia, rash and eosinophilia. Severe jaundice appears three to six days after the initial symptoms. Laboratory investigations reveal grossly elevated serum transaminases, hyperbilirubinaemia and an elevated prothrombin time. Histopathological findings include centrilobular necrosis. All other causes of hepatitis must be ruled out including viral, autoimmune and drug-induced hepatitis. Imaging studies and a liver biopsy may need to be undertaken. Anaesthesia-induced hepatitis is a diagnosis of exclusion. There is no widely available specific assay that will identify the anaesthetic agent as a cause though a few laboratories can measure anti-trifluoroacetylated protein antibodies in plasma. Treatment for AIH is supportive. Over half of cases will progress to fulminant hepatic failure for which the treatment is urgent liver transplantation.

Patients with pre-existing liver disease

One in 700 patients admitted for elective surgery has abnormal liver function tests. Total liver blood flow is 1.5 l/min. The hepatic arterial circulation supplies 25% of total liver blood flow and the portal venous system supplies 75%. The two circulations contribute equally to hepatic oxygenation. In a normal liver the arterial blood flow increases to maintain total liver blood flow and oxygenation if there is a reduction in portal venous flow. In a cirrhotic liver this compensatory response is reduced: the presence of portal hypertension further impairs hepatic blood flow and oxygenation. There is a reduction in liver blood flow and hepatic oxygen uptake in the perioperative period, which impairs the compensatory reciprocal relationship that exists between the hepatic arterial and portal venous circulations. In patients with cirrhotic liver disease this can lead to decompensated liver failure and death.

Investigation

Every patient should be evaluated for the presence of liver disease. The presence or past history of ascites, oesophageal varices, encephalopathy and portal hypertension must be sought. Laboratory investigations are shown in Table 10.1. Quantitative tests of cardiovascular (cirrhotic cardiomyopathy), respiratory (secondary to the mechanical effects of large volume abdominal ascites, pleural effusions or hepatopulmonary syndrome) and renal dysfunction (hepatorenal syndrome) may be necessary. Early involvement of hepatologist is essential for the pre-operative optimization and postoperative care of this high-risk patient group.

Risk prediction

Published evidence demonstrates that the risk of death during the perioperative period in patients with cirrhotic liver disease is between 8 and 70% and increases in proportion to the severity of the liver disease. Liver failure is graded according to the Child–Turcotte–Pugh (CTP) classification (Table 10.2).

Severity of liver disease has more recently been classified by the Model for End-stage Liver Disease (MELD) score. MELD uses the patient's serum bilirubin, serum creatinine and the international normalized ratio for prothrombin time (INR) to predict survival (Table 10.3).

Table 10.1 Laboratory investigations required for the evaluation of a patient with pre-existing liver disease.

Biochemistry	Haematology	Virology
• Liver function tests: ALT, AST, gamma GT, alkaline phosphatase, bilirubin • Albumin • Urea and electrolytes • Estimated GFR • Glucose	• Full blood count • Prothrombin time • Thromboelastography	• Hepatitis viral serology

Table 10.2 Child–Turcotte–Pugh score.

Variable	1 point	2 points	3 points
Biliruin µmol/l	<34	34–50	>50
Albumin g/l	>35	28–35	<28
International normalized ratio	<1.7	1.71–2.20	>2.20
Ascites	None	Mild	Severe
Hepatic encephalopathy	None	Grade I–II (or suppressed with medication)	Grade III–IV (or refractory)

Note: In primary sclerosing cholangitis (PSC) and primary biliary cirrhosis (PBC), the bilirubin references are changed to reflect the fact that these diseases feature high-conjugated bilirubin levels. The upper limit for 1 point is 68 µmol/l and the upper limit for 2 points is 170 µmol/l.

Table 10.3 Model for End-stage Liver Disease score.

MELD score is calculated according to the following formula:

$$MELD = 3.78(Ln\ serum\ bilirubin\ (mg/dL)) + 11.2(Ln\ INR) + 9.57(Ln\ serum\ creatinine\ (mg/dL)) + 6.43$$

A MELD score in the context of risk prediction for surgery of <10, 10 to 14 and >14 can be equated with a CTP class of A, B and C respectively. Individual risk factors (prolonged prothrombin time, hypoalbuminaemia or encephalopathy) are not useful as predictors of mortality and morbidity independently of CTP or MELD.

There are other important factors, in addition to the degree of liver dysfunction, that determine risk in these patients. The type of surgery to be performed is particularly significant. Cardiac surgery, abdominal surgery, emergency surgery and surgery associated with intra-operative blood transfusion requirement all carry a very high mortality of approximately 40 to 60%.

Management

A multidisciplinary approach involving hepatology, surgical, anaesthetic and intensive care teams is necessary. Pre-operative optimization may include treatment of coagulopathy, drainage of ascites, treatment of encephalopathy, electrolyte correction, fluid management and pre-operative antibiotic prophylaxis. Intra-operative care is aimed at maintaining liver blood flow and oxygenation. The anaesthetic technique should include using the least hepatotoxic drugs possible. Hepatic enzyme-inducing drugs must be avoided where possible. The anaesthetic vapours isoflurane and desflurane have minimal effects on liver blood flow so are relatively safe to use. Atracurium is the muscle relaxant of choice as its metabolism is independent of liver function. Morphine can precipitate hepatic encephalopathy and so should be avoided. Fentanyl is an acceptable alternative. Monitoring should include intra-arterial blood pressure and core temperature. Central venous monitoring is indicated for major surgery. Pulmonary arterial catheterization may be necessary, particularly if pulmonary hypertension is suspected. Red blood cells, platelets and fresh frozen plasma should be immediately available. Fluid and patient warming devices should be considered. Postoperative critical care will be required where the common complications of surgery in this patient group (haemorrhage, sepsis, acute liver failure and acute kidney injury) can be managed.

Renal complications

The development of acute kidney injury (AKI) is an ominous event, as it is associated with increases in morbidity, mortality, hospital length of stay and healthcare costs. Acute kidney injury is also associated with an increased risk of gastrointestinal bleeding, respiratory infections and sepsis. Furthermore, recent work has shown that even small increases in serum creatinine levels from baseline are associated with increased mortality. Similarly, transient AKI has been associated with a long-term increase in mortality. The incidence of AKI in hospitalized non-cardiac surgical patients is 1 to 5%. In contrast cardiac surgery has a higher risk of AKI, in the order of 5 to 30%, with an associated mortality of 25 to 50%.

Despite the development of renal replacement therapies that can rapidly correct the metabolic and biochemical derangements of AKI, improvements in AKI-related mortality have not materialized. A recent NCEPOD report described deficiencies in the diagnosis and management of patients with AKI in both medical and surgical inpatients.

As Elderly patients with significant co-morbidities present for major surgery with increasing frequency, it is appropriate to review the role of the anaesthetist in identifying patients at risk of AKI, the steps that can be taken to prevent its development and the initial management once it has occurred.

Causative and associated factors

These can be arbitrarily divided into direct pharmacological and physiological effects of anaesthesia and indirect perioperative risk factors.

Direct factors

Volatile anaesthetic agents

Historically concerns have been voiced regarding the association of low-flow anaesthesia and the generation of the haloalkene compound A. This breakdown product is produced from sevoflurane when carbon dioxide absorbents are used. Compound A has been shown to be nephrotoxic in rats. However, to date no human studies have demonstrated any association with AKI, despite research studies using low-flow anaesthesia for many hours.

Muscle relaxants

The commonly used modern muscle relaxants are not known to cause renal failure. However, care should be taken with their choice in the patient with renal failure as those that depend on renal excretion can accumulate and prolonged neuromuscular blockade can result. Atracurium is recommended due to its metabolism by Hoffman degradation, rendering its duration of action independent of hepatic or renal function.

Antibiotics

- Aminoglycosides are a recognized cause of acute tubular necrosis. The pathophysiology is unclear, but thought to involve intracellular accumulation. As the mechanism of uptake of aminoglycosides is saturable, once-daily dosing is utilized in order to minimize nephrotoxicity.
- Vancomycin has a synergistic nephrotoxic effect with aminoglycosides. Dosing and frequency of administration need careful consideration in those at risk of AKI.
- Acute interstitial nephritis is a hypersensitivity reaction to drugs, most commonly associated with the beta-lactam antibiotics and the fluoroquinolones. It is usually self-limiting, and occurs typically 7 to 14 days after the exposure.

Non-steroidal anti-inflammatory drugs (NSAIDs)

In normal subjects renal prostaglandin synthesis is maintained at a relatively low level and therefore has limited influence on glomerular blood flow and GFR. In patients with underlying renal pathology, these vasodilators (predominantly prostacyclin and prostaglandin E2) become more important, and in these patients NSAID-induced prostaglandin inhibition can contribute to AKI.

Colloids

The hydroxyethyl starches have been shown to double the risk of AKI in patients undergoing major surgery. It has been shown that doses as low as 500 ml can increase the risk of AKI and therefore should be avoided.

Blood transfusion

There is emerging evidence that blood transfusion is predictive of the development of AKI. Whether this is a surrogate for hypovolaemia and impaired perfusion is unclear. There may be a reduction in the incidence of AKI with the use of leukodepleted blood, suggesting an immunogenic mechanism.

Indirect factors

Hypovolaemia

Maintenance of euvolaemia is central to the prevention of AKI. The anaesthetist needs to prevent and treat pre-operative fluid depletion. This can occur as a result of prolonged fasting, bowel preparation and the effects of concomitant pathology, e.g. small bowel obstruction.

Radiocontrast media

As contrast imaging becomes increasingly common, more patients are receiving radio contrast media and so risk developing contrast-induced nephropathy (CIN). Contrast-induced nephropathy has become the third most prevalent cause of AKI in hospitalized patients. Risk factors for CIN are shown in Table 10.4.

Table 10.4 Risk factors for contrast-induced nephropathy.

Procedure factors	Patient factors
High dose of contrast	Diabetes mellitus
Intra-arterial administration	Age >75
Peri-procedural shock	Heart failure
Use of intra-aortic balloon counter pulsation	Hypertension
	Anaemia
	NSAIDS and nephrotoxins
	eGFR <60

Hypotension

Several studies have demonstrated an association between AKI and perioperative hypotension and the resulting reduced renal blood flow. Intravenous and volatile anaesthetic agents cause a decrease in organ perfusion through a reduction in cardiac output and vasodilatation. These effects can lead to a fall in renal blood flow. In addition, a reduction in afferent arteriolar vasoconstriction can disrupt the maintenance of adequate glomerular filtration pressure. Therefore, although these anaesthetic agents do not possess direct nephrotoxicity, their effects on cardiovascular physiology could provoke renal injury if unopposed.

Surgical stress response

The neurohumoral response to surgery causes oliguria. This is mediated by the actions of antidiuretic hormone (water retention), aldosterone and glucocorticoids (salt and water retention) and increased renin activity as a result of reduced blood volume.

Intra-abdominal hypertension

Increased intra-abdominal pressure has become recognized as an important cause of abdominal organ dysfunction. Intra-abdominal hypertension (IAH) has been defined as an abdominal pressure greater then 12 mmHg; abdominal compartment syndrome (ACS) is defined as a pressure greater than 20 mmHg with associated organ dysfunction. Persistently raised intra-abdominal pressures can compromise renal perfusion by impairing renal venous blood flow. Reductions in cardiac output occur due to a fall in venous return. Intra-abdominal hypertension and ACS typically occur after abdominal trauma or due to retroperitoneal haemorrhage from a ruptured abdominal aortic aneurysm. Intra-abdominal hypertension may also occur as a result of vigorous fluid resuscitation. Delayed closure of the abdominal wall after abdominal surgery may be required. The raised intra-abdominal pressure that occurs with laparoscopic surgery can also cause renal injury in the at-risk patient, particularly with prolonged procedures.

Cardiac and aortic surgery

Perioperative AKI occurs more frequently in thoracic aortic surgery, abdominal aortic surgery and cardiac surgery. This is as a result of the interruptions to renal perfusion that can result from vascular cross-clamping or from atheromatous emboli. Equally the patients requiring these operations typically possess significant co-morbidities including hypertension and diabetes mellitus.

Table 10.5 RIFLE classification system.

	GFR criteria	Urine output (UO) criteria
Risk	Serum creatinine x 1.5 Reduction in GFR >25%	UO <0.5 mg/kg/h
Injury	Serum creatinine x 2 Reduction in GFR >50%	UO <0.5 mg/kg/h
Failure	Serum creatinine x 3 Reduction in GFR >75%	UO < 0.3 mg/kg/h or anuria x 12 h
Loss	Peristent ARF = complete loss of kidney function for 4 weeks	
ESKD	End-stage kidney disease (>3 months)	

Positioning

Extremes of patient positioning have been associated with perioperative AKI. These have been most commonly associated with extremes of the lithotomy position maintained for long periods. Rhabdomyolysis can occur as a result of lower limb hypoperfusion.

Antifibrinolytics

Controversy has surrounded the use of these drugs. Aprotinin is associated with AKI; however, it may be a surrogate marker for the higher risk patient, greater operative complexity, increased duration of surgery and increased risk of blood transfusion.

Prediction

Several groups have performed retrospective studies in order to delineate risk factors for AKI. Age, emergency surgery, liver disease, increased body mass index, high-risk surgery, peripheral vascular disease and chronic obstructive pulmonary disease are independent pre-operative predictive factors. Perioperative associated factors include hypotension and the use of vasopressors and diuretics. Ischaemic heart disease and heart failure are also associated with AKI. The Revised Cardiac Risk Index may be useful to predict AKI.

Recognition

The physiological consequences of the acute stress response to surgery are associated with a tendency for the body to retain sodium and water in an attempt to conserve body fluid volumes. Conventional renal biochemical assays (urea and creatinine) are relatively insensitive and delayed markers of AKI. Classification systems have been developed to stratify AKI using current physiological and biochemical measurements to allow earlier diagnosis and highlight the importance of small increases in serum creatinine. The most commonly used systems are the RIFLE criteria developed by the Acute Dialysis Quality Initiative group (Table 10.5) and the subsequent Acute Kidney Injury Network (AKIN) criteria (Table 10.6).

Table 10.6 Acute Kidney Injury Network (AKIN) criteria.

Stage	Serum creatinine criteria	Urine output criteria
1	Increase in serum creatinine of more than or equal to 0.3 mg/dl (26.4 μmol/l) or increase to more than or equal to 1.5- to 2-fold from baseline	Less than 0.5 mg/kg/h for more than 6 hours
2	Increase in serum creatinine to more than 2- to 3-fold from baseline	Less than 0.5 mg/kg/h for more than 12 hours
3	Increase in serum creatinine more than or equal to 4.0 mg/dl (354 μmol/l) with an acute increase of at least 0.5 mg/dl (44 μmol/L) or increase in serum creatinine to more than 3-fold from baseline	Less than 0.3 mg/kg/h for 24 hours or anuria for 12 hours

Prevention

Pre-operative

Steps should be taken to identify the patient at risk of renal failure. Once a patient is identified as being at high risk, efforts should be made to prevent or reduce the severity of potential AKI. Firstly, nephrotoxic medications should be stopped and replaced where necessary. These will include aminoglycosides, vancomycin, NSAIDs and ACE inhibitors. Starch-containing colloids should be avoided. Patients who have received contrast media and are at high risk of developing CIN should be given isotonic fluid loading and N-acetyl cysteine should be considered. If the patient has severe renal dysfunction, a period of renal replacement therapy should be considered after contrast administration. Aggressive fluid resuscitation may be required.

Intra-operative

Adequate hydration, arterial pressure and oxygenation should be achieved. Attention should be paid to fluid balance and invasive monitoring, including arterial and central venous pressure, should be considered. Aortic cross-clamp times in cardiac and aortic surgery should be minimized. Patients should not be left in the lithotomy position for a prolonged period. In laparoscopic surgery attention should be paid to the abdominal insufflation pressure and the duration of the procedure. Cardiac output monitoring should be considered in the high-risk patient.

Postoperative

Care should be taken with postoperative fluid regimes and the drug chart should be scrutinized to prevent administration of nephrotoxic drugs until postoperative recovery is complete. High-risk patients should be recovered in a critical care environment.

Treatment

If AKI develops despite these measures, investigations should be conducted to exclude aetiologies that have specific treatments. Urinalysis should be performed, as the presence of haematuria or proteinuria may signify intrinsic renal disease. Causes such as glomerulonephritis can be amenable to specific treatments and therefore a renal biopsy may be appropriate. A renal ultrasound or CT scan should be obtained early, particularly if surgery could have caused renal tract obstruction. A patient with a dilated renal collecting system requires immediate decompression either by the placement of ureteric stents or nephrostomy tubes. A nephrology opinion should be requested and transfer to a critical care setting should be organized.

Steps should be taken to ensure euvolaemia. Careful fluid balance should include any ongoing losses. Accurate input/output charts should be commenced and central venous pressure monitoring instituted. Care should be taken to ensure an adequate mean arterial pressure (MAP), with a MAP of 65 to 70 mmHg being a reasonable target. Higher MAP may be required in the elderly or in the chronic hypertensive. If this MAP is not achieved despite optimal filling, vasopressor or inotropic support may be required. Cardiac output monitoring should be considered. Diuretics have not been shown to aid renal recovery, but may help treat fluid overload. The timing of renal replacement therapies is a subject of much conjecture, with current opinion suggesting earlier and more aggressive haemodialysis or haemofiltration. Commonly agreed indications to commence RRT include hyperkalaemia, volume overload, metabolic acidosis and symptomatic uraemia. Prescribing should include dosing reductions for renally excreted medications.

Endocrine complications

Endocrine disorders may be unmasked by anaesthesia. Pre-existing endocrine disease may be exacerbated by the demands of the perioperative period and the neurohumoral stress response to surgery. Patients with uncontrolled endocrine disorders may also present for surgery.

Diabetes mellitus

The WHO definition of diabetes is for a single raised glucose reading with symptoms; or raised values on two occasions, of either a fasting plasma glucose ≥ 7.0 mmol/l or with a glucose tolerance test, two hours after the oral dose of a plasma glucose ≥ 11.1 mmol/l. Type 1 diabetes results from the failure of the pancreas to produce insulin. Type 2 diabetes results from reduced insulin secretion, insulin receptor resistance and increased glucose availability.

Poorly controlled diabetes results in hyperglycaemia, electrolyte disturbances, hypovolaemia and acid–base disturbances. The neurohumoral response to surgery also contributes to altered glucose metabolism. As part of this response there is an increase in plasma levels of the following hormones: adrenocorticotrophic growth hormone, thyroid stimulating beta-endorphin, prolactin, gonadotropins, arginine vasopressin, cortisol, aldosterone and glucagon. Insulin and thyroxine levels are reduced. Consequently glucose uptake and use by cells is inhibited.

Diabetic patients must be optimized prior to undertaking a surgical procedure with a thorough pre-operative evaluation and particular attention paid to electrolye and fluid status. Perioperative care must include regular evaluations of serum blood glucose. There is increasing evidence that maintaining relative normoglycaemia over the perioperative period reduces subsequent morbidity and mortality. Care must be taken to avoid hypoglycaemia if an insulin infusion is used peri-operatively.

Table 10.7 Symptoms and signs of hyperthyroidism.

Symptoms of hyperthyroidism
Altered mental status (agitation, anxiety, confusion, coma)
Sweating, heat intolerance
Weight loss, fatigue, muscle weakness
GI symptoms (increased appetite, weight loss, diarrhoea)
Prominent dry eyes
Leg swelling
Signs of hyperthyroidism
Sinus tachycardia, tachyarrhythmias
Goitre, thyroid bruit
Warm, moist skin
Muscle tremor
Systolic hypertension
Exophthalmus, lid lag, lid retraction, periorbital swelling, conjunctival injection
Pretibial oedema
Atrial fibrillation

Hyperthyroidism

Patients with undiagnosed or poorly controlled hyperthyroidism are at risk of the life-threatening condition thyroid storm. The signs and symptoms of hyperthyroidism are summarized by Table 10.7.

Thyroid storm is a severe and sudden exacerbation of thyrotoxicosis. How thyroid storm is precipitated is not well understood. However, the precipitating event is usually a stressful event such as surgery, childbirth, infection, myocardial infarction or trauma. Thyroid storm resembles a severe beta-adrenergic overdose. The diagnosis is clinical. Patients are tachycardic, hypertensive, febrile, may have nausea and vomiting, tremulous, agitated and psychotic. Late in the progression of disease, patients may become stuporous or comatose and hypotensive. Management is summarized in Table 10.8 and relies upon general supportive measures, inhibition of thyroid hormone synthesis, inhibition of beta-adrenergic activity and inhibition of peripheral conversion of T4 to T3. Differential diagnoses include malignant hyperthermia, sepsis, phaeochromocytoma, cocaine or amphetamine overdose, or thyrotoxicosis without crisis.

Prevention relies on the recognition of hyperthyroidism. Mortality with thyroid storm is 20%. Survival depends on early recognition and aggressive treatment both of thyroid storm and its precipitant.

Hypothyroidism

Hypothyroidism is the consequence of reduced synthesis and secretion of thyroxine. Myxoedema is rare and usually presents post-operatively. It is a life-threatening complication of hypothyroidism which can, like thyroid storm, be precipitated by a stressful event such as surgery, childbirth or trauma. It resembles a severe hypometabolic state. Symptoms of hypothyroidism include decreased mental acuity, a hoarse voice, somnolence, cold intolerance,

Table 10.8 Management of thyroid storm.

General supportive measures
Intravenous fluids
Paracetamol
Cooling blankets
Magnesium (for cardiac arrhythmias)

Inhibition of thyroid hormone synthesis (administered orally or nasogastrically)
Methimazole (first-line treatment)
Propylthiouracil (reserved for those intolerant of methimazole or in the first trimester of pregnancy)

Iodide therapy (delay for one hour after beginning methimazole or propylthiouracil)

Inhibition of peripheral beta-adrenergic activity
Propranolol, esmolol, atenolol, metoprolol
Titrate to achieve a heart rate of 80 to 90 beats per minute

Inhibition of peripheral conversion of T4 to T3
Beta-blockade
Dexamethasone 2 mg orally or intravenously every 6 hours

dry skin, brittle hair and weight gain. Signs include hypothermia (from a reduced metabolic rate), facial puffiness, periorbital oedema, hypoventilation (due to respiratory centre depression and poor respiratory muscle function), sinus bradycardia, hypotension and when severe, low-output cardiac failure and cardiomyopathy. The diagnosis of myxoedema is clinical. The treatment is levothyroxine and supportive measures. This group of patients have a reduced intravascular volume so care must be taken when treating hypothermia and cardiovascular depression not to vasodilate the patient without adequate fluid resuscitation. Hypothyroidism often occurs with adrenocortical insufficiency and administration of hydrocortisone is advisable until results of evaluation of the patient's hypothalamic–pituitary–adrenal axis are known.

Adrenocortical insufficiency

The hypothalamic–pituitary–adrenal (HPA) axis regulates the amount of cortisol released by the adrenal glands. This axis can be inhibited by either a primary failure of the HPA or secondary to adrenal atrophy due to exogenous glucocorticoid administration (20 mg of prednisolone or equivalent per day for greater than five days). Both scenarios result in adrenal insufficiency (AI). Whatever the cause, adrenal insufficiency can result in life-threatening haemodynamic instability. The incidence of perioperative adrenal insufficiency is 0.01 to 0.7%. Endocrine evaluation is necessary in any patient with suspected adrenal failure. A short synacthen test is used. Management of acute AI is corticosteroid replacement therapy. Dexamethasone does not interfere with the short synacthen test so can be used if AI is suspected. During an adrenal crisis patients can lose up to 20% of their circulating intravascular volume necessitating intravenous fluid replacement. Prevention of an adrenal crisis includes pre-operative identification of individuals at risk and a structured approach to corticosteroid replacement. Both the dose and duration of steroid supplementation will depend on the nature of the surgery and the pre-existing steroid supplementation.

Phaeochromocytoma

Phaeochromocytomas are secretory tumours of the adrenal gland. 10% are bilateral, 10% are extraadrenal and less than 10% are malignant. These tumours can secrete both epinephrine and norepinephrine. They present as hypertensive crises or cardiomyopathy. Headaches, sweating and palpitations are common symptoms. The diagnosis is made by measuring plasma and urinary levels of catecholamines and their metabolites. Elective adrenalectomy with pre-operative alpha- and beta-blockade is the treatment of choice.

Undiagnosed phaeochromocytomas may present peri-operatively as a hypertensive crisis. Most phaeochromocytomas secrete norepinephrine. This renders the patient hypertensive due to chronic alpha-agonism. Therefore management of hypertension requires alpha-adrenergic antagonists (for example phentolamine). The use of beta-blockers are contraindicated unless preceded by alpha-blockade. This is because beta-2 stimulation causes peripheral vasodilatation and may precipitate a hypertensive crisis from unopposed alpha-1 stimulation by tumour catecholamines.

List of further reading

Anderson, J. S., Rose, N. R., Martin, J. L., Eger, E. I. & Njoku, D. B. Desflurane hepatitis associated with hapten and autoantigen-specific IgG4 antibodies. *Anesth Analg* 2007; **104**(6): 1452–3.

Borthwick, E. & Ferguson, A. Perioperative acute kidney injury: risk factors, recognition, management and outcomes. *BMJ* 2010; **341**: 85–91.

Brienza, N., Giglio, M. T., Marucci, M. & Fiore, T. Does peri-operative haemodynamic optimization protect renal function in surgical patients? A meta-analytic study. *Crit Care Med* 2009; **37**(6): 2079–90.

Kagan, A. & Sheikh-Hamad, D. Contrast-induced kidney injury: focus on modifiable risk factors and prophylactic strategies. *Clin Cardiol* 2009; **33**: 62–6.

Kharasch, E. D., Frink, E. J., Artru, A. *et al.* Long-duration low-flow sevoflurane and isoflurane effects on postoperative renal and hepatic function. *Anesth Analg* 2001; **93**: 1511–20.

Kheterpal, S., Tremper, K. K., Englesne, M. J. *et al.* Predictors of postoperative acute renal failure after noncardiac surgery in patients with previously normal renal function. *Anesthesiology* 2007; **107**(6): 892–902.

Kohl, B. A. & Schwartz, S. How to manage perioperative endocrine insufficiency. *Anaesthesiol Clin* 2010; **28**(1): 139–55.

Muilenburg, D. J., Singh, A., Torzilli, G. & Khatri, V. P. Surgery in the patient with liver disease. *Anesthesiol Clin* 2009; **27**: 721–37.

Neuberger, J. M. Halothane and hepatitis: incidence, predisposing factors and exposure guidelines. *Drug Saf* 1990; **5**: 28–38.

Pannu, N. & Nadim, M. K. An overview of drug-induced acute kidney injury. *Crit Care Med* 2008; **36**(4): S216–22.

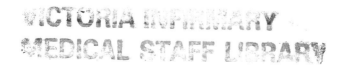

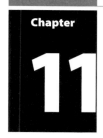

Injury during anaesthesia

David Bogod and Kasia Szypula

Introduction

Injury during the perioperative period refers to inadvertent damage of organs and systems as a result of surgical or anaesthetic intervention. Injury during anaesthesia is an uncommon perioperative complication despite the increasing complexity of surgical practices and techniques, as well as operating on higher risk patients in more advanced age, and with increasingly complex co-morbidities. Many of the injuries occurring are surgery related but these are often intended as a part of surgery. Unfortunately there is a still a wide array of unintentional injuries associated with surgical treatment occurring in the modern practice. In this chapter we will discuss the management of the commonest injuries related to anaesthesia, positioning and invasive procedures.

Dental injury

Dental damage is a frequently reported injury associated with general anaesthesia, with an incidence of 1%. Of these, only 2% require intervention. The severity of the injury ranges from scratching or chipping of teeth to loosening, fractures and avulsions. Dental trauma accounts for between 20 and 50% of litigation claims related to general anaesthesia, but these are generally not expensive to settle. It has to be mentioned that some of the dental injuries are in fact associated with surgical interventions (rigid bronchoscopy or pharyngoscopy).

The maxillary central incisors are most at risk, and the incidence is the highest in patients aged 50 to 70 years. Dental damage is more likely in patients with a difficult airway, periodontal disease, dental prostheses or those undergoing emergency laryngoscopy and intubation. Dental damage is usually sustained during laryngoscopy, but can also be caused by the patient biting down hard on a tracheal tube or other airway device, usually at the time of extubation.

Methods of minimizing dental trauma include patient education and encouraging a visit to the dentist for pre-operative optimization, which may involve restoration work or fitting a protective device. Mouth guards, such as those used during rigid bronchoscopy, may shield the teeth and prevent injury. However, their presence may increase the difficulty of laryngoscopy and cause a paradoxical increase in the risk of dental damage. Anaesthetists can minimize trauma by avoiding pivoting laryngoscope blades on the top incisors. The use of oropharyngeal airways as bite blocks for laryngeal mask airways is controversial.

Anaesthetic and Perioperative Complications, ed. Kamen Valchanov, Stephen T. Webb and Jane Sturgess. Published by Cambridge University Press. © Cambridge University Press 2011.

Patients should be warned about the possibility of dental trauma. Pre-operative assessment and detailed documentation of dentition are essential. Careful inspection of dentition following difficult laryngoscopy is advised.

If a tooth is accidentally removed, it should be reimplanted into its socket and a dental surgeon consulted at the earliest opportunity. In all cases the cause, mechanism and the extent of damage should be clearly documented in the hospital notes. Appropriate locally agreed referral systems should be used. If something has gone wrong and the patient's teeth are damaged, the possibility of legal action should not preclude an apology and explanation of how the damage occurred.

Injury resulting from airway management

Airway injuries are common, and occur in 6 to 20% of anaesthetics. These injuries include trauma to nose, lips and oral mucous membranes and the pharynx, and injury to vocal cords and the tracheobronchial tree. Although airway injuries account for a large proportion of litigation claims in anaesthesia, the severity of injuries and the costs are proportionally small. Pharyngeal injuries include perforation, lacerations, contusions, infection and sore throat. The most common types of laryngeal injuries are vocal cord paralysis, granuloma, arytenoid dislocation and haematoma. Tracheal injuries include perforation, ischaemia and infection. The incidence of sore throat following tracheal intubation is 45%, after laryngeal mask insertion 18% and with facemask anaesthetics 3%.

Airway injuries are usually caused by airway device insertion or removal or by excessive force applied during airway instrumentation. Pharyngeal mucosa can be dissected during nasal intubation. Dissections of the tracheal or bronchial wall through forceful intubation, penetration or perforation with a stylet and rupture from over-inflation of the cuff have all been reported. The incidence of cuff-related ischaemic injuries to the airway mucosa has declined since the move from low-volume, high-pressure cuffs to high-volume, low-pressure ones.

Facemask application, laryngoscopy and laryngeal mask insertion should be done with due attention to vulnerable soft tissues. Tracheal tubes should be appropriately sized and cuffs should not be over-inflated. In patients where tracheal intubation has been traumatic, it is important to watch for signs of pharyngeal dissection, tracheal dissection and rupture.

Most superficial injuries heal spontaneously, but may be distressing to patients. Sore throat is generally self-limiting and can be treated with non-prescription local anaesthetic lozenges. Patients with persistent sore throat or hoarse voice should be referred to ENT for a nasendoscopy. Serious tracheobronchial injuries should be immediately discussed with a thoracic surgeon.

Oesophageal injury

Oesophageal perforation is a serious life-threatening injury that may complicate tracheal or inadvertent oesophageal intubation. Numerous case reports have been published, but the exact incidence remains uncertain.

While oesophageal perforation as a complication of anaesthesia is usually associated with tracheal intubation, it has also been described in the literature as a complication of orogastric or nasogastric tube insertion, use of a Combitube™ or transoesophageal echocardiography. Risk factors include intrinsic pathological changes of the oesophagus or abnormal anatomy, emergency or difficult intubation and anaesthetic inexperience. The most common sites for cervical oesophageal injuries resulting from traumatic or difficult tracheal intubation are the piriform sinus and the posterior oesophageal wall at the tip of the tracheal tube. The ana-tomical vulnerability to injury arises from the absence of a reinforcing longitudinal muscle layer in these areas. Furthermore, the use of cricoid pressure and hyperextension of the neck compresses the cervical oesophagus against the bodies of the sixth and seventh cervical ver-tebrae, which increases the risk of injury.

The recent increase in the use of transoesophageal echocardiography (TOE) during sur-gery and in intensive care has unfortunately also added to the increase of oesophageal injur-ies. The estimated incidence of serious oesophageal injury following TOE is 0.2% based on case series of gastro-oesophagoscopy for pathology of the gastrointestinal tract. Although the use of TOE is now recommended in all cases of cardiac surgery, judicious use should be considered. High-risk category patients include the elderly, patients with small body size, difficulty in swallowing, oesophageal varices and previous oesophageal and gastric surgery. However, there are times when the benefit from TOE exceeds the risk of oesophageal injury (Type A aortic dissection, haemodynamic instability, peri-arrest situations) and then the investigation should be undertaken with caution.

Whenever there is a traumatic intubation with or without inadvertent oesophageal intubation, the possibility of oesophageal injury should be considered. Early diagnosis of this complication, although sometimes difficult, is vital to successful treatment and requires a high index of suspicion because the symptoms are often non-specific and may be delayed. It should be suspected in a patient with cervical subcutaneous emphysema, pneumothorax, cyanosis, fever, dysphagia, throat pain and a history of difficult intubation. Definitive diag-nosis of an oesophageal tear is made either by endoscopy or radiographic techniques using water-soluble contrast media. Delay in diagnosis results in high mortality from mediastinitis and its complications.

Management of the injury includes conservative (antibiotics, total parenteral nutrition and nasogastric suction) and surgical management (primary repair, drainage, oesophageal exclusion and oesophagectomy). The choice of treatment depends on the location, extent of the injury, the time interval between the incident and the diagnosis, the presence of oesopha-geal pathology, presence of sepsis and the patient's medical condition. Mortality is high, and for full-depth oesophageal tear, exceeds 50%.

Peripheral nerve injury unrelated to regional anaesthesia

Peripheral nerve injury is reported in approximately 0.4% of general and 0.1% of regional anaesthetics. However, it is possible that the true incidence is higher due to under-report-ing. Many cases of peripheral nerve damage have no identifiable aetiology. During general anaesthesia, the commonest causes are mechanical, such as stretch and compression, and ischaemic, usually related to poor patient positioning. The ulnar and common peroneal nerves are the most susceptible because they lie in a very superficial position close to bony prominences. The brachial plexus can be injured if the arm is placed in any extreme pos-ition, but most commonly if externally rotated and abducted. Damage to the radial nerve usually occurs as a result of compression. The sciatic nerve is at risk in slim patients on a hard operating table, or from stretching in the lithotomy position. Nerves less commonly injured include the tibial, femoral, obturator, saphenous, pudendal, facial and supraorbital (Table 11.1).

Awareness of the sites vulnerable to compression and stretch, and meticulous patient positioning and padding, are key to prevention of nerve injuries during general anaesthesia.

Table 11.1 Common peripheral nerve injuries unrelated to regional anaesthesia.

Nerve	Common aetiologies
Brachial plexus	Excessive stretching, particularly induced by arm abduction, external rotation and posterior shoulder displacement.
	Compression, in the lateral decubitus position, with the cord compressed against the thorax by the humeral head.
Ulnar nerve	Compression at the medial epicondyle of the humerus.
	Stretch during extreme flexion of the elbow across the chest.
Radial nerve	Compression between the operating table edge and the humerus, or in the lateral position with the uppermost arm abducted beyond 90° and suspended from a vertical support.
Sciatic nerve	Compression, especially in thin patients on a hard table and when the opposite buttock is elevated.
	Stretch in the lithotomy position with maximal external rotation of the flexed thigh.
Common peroneal	Compression against the head of the fibula in the lithotomy position or between the fibula and the operating table in the lateral position.

Particular attention should be paid to operating table extensions, arm boards and leg stirrups. Padding at the elbows and the fibular head may reduce the risk of upper and lower extremity neuropathies respectively. Extreme flexion and extension as well as pronation and supination joint positions should be avoided. Arm abduction should be limited to 90 degrees for short periods in supine patients, or 70 degrees if prolonged abduction is anticipated. Prone patients may tolerate arm abduction greater than 90 degrees. Thorough history taking, examination and documentation of any pre-existing nerve lesions are essential.

Symptoms usually occur within a few days but may occasionally not present for two to three weeks. The spectrum and severity of symptoms varies and includes painless or painful paraesthesiae, sensory or motor loss. All patients with suspected nerve injury should be referred to a neurologist for assessment. Electromyography, nerve conduction studies and MRI can aid the diagnosis.

Most perioperative nerve injuries recover within a few months of surgery. However, treatment and prognosis depend on the nature and severity of the lesion and patients should be advised on these by a specialist.

Visual loss

Perioperative eye injuries and blindness are rare but important complications of anaesthesia, and vary in severity from transient diplopia or blurring of vision to irreversible blindness. The incidence of ocular injuries during anaesthesia is 1:1,000 (0.1%) and of blindness is 1:125,000 (0.0008%). Although constituting a small proportion of legal claims, eye injuries are associated with significantly greater monetary settlements than claims for non-ocular injuries. The most frequent ocular complication of general anaesthesia is corneal abrasion. The three causes of postoperative blindness are ischaemic optic neuropathy, central retinal artery thrombosis and cortical blindness.

General anaesthesia reduces tear formation and stability, increases the frequency of lagophthalmos (failure of the eyelids to close fully), abolishes the blink reflex and inhibits

Bell's phenomenon (eyeball turns upwards during sleep, protecting the cornea). Corneal abrasions are usually the result of the lagophthalmos and the cornea drying during anaesthesia, or trauma from the anaesthetic facemask, laryngoscope or surgical drapes. There is an increased risk of injury in patients undergoing tracheal intubation, as compared with mask ventilation. Other associated factors include duration of surgery of more than 90 minutes, prone positioning and head and neck surgery. Chemical injury can occur through contact with antiseptic skin preparation.

Blindness is usually caused by ischaemic optic neuropathy, which involves damage to the posterior segment of the eye (retina or optic nerve) or may be related to damage to the visual cortex. Mechanisms possibly responsible for these injuries include compression, hypotension, hypoxia, embolism and anaemia. Patients at higher risk of ischaemic optic neuropathy include those with diabetes, hypertension, smoking and polycythaemia. Retinal detachment has been reported with extreme Trendelenburg and prone positioning.

Meticulous eye care during anaesthesia is vital. Strategies recommended for the perioperative protection of the eye include simple manual closure of the eyelids, taping the eyelids closed, instillation of paraffin-based ointments into the conjunctival sac, instillation of aqueous solution or viscous gels into the eye and the use of hydrophilic contact lenses. All patients should have their eyes taped closed immediately after induction of anaesthesia. Patients undergoing anaesthesia in the prone position should have their eyes taped closed and the head maintained in the neutral position avoiding pressure on their eyes. Providone-iodine 10% aqueous solution should be used if skin preparation on the face is required, as it is non-toxic to the cornea. Mechanical pressure to the eyes should be avoided and adequate mean arterial pressure maintained. Horseshoe headrests should not be used for prone patients as they have been implicated in nearly all cases of pressure damage in the prone position.

Presence of corneal abrasion is suggested by clinical symptoms including excessive tear production, miosis, photophobia, foreign body sensation in the eye and pain. Ischaemic optic neuropathy should be suspected in any patient with sudden loss of vision, visual field defect or reduced visual acuity.

All patients complaining of postoperative visual disturbance should be promptly reviewed by an ophthalmologist. Treatment of corneal abrasions is aimed at reducing pain and preventing conjunctivitis. Vision rarely returns after ischaemic optic neuropathy. However, treatment may improve the visual field defect caused by central retinal artery occlusion.

Acoustic loss

Perioperative hearing loss is a rarely reported phenomenon. It is often subclinical and may go unnoticed unless audiometry is performed. Following spinal anaesthesia 10 to 50% of patients experience an audiometrically measurable hearing loss, although only 25% of these are symptomatic. The precise incidence of hearing loss after general anaesthesia is estimated at 0.01%. It is more frequently associated with surgery in which cardiopulmonary bypass is used than other types of surgery, with an incidence of permanent hearing impairment estimated to be 0.1%.

Perioperative hearing impairment can be conductive or sensorineural, unilateral or bilateral, transient or permanent in nature. It has been reported following many different anaesthetic techniques including neuraxial blocks, general anaesthesia and interscalene nerve blocks. Aetiology often cannot be ascertained but possible causes include mechanical, trauma, noise-induced, changes in CSF pressure, nitrous oxide, embolism and ototoxic drugs. In cardiopulmonary bypass surgery it is thought to be predominantly embolic in origin. In general anaesthesia for non-cardiopulmonary bypass surgery it is most likely to be due to excessive or sudden changes in the middle ear pressure, administration of nitrous oxide causing oscillation in the middle ear which can lead to tympanic perforation, vascular pathology and ischaemic damage to hair cells, and excessive noise from surgical power equipment. After spinal anaesthesia the hearing loss correlates with the design of the spinal needle tip and the needle size, and age – the same factors that are implicated in post-dural puncture headache.

In patients undergoing general anaesthesia care should be taken to avoid excessive or prolonged pressure on the external ear, and spillage of cleaning solutions into the ear canal. Potential foreign bodies such as syringe caps should not be kept on the pillow. When administering ototoxic drugs such as diuretics, anti-inflammatory agents and aminoglycoside antibiotics, attention should be paid to the appropriate dose and the speed of administration. When performing neuraxial blocks and lumbar punctures, a small-gauge pencil-point needle should be used.

Specific presentation and onset of hearing impairment can vary, especially following neuraxial blockade. Patients presenting with clinical hearing impairment complain of unilateral or bilateral hearing loss or reduction in acoustic acuity. Subclinical hearing impairment following anaesthesia may occur more frequently than appreciated.

When hearing impairment is noticed a history of previous hearing problems, recent upper respiratory tract infections, type of anaesthetic and use of ototoxic drugs should be documented by the anaesthetist and an external examination performed looking for evidence of trauma, foreign body, erythema or oedema. Weber and Rinnie's tests can be performed at the bedside. ENT consultation and audiometric testing may help further management. If a specific aetiology can be found, treatment can be effective in certain cases. Prognosis for hearing impairment after cardiopulmonary bypass is poor, whereas for non-cardiopulmonary bypass surgery it is relatively good, with at least 50% of patients achieving partial recovery or better. Most patients with hearing impairment after spinal anaesthesia recover without intervention, although some respond well to epidural blood patch.

Pressure injury

Pressurized pneumatic cuffs can be used to prevent the central spread of local anaesthetic during intravenous regional anaesthesia or to reduce bleeding and improve the surgical field when operating on an exsanguinated limb.

The incidence of complications is related to the inflation pressure and the duration of inflation, with limb ischaemia being the most serious. Excessive pressure can also damage underlying vessels, increasing the incidence of microemboli formation in the exsanguinated limb. This increases the risk of pulmonary microvascular injury.

The cuff should be wider than half the limb diameter and should be applied over smooth padding. The edges of the cuff must overlap to ensure it exerts even pressure all around the limb. When applied to the leg, the tourniquet is usually inflated to a pressure 100 mmHg above systolic arterial blood pressure. On the arm, 50 mmHg above systolic blood pressure is used. Tourniquet time should not exceed two hours with a reperfusion time of at least 20 minutes.

Cutaneous injury

Cutaneous injuries are a common but usually minor complication of anaesthesia. The vast majority of cutaneous injuries result from pressure-induced reduced skin perfusion resulting in ischaemia and tissue necrosis. Patients at particular risk of pressure ischaemia are those with advanced age, poor nutritional state, chronic illness, immobility and incontinence. Another common cause is irritant dermatitis caused by adhesive dressings, tape and ECG electrodes, and other topical materials. Tissued intravenous drug infusions may result in damage to skin. Skin necrosis may occur if irritant drugs intended for deep intramuscular injection are delivered instead into the subcutaneous tissues. Anaesthetized patients are also susceptible to burns from faulty diathermy or patient warming devices. Postoperative alopecia is rare but can be very disfiguring, and is caused by pressure-induced ischaemia. Risk factors include prolonged period of unconsciousness, hypotension, massive blood loss and the use of vasoconstrictor agents.

Careful patient positioning, meticulous pressure-point care and continuous vigilance during the intra-operative period are key to prevention of cutaneous injuries. Any previous adverse reactions to commonly used adhesive dressings and disinfectants should be noted at the pre-operative visit, and these should be avoided. The risk of alopecia can be reduced by occasional intra-operative head repositioning.

Cutaneous injuries are usually recognized at the end of surgery. In pressure injuries, persistent redness is usually the first sign of prolonged poor perfusion. In irritant dermatitis, erythema or a macular rash may be present upon removal of adhesive dressings and electrodes. Patients with alopecia initially present with occipito-parietal pain and tenderness within 24 hours, followed by oedema, crusting and ulceration. Hair loss occurs within 3 to 28 days of surgery.

Any cutaneous injuries or suspected injuries should be noted and closely observed. Referral to a tissue viability team or to dermatology should be considered in patients with more severe or persistent injuries. Most injuries are self-limiting. In alopecia, hair regrowth is usually within 12 weeks.

Muscular injury

Compartment syndrome is a potentially devastating perioperative complication, with an incidence of 2.3 per 100,000. A higher proportion of cases have been reported in patients in the lithotomy or lateral decubitus position than in the supine position. If undiagnosed, or diagnosed late, it can result in rhabdomyolysis, renal failure, irreversible neurological deficit, loss of limb or even death.

Compartment syndrome in the perioperative setting usually occurs from increased compartment pressure resulting from poor positioning for prolonged periods or from reduced limb perfusion from elevation of the limb above the level of the heart. Excessive joint flexion can also cause vessel occlusion and reduced perfusion. Other causes include hypotension (related to anaesthetic agents, inadequate fluid administration or sympathetic block), peripheral vascular disease and surgical retraction on major vessels.

The risk of compartment syndrome can be reduced by appropriate positioning and padding of pressure areas, and occasional repositioning during long surgical procedures. Blood pressure should be maintained within the normal range for the patient. However, the use of vasoconstrictor drugs may further reduce compartment blood flow.

The main presenting symptom of compartment syndrome is pain. Although there have been suggestions that the use of PCA opioids or regional analgesia can delay the diagnosis of compartment syndrome, there is no evidence to support this. There is an average delay of 15 hours to diagnosis and surgical treatment. A high index of clinical suspicion, regular review of the patient and measurement of compartment pressures are essential in aiding early diagnosis.

The treatment of compartment syndrome is decompression by fasciotomy. Early aggressive fluid replacement guided by CVP monitoring is recommended. Urinary pH should be monitored and maintained as near normal as possible to prevent precipitation of myoglobin and urate. The quality of functional result is directly related to the interval between injury and decompression. The frequency and severity of complications, including neuromuscular damage and renal failure due to myoglobinuria, are inversely proportional to the promptness of decompression.

Skeletal injury

Fractured ribs and other injuries can result from patients being dropped or falling from the operating table onto the floor. Joint dislocations can occur as a result of extreme non-anatomical limb positioning, particularly in patients with underlying joint dysfunction or replacement. The cervical spine can be damaged by excessive hyperextension of the neck during laryngoscopy or other airway manoeuvres. Temporo-mandibular joint (TMJ) dysfunction is a recognized complication associated with airway instrumentation. Interestingly, many patients developing this complication have a past history of TMJ dysfunction or subluxation.

Vascular injury

Injuries associated with arterial cannulation include ischaemia, vasospasm, pseudo-aneurysm, arterio-venous fistula formation, haematoma, thrombosis, embolism and infection. There is a high incidence of early occlusion of the radial artery post cannulation (20%). Recannulation of the occluded artery usually occurs, but may take several weeks. Permanent ischaemic damage is rare. Less than 1% of arterial line complications are clinically significant.

Factors associated with an increased risk for arterial line-associated ischaemia include long and wide-bore catheters, presence of shock, use of vasoconstrictor drugs, female gender, hyperliporoteinaema and peripheral vascular disease. Multiple attempts and haematoma formation are predictive of an adverse outcome. Cannulation should be as atraumatic as possible, minimizing the number of arterial punctures and avoiding haematoma formation. A short 20-gauge Teflon cannula should be used. Decannulation should occur as early as possible. The level of experience of the operator reduces the risk of complications.

The patient's limb should be examined on a regular basis for signs of decreased hand perfusion. If ischaemia is suspected, the cannula should be removed. For patients with persisting symptoms brachial plexus or stellate ganglion block, as well as surgical exploration, could be considered.

The incidence of accidental arterial puncture with CVC insertion varies from 0.9 to 19%. Haematoma is reported to occur in up to 4.4% and haemothorax in 0.6%. Overall, internal jugular catheterization and subclavian venous catheterization carry similar risks of mechanical complications. Subclavian cannulation is associated with the highest incidence of pneumothorax and haemothorax. Internal jugular cannulation is more likely to be complicated by arterial puncture. Haematoma and arterial puncture are common during femoral venous catheterization. The risk of vascular complications is higher in catheters inserted in the upper limb compared with femoral. Less common vascular complications include false aneurysms and arterio-venous fistulas. The use of ultrasound has been shown to reduce the number of mechanical complications for central venous catheters compared with the anatomical landmark techniques. This has been reflected also in the NICE guidance in 2002 for routine use of ultrasound imaging during central venous cannulation.

Blood exposure incidents (non-patient injury)

Needlestick injury is relatively common amongst healthcare workers, including anaesthetists, who regularly perform invasive procedures. The true incidence of inoculation injuries in the UK is unknown, but is thought to be in excess of one million per annum. The blood-borne viruses (BBVs) that present most cross-infection hazard include HIV and several hepatitis viruses. Occupational exposures include percutaneous exposures, human scratch or bite and mucocutaneous exposures, where the mucous membranes (mouth, nose or eyes) or non-intact skin have been contaminated. A significant exposure is a percutaneous or mucocutaneous exposure to blood or other body fluids from a source that is known to be, or as a result of the incident found to be, HBV surface antigen (HBsAg), HCV or HIV positive (Table 11.2).

Mucocutaneous exposures carry a lower risk of BBV infection, estimated at 1 in 1,000 for HIV. There is currently no information on the risk of transmission for HBV and HCV following mucocutaneous exposure.

Factors that may increase the risk, and influence management, of the incident are:

- percutaneous injury rather than mucous membrane or broken-skin exposure
- injury with a device from a source patient's artery or vein
- blood exposure rather than exposure to blood-stained fluid, diluted blood or other body fluid
- injury from hollow-bore rather than solid-bore needle
- deep rather than superficial injury
- visible blood on the device
- no protective equipment used (e.g. gloves, double gloves, eye protection)
- first aid measures not implemented (e.g. washing, bleeding)
- HCV RNA detectable in source patient on most recent blood test
- high viral load of HIV in source patient
- HBeAg detectable in source patient blood
- exposed person not or inadequately immunized against hepatitis B
- source patient co-infected with more than one BBV.

Many inoculation injuries result from a failure to follow recommended procedures, and from careless disposal of waste. Every effort should be made to avoid blood and body fluid exposures occurring, through safe systems of work. All exposure incidents should be reviewed to consider how recurrence might be prevented. Measures to avoid exposure to blood-borne viruses should include: immunization against hepatitis B, the wearing of gloves

Table 11.2 Incidence and seroconversion rates for blood-borne viruses.

	UK population prevalence	Prevalence in UK IVDUs	Average seroconversion risk after percutaneous exposure to known infected source
HIV	0.08%	London 3% Elsewhere 0.5%	0.3%
HCV	0.4–0.5%	41%	0.5–1.8% (if detectable RNA)
HBV	0.5% HBsAg carriers	22%	30% (non-immune individual exposed to HBeAg positive source)

and other protective clothing, the safe handling and disposal of sharps, including the provision of medical devices incorporating sharps protection, and measures to reduce risks during surgical procedures. Cuts and grazes should be covered with waterproof dressings. Trusts should include personal protection training for all staff at induction.

When a blood exposure incident occurs, if the mouth or eyes are involved, they should be washed thoroughly with water. If skin is punctured, free bleeding should be gently encouraged and the wound should be washed with soap or chlorhexidine and water, but not scrubbed or sucked. If there is any possibility of HIV exposure, urgent advice should be sought about the relative indications for anti-retroviral post-exposure prophylaxis (PEP). Where indicated, HIV prophylaxis (PEP) should be initiated as soon as possible after the exposure, ideally within an hour following a careful risk assessment. Post-exposure prophylaxis is now generally not recommended if 72 hours has elapsed. Recommended follow-up period after occupational exposure to HIV, as a minimum, is now for at least 12 weeks after the incident, or if PEP was taken, for at least 12 weeks from when PEP was stopped.

List of further reading

Aitkenhead, A. R. Injuries associated with anaesthesia. A global perspective. *Br J Anaesth* 2005, **95**(1): 95–109.

Chopra, V., Bovill, J. G. & Spierdijk, J. Accidents, near accidents and complications during anaesthesia. A retrospective analysis of a 10-year period in a teaching hospital. *Anaesthesia* 1990; **45**: 3–6.

Contractor, S. & Hardman, J. G. Injury during anaesthesia. *Cont Educ Anaesth Crit Care Pain* 2006; **6**(2): 67–70.

Cook, T. M., Scott, S. & Mihai, R. Litigation related to airway and respiratory complications of anaesthesia: an analysis of claims against the NHS in England 1995–2007. *Anaesthesia* 2010; **65**: 556–63.

Domino, K. B., Posner, K. L., Caplan, R. A. & Cheney, F. A. Airway injury during anesthesia: a closed claims analysis. *Anesthesiology* 1999; **91**: 1703–11.

Health and Safety Executive. Blood-borne viruses in the workplace. Guidance for employers and employees. www.hse.gov.uk/pubns/indg342.pdf (accessed 15 April 2010).

Roth, S., Thisted, R. A., Erickson, J. P., Black, S. & Schreider, B. D. Eye injuries after nonocular surgery: a study of 60,965 anesthetics from 1988 to 1992. *Anesthesiology* 1996; **85**(5): 1020–7.

Sawyer, R. J., Richmond, M. N., Hickey, J. D. & Jarratt, J. A. Peripheral nerve injuries associated with anaesthesia. *Anaesthesia* 2000; **55**: 980–91.

Sprung, J., Bourke, D. L., Contreras, M. G., Warner, M. E. & Findlay, J. Peri-operative hearing impairment. *Anesthesiology* 2003; **98**: 241–57.

UK Health Departments. Guidance for clinical health care workers: protection against infection with blood-borne viruses. www.dh.gov.uk/prod_consum_dh/groups/dh_digitalassets/@dh/@en/documents/digitalasset/dh_4014474.pdf (accessed 15 April 2011).

Warner, M. E., LaMaster, L. M., Thoeming, A. K. *et al.* Compartment syndrome in surgical patients. *Anesthesiology* 2001; **94**(4): 705–8.

White, E. & Crosse, M. The aetiology and prevention of peri-operative corneal abrasions. *Anaesthesia* 1998; **53**: 157–61.

Chapter

12

Regional anaesthesia complications

Tim M. Cook and Mike Coupe

Generic complications

There is evidence that regional anaesthesia (RA), when performed well, can improve the patient experience and in some circumstances outcome. It can reduce the overall cost of an operative procedure and may improve theatre efficiency. However, there are a number of complications associated with RA that require thorough understanding by any anaesthetist aspiring to be competent in the field.

Major complications of RA are relatively infrequent and range from temporary and minor to devastating and permanent. Knowledge of the incidence and causative factors of RA complications is vital if they are to be avoided and is central to sensible patient selection and the process of consent. Such complications are particularly important to anaesthetists and their patients for several reasons. Firstly, they can be considered 'active complications' because there is usually a choice as to whether RA is performed or omitted: thus RA complication only follows after the active choice to use RA. Secondly, they may be clearly identified as 'anaesthetic' rather than perioperative or surgical. Thirdly, they lead to a disproportionately high rate of litigation.

Frequency and severity of complications of regional anaesthesia

Minor complications (pain on injection, minor bruising, brief neuropraxia) may occur in up to 5% of cases. The incidence of major complications of RA is unknown. The best estimate of the incidence of permanent harm following central neuraxial blockade (CNB) comes from the *Third National Audit Project of the Royal College of Anaesthetists* (NAP3), which will be discussed in detail later. This project led to an estimate of permanent harm following CNB of 4.2 in 100,000, if judged pessimistically, or 2.0 per 100,000, if judged more optimistically. Estimates of permanent harm after peripheral neuraxial blockade (PNB) at 1.87 per 10,000 to 4 per 10,000 are approximately ten-fold lower. These estimates hide a spectrum of risk depending on the specific form of block performed and the clinical context. For example epidural catheter placement in an elderly perioperative patient has perhaps a 100-fold higher risk of harm than obstetric spinal anaesthesia.

Litigation after regional anaesthesia

Several recent studies suggest that in the UK over 1 million episodes of RA take place every year including 700,000 episodes of CNB. These represent approximately 20 to 25% of all

Anaesthetic and Perioperative Complications, ed. Kamen Valchanov, Stephen T. Webb and Jane Sturgess.
Published by Cambridge University Press. © Cambridge University Press 2011.

anaesthetic interventions. In contrast, litigation related to RA accounts for 44% of all litigation against anaesthetists. Litigation after RA can be summarized as follows:

- Injuries are generally of a lower severity than in non-RA claims (RA <20% of claims based on permanent harm; non-RA 38%).
- Central neuraxial blockade accounts for >80% of all RA claims, with epidurals prominent (epidural 72% of RA claims; spinal 15%; combined spinal anaesthesia, CSE, 2%).
- Peripheral neuraxial blockade is an infrequent cause of litigation accounting for as little as 15% of RA claims (20% of these follow ophthalmic RA).
- Approximately half of claims are obstetric with the severity of injuries leading to obstetric RA claims being less severe on average than non-obstetric RA claims.
- The 'presenting complaint' for RA claims include (in order of frequency) nerve damage, pain from inadequate blockade, back pain, secondary injury to an insensate area of the body following RA, accidental dural puncture, infection, drug error, ophthalmic globe perforation and epidural haematoma. Nerve damage and pain from inadequate block are the presenting complaint for almost half of RA claims.
- Comparing obstetric to non-obstetric RA claims the presenting complaint is more commonly inadequate block leading to pain (31% vs. 4%) and less commonly nerve injury (21% vs. 37%).
- The cost of litigation following RA is about one-third of the cost of all litigation against anaesthetists and comprises a few very costly cases and a much larger number with small or no cost.

Peripheral nerve injury

Mechanisms

Nerve injury may be classified by the degree of anatomical disruption and, by extension, the likely clinical course and potential for recovery:

- **Neurotmesis** – all essential structures of a nerve are severed, spontaneous recovery is highly unlikely.
- **Axonotmesis** – the conducting fibres are severely damaged and complete peripheral degeneration follows. In contrast to neurotmesis, the epineurium and supporting structures are preserved, and there is good potential for spontaneous recovery as regenerating conducting fibres are guided by the intact architectural structure.
- **Neurapraxia** – interruption of nerve function in the absence of peripheral degeneration, loss of function may be prolonged but recovery is complete.

Pathophysiology

Applying local anaesthetic to a nerve can cause damage in a number of ways. Although the relative contribution of each of these in the genesis of a peripheral nerve injury is rarely clear, understanding the mechanisms may aid avoidance.

Direct cytotoxicity

Local anaesthetics have several cytotoxic effects, generally proportional to their concentration and the duration of exposure. Solutions with concentrations in the clinical range are

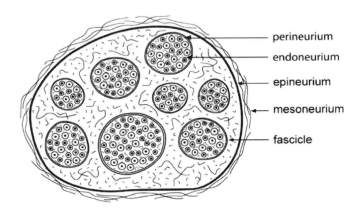

Figure 12.1 Nerve structure (copyright Paul Bigeleisen, reproduced with permission).

perineurium
endoneurium
epineurium
mesoneurium
fascicle

cytotoxic in vitro. In vivo studies show that deposition within the nerve fascicles increases toxicity, bypassing the normal regulatory function of the perineurium and blood vessel endothelium, both of which act to protect delicate neural tissue (Figure 12.1).

Mechanical damage

Prior to the advent of ultrasound imaging, it was commonly assumed that puncture of the epineurium and entry of a needle into a peripheral nerve would be likely to cause neural damage. However, it is clear that nerve penetration and even intraneural injection of local anaesthetic solution does occur during PNB, but does not commonly result in neuropathy. This clinical finding is mirrored in animal models, where injection of local anaesthetic beneath the epineurium but outside the perineurium, the tougher membrane that surrounds the fascicles, results in histological changes associated with inflammation, including lymphocytic infiltration and the granulation tissue formation, but not functional loss. Perineural puncture seems to be more important in generating a significant nerve injury than puncture of the epineurium alone, and is related to:

- location along the nerve (more common proximally, where the proportion of loose connective tissue to neural tissue is lower)
- type of needle used (more common with sharp-rather than blunt-tipped needles).

Once the perineurium is punctured, injection of fluid increases the chance of a nerve injury.

Ischaemia

Inadequate blood flow to a nerve is, perhaps, the final common pathway for the generation of a nerve injury. Local anaesthetics directly reduce nerve blood flow, by affecting endothelial processes regulating vascular tone. This effect is not linearly related to dose: for example, application of bupivacaine at higher doses increases blood flow. The production of high intraneural pressure is likely to reduce blood flow to the nerve, and may be more common with injections within the perineurium, where the compliance of the compartment is lower, than injections within the epineurium only.

Local anaesthetic toxicity

One of the most feared complications of RA is local anaesthetic systemic toxicity (LAST) due to injection into a blood vessel or excessive systemic absorption of local anaesthetic.

The most serious cases of LAST generally involve the long-acting local anaesthetic, bupivacaine. Most cases of LAST present within five minutes of local anaesthetic injection, with 25% of cases being delayed, sometimes for up to an hour after injection. Around 90% of episodes of LAST result in central nervous system (CNS) toxicity, approximately half of which are accompanied by cardiovascular (CVS) toxicity. Approximately 10% of patients present with CVS toxicity alone. Due to direct cardiac effects, bupivacaine and related drugs are more likely to present with CVS toxicity, even without preceding CNS toxicity.

Clinical features

Central nervous system toxicity

High levels of local anaesthetic in the brain are thought to selectively block inhibitory pathways in the cerebral cortex, probably by blocking voltage-gated sodium channels. The removal of cortical inhibition of subcortical excitatory pathways leads to an excitatory state and the clinical picture of CNS toxicity: agitation, loss of consciousness and seizure. Patients may report or display prodromal features including dysarthria, perioral numbness or tingling, reduction in conscious level or confusion. Report of these symptoms should result in cessation of local anaesthetic injection, and consideration of the possibility that significant CNS or CVS toxicity may develop.

Cardiovascular toxicity

CVS toxicity can lead to rapid cardiovascular collapse and death. The mechanisms involved have not been elucidated fully, but are likely to involve the action of local anaesthetics on several cardiac voltage-gated and ligand-gated channels, resulting in profound electrophysiological disturbance and negative inotropy. Until recently, significant CVS toxicity carried a poor prognosis, as standard resuscitation protocols were often ineffective. However, robust evidence from case reports and animal studies supports the use of lipid emulsion in the treatment of cardiovascular collapse from LAST. The mechanism of action is as yet unknown but may include simply acting as a circulating 'sink' for local anaesthetic, rapidly reducing the concentration of local anaesthetic in the myocardium or beneficial effects on the myocardial fatty acid pathways that are disturbed by local anaesthetics.

Prevention

Maximum dose

Minimizing the dose of local anaesthetic administered seems likely to reduce the risk of LAST. This has prompted the concept of the 'maximum dose' of local anaesthetic, (lidocaine 3 mg/kg, racemic bupivacaine 2 mg/kg). In practice systemic blood levels of local anaesthetic vary widely in different patients, and LAST can occur after smaller doses of local anaesthetic. Nevertheless use of the minimum necessary dose of local anaesthetic is a logical way to reduce the risk of LAST. Ultrasound guidance may have benefits as it enables reduced doses of local anaesthetic whilst maintaining a high block success rate and early recognition of intravascular injection. However, there is, as yet, no robust evidence that ultrasound guidance does indeed reduce the incidence of LAST.

Test dose

Intravascular injection of 10 to 15 µg of adrenaline can be used to identify intravascular placement of needle or catheter by:

- increase in heart rate of ten beats per minute
- increase in systolic blood pressure of 15 mmHg
- increase in T-wave amplitude of 25%.

These responses should prompt a change in needle or catheter position before further injection of local anaesthetic. The combination of heart rate and blood pressure changes, or T-wave changes alone, has 80% sensitivity and positive predictive value in the non-pregnant population. The test is less reliable in the elderly and in patients taking beta-blockers in whom the heart rate and blood pressure response may be attenuated.

Incremental dosing

Injecting aliquots of local anaesthetic leaving enough time between injections to ensure there are no signs or symptoms of LAST has intuitive appeal, but is limited by practical problems, particularly difficulty keeping the block needle still for the 30 to 45 seconds required for local anaesthetic to reach the heart or brain.

Use of less toxic local anaesthetic agents

The R-enantiomer of bupivacaine, found in racemic bupivacaine, has a relatively high cardiac toxicity potential. This may be avoided by use of the chiral drugs levobupivacaine (the L-(S) enantiomer of bupivacaine) or ropivacaine (also an S-enantiomer). These drugs are therefore recommended, particularly for large volume blocks.

Treatment

This includes recognition of the clinical signs of LAST, cessation of injection, cardiopulmonary resuscitation and specific treatment with intravenous lipid. This is a medical emergency and as such is best treated following an evidence-based protocol, such as that published by the Association of Anaesthetists of Great Britain and Ireland (AAGBI) (Figure 12.2).

Wrong route errors

A wrong route occurs when a drug intended for intravenous administration is inadvertently administered via an RA route or vice versa. Unique amongst complications of RA they are completely avoidable. A well recognized wrong route error occurs when vincristine is inadvertently injected into the subarachnoid space (instead of methotrexate). This is universally damaging and often fatal. In oncology many safety mechanisms are now in place to prevent this occurrence, but sporadic cases still occur.

This type of wrong route error seems to be very rare in anaesthesia. Wrong route errors in RA generally involve inadvertent administration of local anaesthetic intravenously and can be divided into five types:

A – Migration of a continuous infusion of local anaesthetic (placed for RA) into a vein

B – Connection of the distal part of an infusion (intended for RA) to a venous cannula

C – Injection of a large volume of local anaesthetic into a vein during early establishment of a high-volume block

AAGBI Safety Guideline

Management of Severe Local Anaesthetic Toxicity

1
Recognition

Signs of severe toxicity:
- Sudden alteration in mental status, severe agitation or loss of consciousness, with or without tonic-clonic convulsions
- Cardiovascular collapse: sinus bradycardia, conduction blocks, asystole and with or without tonic-clonic convulsions
- Local anaesthetic (LA) toxicity may occur some time after an initial injection

2
Immediate management

- Stop injecting the LA
- Call for help
- Maintain the airway and, if necessary, secure it with a tracheal tube
- Give 100% oxygen and ensure adequate lung ventilation (hyperventilation may help by increasing plasma pH in the presence of metabolic acidosis)
- Confirm or establish intravenous access
- Control seizures: give a benzodiazepine, thiopental or propofol in small incremental doses
- Assess cardiovascular status throughout
- Consider drawing blood for analysis, but do not delay definitive treatment to do this

3
Treatment

IN CIRCULATORY ARREST
- Start cardiopulmonary resuscitation (CPR) using standard protocols
- Manage arrhythmias using the same protocols, recognising that arrhythmias may be very refractory to treatment
- Consider the use of cardiopulmonary bypass if available

GIVE INTRAVENOUS LIPID EMULSION
(following the regimen overleaf)
- Continue CPR throughout treatment with lipid emulsion
- Recovery from LA-induced cardiac arrest may take >1 h
- Propofol is not a suitable substitute for lipid emulsion
- Lidocaine should not be used as an anti-arrhythmic therapy

WITHOUT CIRCULATORY ARREST
Use conventional therapies to treat:
- hypotension,
- bradycardia
- tachyarrhythmia

CONSIDER INTRAVENOUS LIPID EMULSION
(following the regimen overleaf)
- Propofol is not a suitable substitute for lipid emulsion
- Lidocaine should not be used as an anti-arrhythmic therapy

4
Follow-up

- Arrange safe transfer to a clinical area with appropriate equipment and suitable staff until sustained recovery is achieved
- Exclude pancreatitis by regular clinical review, including daily amylase or lipase assays for two days
- Report cases as follows:
    in the United Kingdom to the National Patient Safety Agency (via www.npsa.nhs.uk)
    in the Republic of Ireland to the Irish Medicines Board (via www.imb.ie)
- If Lipid has been given, please also report its use to the international registry at www.lipidregistry.org. Details may also be posted at www.lipidrescue.org

Your nearest bag of Lipid Emulsion is kept...

This guideline is not a standard of medical care. The ultimate judgement with regard to a particular clinical procedure or treatment plan must be made by the clinician in the light of the clinical data presented and the diagnostic and treatment options available. Association of Anaesthetists of Great Britain & Ireland 2010.

Figure 12.2 Evidence-based protocol (reproduced with the permission of the Association of Anaesthetists of Great Britain and Ireland).

D – Connecting an infusion bag of local anaesthetic (instead of intravenous fluids) to an intravenous-giving set

E – Incorrect administration of a drug into an epidural (or other RA) infusion catheter

In types A and B plasma concentrations of local anaesthetic rise slowly and prodromal signs of LAST will generally be detected well before major CNS or CVS complications. Types A and B probably occur most frequently but type D appears to be the most likely to be fatal. Types B to E all involve human error. Types B and D appear most commonly to be the result of an error by a nurse or midwife, while types C and E usually involve anaesthetist error. Type C can be made far less likely by use of test doses and incremental injection. Fatality from type D is most likely when a large volume of fluid is administered rapidly, for example to treat CNB-induced hypotension. Type E is most commonly performed by anaesthetists who are either distracted at the start of a case (antibiotics, suxamethonium) or during times when a drug must be given promptly (vasopressors, syntocinon). Case examination suggests types D and E frequently occur when CNB-induced hypotension is being treated urgently and this may represent a high-risk period for wrong route error.

There are numerous strategies to prevent wrong route errors and these include:

- segregation of intravenous fluids away from all local anaesthetics (including bags for infusion)
- improved marking of bags of local anaesthetic to distinguish them from intravenous fluids
- double checking of all drug administration involving RA
- engineered solutions have great appeal and considerable potential but may not be as easy to manufacture as might be expected:
  - needle and syringe connectors that do not fit intravenous (Luer) connectors (making types B and D impossible)
  - an alternative spike and bag system that prevents connection of a local anaesthetic bag to an intravenous-giving set, and vice versa (making type D impossible)
- ultimately wrong route errors are a form of drug error – training, awareness of the possibility and vigilant practice remain key to prevention.

Injury secondary to insensate areas

Research is ongoing to identify selective local anaesthetics capable of blocking only nerves encoding pain information: either by targeting subsets of the sodium-channel family, or of alternative channels only present on pain nerves. However, at present all sensory blockade is accompanied by numbness and weakness: this leaves the limb in particular prone to inadvertent injury by unrecognized heat or mechanical trauma. After PNB patients should be advised about the need to protect their limb whilst it lacks sensation and good motor control. Continuing motor block following PNB is an unwelcome accompaniment to analgesia, but as long as it is recognized and managed appropriately it should not be a reason for delayed mobilization or discharge. After CNB, pressure area protection and surveillance minimizes risk of harm. Where compartment syndrome may be a risk CNB may need to be avoided altogether.

Bleeding

Bruising may occur whenever a needle enters the tissues. This is predictable, short-lived and generally unimportant. Prolonged bleeding can cause problems due to haematoma formation. This can lead to nerve injury due to nerve compression and ischaemia. The site of the block dictates to what extent the bleeding can be limited by direct compression: bleeding is rarely a problem in PNB, except when the bleeding occurs in a rigid compartment such as the vertebral canal. Thus, vertebral canal haemotoma is one of the most feared complications of CNB.

Consent issues

All decisions about aspects of medical care require a robust process of informed consent. Informed consent for RA must involve an open explanation of the risks of the block and its benefits, as well as the risks and benefits of not performing it. Information should include numerical estimates of the extent of risk and benefit for that particular patient, where they exist. Although this may be difficult it is pertinent that complaints about the process of consent are prominent in up to 10% of cases of litigation after RA. Adequate time must therefore be taken to gain informed consent and coercion to accept RA is not acceptable.

Complications of central neuraxial block

The Third National Audit Project of the Royal College of Anaesthetists

The Third National Audit Project of the Royal College of Anaesthetists: Major Complications of Central Neuraxial Block (NAP3) is probably the most definitive study of complications of CNB. Using an investigator in every hospital in the UK a census of activity was performed and all major complications of CNB were notified for one year. The project thus effectively followed a prospective cohort of 707,000 patients undergoing CNB. Case review was in depth and the final report acknowledged the uncertainty in determining causation of complications: therefore reporting all results with both optimistic and pessimistic interpretation (as well as confidence intervals reflecting statistical uncertainty). The project produced a large amount of new knowledge to build on several excellent previous studies. The main finding of NAP3 was that the incidence of major complications was lower than several recent smaller publications that had raised concern within the specialty.

Most notably the study's size enabled incidences of complications to be computed by block type (epidural, spinal, caudal and CSE) and by clinical indication (adult perioperative, obstetric, chronic pain and paediatric). Further analyses showed clearly the marked differential risk for different blocks and indications. Of note all obstetric and paediatric CNB fell into a low-risk category. Central neuraxial blockade in the adult perioperative period held the highest risk of harm. The results suggest that it is likely that factors influencing risk of major complications of CNB include patient factors and clinical circumstance as much as block type. The point estimates of risk reported in NAP3 are summarized in Table 12.1.

In addition to quantitative analysis there was considerable qualitative analysis. The full report contains in-depth analysis of all subjects described here with illustration through real case summaries. The report is available in full or as a slideshow summary. A follow-up survey indicates NAP3 has changed departmental practice in more than half of UK hospitals and the individual practice of up to two-thirds of anaesthetists.

Table 12.1 NAP3: point estimates of incidence for cases of permanent harm after CNB.

Indications	Pessimistic[1]	Optimistic[2]
Overall	1 in 23,500	1 in 50,500
Paraplegia and death	1 in 54,500	1 in 141,500
Overall death	<1 in 100,000	<1 in 200,000
Perioperative	1 in 12,500	1 in 24,000
Obstetric	1 in 80,000	1 in 320,000
Chronic pain	1 in 40,000	had full recovery
Paediatrics	no permanent harm	no permanent harm
Cases with permanent harm with perioperative epidural		
Overall	1 in 5,800	1 in 12,000
Paraplegia and death	1 in 16,000	1 in 98,000
Cases with permanent harm with perioperative spinal		
Overall	1 in 38,000	1 in 63,000
Paraplegia and death	1 in 47,000	1 in 95,000
Cases with permanent harm with perioperative CSE		
Overall	1 in 5,500	1 in 8,300
Paraplegia and death	1 in 8,300	1 in 8,300

[1] Pessimistic: all reported complications deemed to be related to CNB.
[2] Optimistic: some reported complications deemed unlikely to be related to CNB and therefore excluded from analysis.

Specific complications of CNB

These include the following:

- spinal cord ischaemia
- vertebral canal haematoma
- vertebral canal abscess
- infective and non-infective meningitis
- cauda equina syndrome and adhesive arachnoiditis
- direct spinal cord and peripheral nerve injury
- cardiovascular collapse and perioperative hypotension
- post-dural puncture headache
- back pain
- complications of neuraxial drugs.

Spinal cord ischaemia

Spinal cord ischaemia is a devastating injury. Understanding it requires an understanding of the basics of spinal cord blood supply.

The anterior spinal artery supplies the anterior two-thirds of the cord. Superiorly it is formed by the vertebral arteries joining together; lower down-flow is augmented by a number of radicular arteries in the cervical, thoracic and lumbar regions. These vary in size and one may become dominant but there is much variation. The posterior third of the cord is supplied by one or two smaller posterior spinal arteries, augmented by radicular arteries. The vertebral arteries are end arteries so occlusion of an artery may lead to death of that part of the spinal cord.

Ischaemic injury at any level of the cord may be complete or partial. With damage in the anterior spinal artery territory symptoms are typically limb weakness (corticospinal tract), loss of bowel and bladder function (autonomic outflow) and loss of pin-prick and temperature sensation (spinothalamic tract). Joint position sense and vibration sense are largely spared, as these sensations are carried in nerves travelling within the dorsal columns in the posterior cord. Ischaemic injury may occur at any level from the cervical cord to the conus medullaris. The resultant neurological pattern is akin to a cord transection at the level of ischaemia. Occasionally ischaemia may be unilateral. In the acute phase all functions may be affected, but later some muscle tone returns with extensors stronger than flexors. If the posterior spinal arteries are damaged there is loss of joint position and vibration sense and some loss of motor power and/or sphincter function.

Spinal cord ischaemia develops if the blood flow to the spinal cord is inadequate for the tissues' metabolic needs. Anything that interrupts spinal cord arterial blood flow can lead to ischaemia, including a sustained fall in systemic arterial blood pressure or marked rise in venous blood pressure. Local factors may also be important, and arterial disease (diabetes, smokers), high blood pressure or spinal cord stenosis are all considered to be risk factors. Surgical risk factors include operations on the spine, aorta (especially cross-clamping or stenting in the thoracic region), thorax, those involving dissection in the retroperitoneal or paravertebral areas and those in which the back is extended when positioning. Intraspinal lesions (stenosis, disc-prolapsed, tumour) may increase risk of cord ischaemia by reducing venous drainage or spinal canal compliance.

The role of an epidural (or spinal) in increasing the risk of spinal cord ischaemia is unproven and the number of patients who develop spinal cord ischaemia with and without an epidural during surgery is unknown.

Central neuraxial blockade may theoretically increase the risk of spinal cord ischaemia by:

1. causing arterial hypotension (any CNB)
2. raising intraspinal pressure (epidural infusion and especially bolus).

It is known that when fluid is injected into the epidural space it raises the pressure in the vertebral canal and this can theoretically reduce blood flow to the spinal cord. If this does occur the effect is transient, lasting a matter of minutes.

In major thoracic and intra-abdominal surgery it is likely that surgical factors affect spinal blood flow to a far greater extent than the presence of CNB.

When spinal cord infarction occurs the likelihood of recovery is very low and the resulting disability is likely to be profound. In the acute phase atypical neurological deficit may lead to diagnostic confusion. Magnetic resonance imaging (MRI) in the early phase is often unremarkable with any changes taking several weeks to develop.

The major importance of spinal cord ischaemia and CNB is two-fold.

Firstly, CNB may complicate or delay the diagnosis of spinal cord ischaemia. If the diagnosis is considered every effort must be made to exclude treatable causes (vertebral canal haematoma, other space-occupying lesions) before the diagnosis is accepted.

Secondly, when cord injury occurs in the presence of CNB it is highly likely that the CNB will immediately be implicated. The anaesthetist, therefore, should consider the necessity for CNB carefully where there is thought to be a high risk of spinal cord ischaemia. The anaesthetist should routinely ensure that blood pressure is maintained during major surgery with CNB. Avoidance of hypotension should extend into the postoperative period and this may require appropriate cardiovascular support with fluids of vasopressors if necessary. This remains a major challenge in delivery of safe postoperative CNB.

The use of lumbar cerebrospinal fluid drains in patients with identified high risk to reduce the risk of spinal cord ischaemia is controversial, but if employed is more likely to be effective in prevention than treatment.

Vertebral canal haematoma

Vertebral canal haematoma (VCH) is a very important complication of CNB. It is very rare (estimates are around 1 in 100,000) but failure to detect it within a few hours of occurrence is likely to condemn the patient to permanent paraplegia.

When bleeding occurs within the enclosed space of the vertebral canal this can lead to cord compression. This in turn leads to neural ischaemia, which, if not promptly treated, causes permanent loss of function. Vertebral canal haematoma is therefore a medical emergency.

Due to its rarity it is a poorly studied phenomenon. It is strongly associated with coagulopathy, especially with the concomitant use of anticoagulants, and its risk seems to be greater in the elderly or infirm, and when CNB is used for major surgery rather than other indications. Renal impairment may delay elimination of several drugs (including heparin) thereby increasing risk of VCH.

In NAP3 all VCH followed major elective surgery and many cases involved thoracic epidurals. In the thoracic spine, the ratio of canal to nerve tissue is lowest and this may increase risk. Epidural catheter removal appears at least as high a risk for VCH as insertion and this mandates neurological monitoring that continues for 24 hours after cessation of CNB.

Vertebral canal haematoma classically presents, after technically difficult CNB, with back and radicular pain, increasing bilateral leg weakness and progressive paraplegia. In reality VCH may occur without trauma at insertion. It occurs more often after epidurals than spinals, but not invariably. Each of the classic symptoms may be absent and although leg weakness or numbness appears ubiquitous, even this may be unilateral. Similarly motor block of the legs occurring in the presence of a thoracic epidural should immediately raise suspicion as should any inappropriately dense block.

Cessation of local anaesthetic infusion should lead to a demonstrable return of power within no more than four hours. Failure for this to occur mandates further investigation (MRI scan). If initial cessation leads to recovery of motor function but restarting the epidural again causes excessive motor block this is not reassuring. An MRI scan should be performed.

Once diagnosed, decompression may be necessary to prevent paraplegia. It is generally considered that this must take place within eight hours of the onset of symptoms, though the evidence to support this is weak. Treatment should be as prompt as is possible.

In NAP3, VCH was particularly associated with thoracic epidural anaesthesia in elderly infirm patients undergoing major surgery. Vertebral canal haematoma occurred in about 5 per 100,000 perioperative epidurals. All received drugs affecting coagulation and VCH developed after catheter removal in half of the cases. Several VCH diagnoses were delayed because unilateral motor weakness was assumed to be due to epidural drugs and weak legs during thoracic epidural analgesia were ignored. Once suspicion was raised there were numerous local and neurosurgical delays before treatment. Permanent paraplegia was almost ubiquitous and in several cases this might have been avoided by quicker actions. The one patient whose VCH was diagnosed and treated very promptly made a full recovery.

Strategies to avoid VCH and its consequences include:

- full history of drugs affecting coagulation
- avoidance of CNB in patients with particularly high risk (especially those taking more than one drug affecting coagulation or with other causes of impaired blood clotting) unless benefit clearly exceeds risk
- strict adherence to policies regarding timings of drug and CNB, and CNB catheter removal
- careful atraumatic technique
- a high-quality acute pain team – not only providing expert review of patients, but more importantly educating ward staff to detect these rare emergencies and communicate concerns effectively
- careful monitoring of leg motor function for all patients with CNB
- adherence to strict protocol for escalation of review/investigation in cases of suspected VCH:
    - early senior anaesthetist review (other clinicians may misinterpret)
    - low threshold for stopping CNB infusion to assess recovery of function
    - early MRI when VCH clinically suspected (available 24 hours a day)
    - predefined mechanism to ensure patients with confirmed VCH get early appropriate neurosurgical referral and timely treatment.

(See Figure 12.3).

The increased range and complexity of drugs used to provide thromboprophylaxis in the perioperative period and anticoagulation following vascular stenting is becoming a major area of risk in anaesthesia. Inevitably, there is an ever-increasing opportunity for error in the timing of CNB and CNB catheter removal in relationship to anticoagulation. More than ever, there is a requirement for local protocols to be developed mandating timings of administration of anticoagulants with respect to CNB administration and CNB catheter removal. Several new anticoagulants specifically state that continuous CNB should be used with caution (Rivaroxaban) or not at all (Dabigatran) and this adds a further level of complexity. The benefit of such drugs may not be as well proven as some believe and in some cases this may lead patients to miss out on the benefits of CNB for major surgery.

It is important to remember that VCH is very rare and the vast majority of patients (even with increased risk factors) will not suffer this complication. These same patients may have most to gain from (particularly perioperative) CNB. Safe delivery of CNB requires careful individualized assessment of both absolute and relative risk before its performance. Despite the rarity of VCH, processes should be in place wherever CNB is used to ensure every case is identified early and managed as an emergency.

Management of leg weakness with epidural analgesia

All patients receiving epidural analgesia must have leg strength assessed regularly using the 'leg strength score'(see below) that appear on the epidural observation form. Thoracic epidural analgesia should not cause profound leg weakness. Increasing leg weakness usually means the infusion rate is too high. However it may mean that the patient is developing an epidural haematoma or epidural abscess. If not diagnosed and treated promptly, this will lead to paraplegia. Use this algorithm to help differentiate.

Increasing leg weakness? Leg strength score 3 or 4?

YES

Increasing leg weakness? Leg strength score 3 or 4? Painful, swollen or pus at site?

Switch off epidural infusion. Contact the Acute Pain Team and inform them of the situation

NO ← Discuss if catheter is to be removed? → YES

Reassess leg strength every 30 minutes

Recommence epidural infusion and routine observations

Send catheter tip, site swab and blood cultures to microbiology. If pus is present send urgent sample to lab. Apply dry dressing to site. Inform microbiologist (bleep 7599). Start recommended antibiotic cover

Leg strength improving? — YES — Patient comfortable?

NO

NO

More than 4 hours since stopping epidural infusion? NO

Reassess leg strength every 30 minutes

YES

Contact the Acute Pain Team to reassess the patient's analgesia ← YES — Leg strength improving?

Suspect an epidural haematoma. Proceed as follows

NO

More than 4 hours since stopping epidural infusion? NO

During weekday office hours contact a member of the Acute Pain Team (bleep 7113 or 7222) who will arrange an urgent spinal MRI scan through the radiology department and contact the spinal surgical team. After hours and weekends contact the anaesthetist on call (bleep 7113) who will arrange an urgent spinal MRI scan through the on-call radiologist and neurosurgical teams. An epidural haematoma or abscess has to be evacutated within 8 hours of the onset of symptoms for your patient to have the best chance of recovery of neurological function. Do not delay

YES

Suspect an epidural abscess. Proceed as follows

Grade Criteria Degree of Block (Bromage Scale)

score 1	Free movement of legs and feet. Nil(0%)	
score 2	Just able to flex knees with free movement of feet. Partial (33%)	
score 3	Unable to flex knees, but with free movement of feet. Almost Complete (66%)	
score 4	Unable to move legs or feet. Complete (100%)	

Figure 12.3 Management of leg weakness with epidural analgesia. (Courtesy of Royal United Hospital, Bath. In turn adapted from work at Derriford Hospital, Plymouth.)

Vertebral canal abscess

Vertebral canal abscess (VCA) is, like VCH, a cord-threatening complication of CNB. Investigation and treatment (often non-surgical) in the absence of progressive neurology should be urgent. Where the patient has neurological deficit the need to exclude VCH requires emergency management.

Vertebral canal abscess is at one end of a spectrum of local infective complications of CNB, which includes local infection, deep (extravertebral) tissue infection and VCA. While local infection is common (and catheter colonization even more frequent), VCA is rare.

Vertebral canal abscess is more likely in patients with compromised immunity (malnutrition, cancer, diabetes mellitus, HIV, steroids, etc.). Many of these risk factors will be present either recognized or unrecognized in the elderly perioperative patient. The presence of an epidural catheter, especially for a prolonged period, is a recognized risk factor as are multiple steroid epidural injections.

It has been suggested that a prelude to a VCA may be a subclinical haematoma, which acts as a focus for infection, but this is unproven. Although the epidural tract creates a route for ingress of infection haematogenous spread may also occur, leading to controversy over the use of epidurals in patients with (or at risk of) sepsis.

The major challenge with VCA is diagnostic: firstly, it can be difficult to differentiate it from more minor infections; and, secondly, because it may present at a time and site that is distant from the original CNB. Classically, back pain, signs of local and generalized sepsis and worsening neurological deficit are seen. Vertebral canal abscess may present with several of these symptoms or none. While many VCAs will present with local signs of sepsis during or soon after CNB, VCA should also be excluded in any patient with signs of sepsis or neurology after recent CNB. In NAP3, two patients presented with abscesses more than one month after the procedure and several were at sites considerably distant to the CNB insertion site.

Diagnosis is by a combination of microbiological screening and radiological imaging (MRI scan). The value of triple screening (site, catheter tip and blood cultures) in making a diagnosis is unproven.

The infective organism is most commonly *Staphylococcus aureus* but many other bacteria may be isolated. Treatment may be conservative (high-dose prolonged antibiotic therapy) or surgical (washout and decompression as indicated). There is no strong evidence of which approach is the most effective.

Prevention of VCA (and other CNB-associated infections) relies on two principles:

1. Central neuraxial blockade should only be performed with the highest levels of aseptic technique. Where this cannot be achieved CNB should be avoided. Infection occurring after incomplete asepsis is likely indefensible. Where there is the possibility of pre-existing infection, antibiotic treatment should be initiated before performing CNB.

2. Prolonged use of catheters for CNB increases the risk of VCA. While this is accepted, the appropriate duration of use is undefined (and logically differs for individual patients and circumstances). The incidence of VCA after labour epidural is very low and also when a perioperative catheter is in place for up to 48 hours. As a general principle a CNB catheter should be left in for the minimum time consistent with clinical benefit. If it is left in place beyond 72 hours it demands a high level of surveillance and daily assessment of the risk and benefit of it remaining. In the perioperative period, the need for an epidural catheter beyond four to five days is likely to be very rare. Transparent 'breathable' dressings enable daily inspection of the entry site and minimize fluid collections. There is some evidence that redressing or repositioning epidural catheters is likely to increase the frequency of infections: it should be avoided. There is no robust evidence that tunnelling CNB catheters reduces risk of infection.

Large series of VCA are not reported, so NAP3 is informative regarding outcome. In NAP3, VCA was three times as common as VCH (approximately 2 per 100,000) with permanent harm in half to a quarter of these patients (depending on case interpretation). The incidence in the perioperative group was six-fold higher and included mostly patients who were notably debilitated before the CNB and received prolonged epidural catheterization. There were significant delays in diagnosis in several cases. Half of patients with VCA made a full recovery, in several cases over many months: of those who did not there were cases of death, tetraplegia and paraplegia, so VCA must not be regarded as an unimportant injury. One interesting observation was that VCA diagnosed as a result of local signs had a better outcome than VCA presenting with no local signs.

Infective and non-infective meningitis

Infective meningitis is a rare complication of CNB with previous estimates of 2 per 100,000 and a point estimate in NAP3 of 0.5 per 100,000.

Risk factors for bacterial meningitis following CNB, as with abscess, include immunosuppression and poor aseptic technique. Bacterial meningitis may follow spinal or epidural anaesthesia.

When following spinal anaesthesia, bacterial meningitis is most likely to present within 24 hours and the infective organism is usually a nasal commensal (streptococcal species). Two recent separate 'mini-epidemics' of post-spinal bacterial meningitis were both traced to the anaesthetist's nasal fauna. Though one of the relevant anaesthetists wore a facemask these cases emphasize the obligation to maintain full asepsis while performing all CNB. Delay in diagnosis may arise because persistent headache (often the only symptom initially) is diagnosed as post-dural puncture headache. Persisting or severe headache should prompt consideration of other diagnoses. Early diagnosis and prompt targeted antibiotic treatment should lead to full recovery. Delay in diagnosis and treatment has the potential for permanent sequelae.

Bacterial meningitis after epidural in contrast often occurs later, is associated with prolonged use of an epidural catheter and the causative organism, as in VCA, is commonly *Staphylococcus aureus*.

Differential diagnosis of bacterial meningitis (also see Post-dural puncture headache) includes 'aseptic meningitis', which is a rather elusive condition. It is variously described as being due to chemical irritation (due to microscopic amounts of antiseptic) or introduction of microscopic metal shards during subarachnoid injection. Presentation and investigations mimic bacterial meningitis, but the CSF is sterile. Treatment is conservative and the condition self-limiting.

Cauda equina syndrome and adhesive arachnoiditis

The rare conditions cauda equina syndrome and adhesive arachnoiditis may present following spinal anaesthesia. In the 1990s a spate of cases of cauda equina syndrome in the USA was attributed to repeated dosing with hyperbaric 5% lidocaine via intrathecal catheters. This led to excessive doses of local anaesthetic bathing the caudal nerves and widespread nerve damage. Avoidance of this combination should prevent recurrence. Very rare cases of adhesive arachnoiditis can occur after spinal anaesthesia. While some interpret this as being caused by introduction of small quantities of chlorhexidine, the evidence for this is absent. Notwithstanding that, it is currently advisable to use only 0.5% chlorhexidine for CNB, to ensure this completely dries and for the anaesthetist's gloved hands to avoid all direct contact with the fluid while performing the block.

Direct spinal cord and peripheral nerve injury

Direct nerve injury (whether to spinal cord or peripheral nerves as they leave the spinal cord) can occur with similar mechanisms to those described earlier. The incidence of such injuries has previously been estimated as between 1 in 1,000 to 1 in 100,000, and 0.6 per 10,000 in obstetric CNB. In NAP3 the pessimistic and optimistic point estimates of permanent harm were considerably lower at 1 per 100,000 and 0.4 per 100,000 respectively.

The most important cause of direct cord and nerve injury during CNB is likely direct needle injury. No location devices are routinely used for CNB and bony landmarks are the mainstay. Sonographic location of the neuraxis is in its infancy and little used clinically. The potential for direct cord or nerve injury is recognized during CNB by pain (paraesthesia) during needle placement, catheter placement or drug injection. When such paraesthesia is elicited it is routine practice to stop injection and if paraesthesia does not settle immediately to remove and reposition CNB. It is a fundamental principle of CNB not to proceed when the procedure is causing pain. Direct cord or nerve injury is also recognized 'after the event' when motor block, anaesthesia, dysaesthesia or neuropathic pain persists after block regression.

Management ideally involves careful clinical assessment by several specialties (neurology, anaesthesia and obstetrics where indicated) as each will lack some of the other's knowledge. Investigation will likely include MRI and electrophysiological studies in an attempt to exclude other causes, gauge the site and extent of injury, and so assess causation and enable broad prognostication. It is important to note the information derived from electrophysiological testing is very dependent on the interpretation of the person performing it and their expertise will go a long way in determining the value of the test. Delaying these tests by two to three weeks after the injury enables the extent of axonal loss to be estimated, aiding prognostication.

There are no specific treatments that improve recovery but support of physiotherapy, occupational therapy and pain management may mitigate the extent of any disability.

One finding of NAP3 was that more than 60% of the cases of direct spinal cord or nerve injury deemed serious enough to report to the project made a confirmed full recovery, mostly within two months. As milder cases were likely not notified and that all cases lost to follow-up were assumed to have made no improvement, it is highly likely that well in excess of 75% of cases of direct cord and nerve injury recover.

Determining causation is the most difficult part of assessing these injuries. This may be easy when the nerve injury follows significant paraesthesia that is in the same or similar neurological distribution. For other direct injuries several other causes must be excluded. This is particularly pertinent to nerve injury in association with obstetric CNB: here nerve injury may be caused by pregnancy itself, cephalopelvic disproportion, prolonged or obstructed labour, patient positioning in stirrups and instrumental delivery.

Direct nerve damage may occur after spinal, epidural or CSE: with significant concerns that the needle-through-needle CSE technique is associated with the highest incidence.

Occasionally concerns may be raised of chemical injury to nerves. Antiseptic solutions are most commonly implicated, sometimes without evidence. This is discussed above (arachnoiditis).

The fact that significant nerve injury is often preceded by painful paraesthesia and that this mandates cessation of needle placement or injection in awake patients, supports the argument that it is logical to perform CNB in the awake patient (accepting light conscious sedation). Cases in NAP3 where CNB needles appear to have been placed into the thoracic or lumbar cord of asleep patients tends to reinforce this belief. However, the fact that patients with bilateral severe parasthesiae at the time of needle placement, fared less well than those with lesser immediate symptoms, might suggest the damage is already done when the paraesthesia occurs. The arguments will continue.

A further unanswered question is whether surgery should proceed after suspicious paraesthesia has occurred. The possibility of surgery (stress response, positioning, retraction, hypotension) leading to a 'second hit' to the injured nerve suggest the cautious approach is to defer major surgery in such cases.

Cardiovascular collapse and perioperative hypotension

Early hypotension

Sudden hypotension, most commonly after spinal blockade, may be caused by vaso-vagal fainting or sympathetic blockade from the CNB. In the case of a high block, bradycardia may also develop. Hypotension is almost inevitable during obstetric spinal for caesarean section and rarely causes problems provided it is anticipated and promptly treated. Severe hypotension in the elderly and those with severe cardiovascular disease following spinal anaesthesia may be more problematic as the patient may tolerate it less well, and the drugs used to treat it may cause secondary problems (arrythmia, coronary vasoconstriction). Hypotension may be exacerbated by pre-existing hypovolaemia, co-morbidities (hypertension, ischaemic heart disease, valvular disease, diabetes mellitus) or drug treatment (antihypertensives, alpha- and beta-blockers). While the value of volume preloading is very limited pre-operative optimization, anticipation, prompt diagnosis and early treatment including head-down positioning will minimize the sequelae of early hypotension. In some countries leg binding is also used for this role. Use of a test dose prior to loading an epidural is also important in preventing total spinal block and profound hypotension.

One French study reported a rate of six cardiac arrests and one death per 10,000 spinals. In NAP3, three deaths (half of all CNB-related deaths, even on pessimistic assessment) occurred from cardiovascular collapse after spinal anaesthesia: a rate of 0.6 per 100,000.

Late hypotension

Late hypotension is a particular feature of epidurals, both peri- and post-operatively, but may also be seen in the first 24 hours after spinal anaesthesia. An element of remaining sympathetic blockade combined with intravascular depletion (dehydration, blood loss, starvation, third-space fluid shifts, systemic inflammatory response) is likely to be causative.

It will be appreciated from the preceding section on spinal cord ischaemia (as well as for many other reasons) that this prolonged hypotension must be avoided. Whilst in the operating theatre environment it is commonplace to administer a combination of fluids and vasopressors to maintain normotension, this tends to lapse on the wards, with only fluid available and vasopressors restricted to high-care areas. This remains a challenge for many hospitals. Development of protocols whereby vasopressors in modest doses may be used to reverse the sympathetic blockade caused by CNB (which has greater physiological logic than pouring in more fluid) would likely be of potential benefit to patients.

Post-dural puncture headache

Post-dural puncture headache (PDPH) occurs predictably after spinal blockade in 0.5 to 1% of young pregnant patients. The rate is less in older and non-pregnant patients.

Post-dural puncture headache is usually only of modest severity and is a self-limiting condition. Simple treatment (adopting the supine position, regular analgesia, good hydration and perhaps caffeine or sumatriptan) are usually effective and resolution occurs within a few days. Occasionally isolated cranial nerve palsy (self-limiting) presents as part of PDPH: the sixth cranial nerve is most commonly affected. When PDPH occurs after inadvertent dural puncture (0.5 to 2% of obstetric epidurals) an epidural blood patch may be needed (in 50 to 70% of cases). This is an invasive procedure, with the risk of introducing neuraxial infection. It may also cause severe radicular pain during injection and prolonged backache. It should not be undertaken lightly.

Differential diagnoses of PDPH should be considered if it is severe, prolonged, atypical or where there are unexplained additional symptoms or signs. Differential diagnoses include:

- bacterial meningitis
- aseptic meningitis
- subdural haematoma
- subarachnoid or other intracranial bleeds
- venous sinus thrombosis.

Subdural haematoma may uncommonly complicate PDPH. Severe headaches and cranial nerve palsy should raise the possibility of the diagnosis. Most are self-limiting and require careful observation. Neurosurgical evacuation may occasionally be required.

Back pain

There is no robust evidence of CNB, especially in the obstetric setting, being a cause of prolonged backache: the more frequent cause is pregnancy and childbirth or constitutional elements.

Complications of neuraxial drugs

There are numerous complications of neuraxial drugs and these include:

- high spinal (too much spinal local anaesthetic)
- high epidural (too much epidural local anaesthetic)
- subdural block (local anaesthetic in the subdural space)
- total spinal (too much spinal local anaesthetic or unrecognized intrathecal placement of an intended epidural catheter)
- respiratory depression (excessive neuraxial opioid, excess of other neuraxial adjuncts).

These all lead to variably high segmental blockade, in keeping with the type of block described (subdural block is patchy but dense and unexpectedly high for the dose of local anaesthetic). Consequent on the high block there is extensive sympathetic block leading to vasodilatation and hypotension. If autonomic blockade (which may be six segments above sensory block) is above T4, the heart is exposed to unopposed vagal action, leading to the risk of severe bradycardia. In total spinal, flaccid respiratory paralysis occurs with or without unconsciousness.

A main principle of management of all these complications is to maintain blood pressure with fluids and drugs as indicated. In total spinal, the airway must be secured and general anaesthesia is recommended to ensure lack of awareness. Recovery usually takes one to three hours.

Respiratory depression is most frequently from injection of the wrong dose in the right place (relative opioid overdose) or the right dose in the wrong place (e.g. intended epidurally, administered subarachnoid).

Amongst the opioids morphine poses a particularly high risk in the neuraxis. Lipophilic drugs such as fentanyl and diamorphine generally cross between the epidural and subarachnoid space with relative ease and once in the subarachnoid space they enter the neuraxis, rapidly producing a segmental block. In contrast hydrophilic drugs such as morphine cross the intact dura poorly. A hole in the dura dramatically increases drug flux. Once in the subarachnoid space morphine may remain in the CSF and migrate cephalad to the brainstem where it can cause respiratory depression by affecting the respiratory centre. After spinal injection of morphine, respiratory depression may occur six hours and rarely 24 hours later. Epidural morphine in the presence of a dural puncture (e.g. unrecognized dural puncture or intended dural puncture during CSE) passes from epidural to subarachnoid space in a much higher dose than normal. The cephalad migration of morphine may also be accelerated by patient movement. A typical case might follow a CSE with epidural morphine, the patient is fine until returning to the ward where transfer onto the bed is followed by 'unexplained' respiratory arrest. Use of only lipophilic opioids in the neuraxis lessens the risk of such events.

Complications of peripheral nerve blockade

The application of local anaesthetic directly on to peripheral nerves (peripheral nerve blockade, PNB) has been a staple of anaesthetic practice since the late nineteenth century. Following a loss of popularity in the latter half of the twentieth century, recent years have seen a resurgence of interest in PNB partly driven by new technology that holds the promise of safer, better and perhaps quicker nerve blocks.

Well performed PNB improves the patient experience and may positively affect outcome. Other advantages applicable to PNB and CNB are described earlier. However, poorly performed PNB may lead to ineffective blockade and an increase in local or distant complications. A fundamental principle of PNB, even when using various nerve localization devices, is that the operator must have a good understanding of the anatomy of the block site and the functional anatomy of the area requiring blockade.

Peripheral nerve injury

The reported incidence of nerve injury following PNB depends on the stage at which evidence is sought. Reports of early nerve injury inevitably include neurapraxias that in time will resolve completely, whereas late surveys may miss temporary nerve dysfunction that has already resolved. Temporary nerve dysfunction probably occurs in around 3% of PNB but permanent nerve injury is very rare. The best contemporary estimates of risk of permanent nerve injury following PNB come from two large prospective studies from France and Australia, which suggested risks of 2.38 per 10,000 (95% CI not stated) and 4 per 10,000 (95% CI 0.8 to 11 per 10,000) respectively. It is clear that of those patients who are initially suspected of having an important nerve injury, only a very small proportion eventually turn out to have a demonstrable anatomical or functional nerve lesion.

Prevention

The risk of permanent nerve injury is so low that there has not yet been a study with enough power to detect a significant reduction in incidence as a result any one particular intervention.

However, the following, either alone or more likely in combination, may reduce the risk of nerve injury:

- thorough knowledge of anatomy (and sonoanatomy when ultrasound location is used)
- the use of ultrasound in skilled hands
- good aseptic technique
- avoidance of parasthesia
- pressure-limiting injection lines.

Investigation and management

Mild and resolving symptoms often require no further investigation providing improvement continues: the prognosis for full recovery is very good. If symptoms are more severe or progressive then full assessment by a neurologist in combination with an anaesthetist is advised. Electrophysiological testing and MRI imaging of the nerve may identify the precise position along the nerve where the injury has occurred and may serve to distinguish nerve damage due to PNB from other causes. The differential diagnosis may include:

- compressive injuries from patient positioning
- compressive injuries from prolonged tourniquet use
- coincidental or pre-existing neurological disease
- surgical nerve injury.

Evidence of a complete nerve transection should prompt referral to a neurosurgeon for consideration of nerve repair. Pain should be actively managed by a pain specialist with expertise in the treatment of neuropathic pain.

Infection

Infective risks following PNB have not been fully quantified. Infection following single-shot PNB is rare, but is more common after insertion of a peripheral nerve catheter. In one study, 57% of femoral nerve catheters were colonized with bacteria 48 hours after insertion: most commonly with *Staphylococcus epidermidis*, but also *Entercoccus* species and *Klebsiella*. While colonization does not commonly lead to invasive infection, it is accepted practice that full aseptic precautions should be taken during PNB. Current recommendations from the Association of Anaesthetists of Great Britain and Ireland does not distinguish between single-shot peripheral nerve blocks and the insertion of peripheral nerve catheters, recommending the use of sterile gloves and drapes for all PNB. Given the propensity for peripheral nerve catheters to become colonized with skin flora, it would nevertheless seem sensible to take full aseptic precautions (gown, gloves, mask, drapes) during their insertion.

Misplaced needle injuries

These arise when the needle is intended to be placed close to a nerve but enters or injures other local structures.

Respiratory system

Care should be taken when performing these blocks in patients with pre-existing respiratory disease for two reasons. Firstly, the upper brachial plexus blocks (interscalene and supraclavicular) are associated with a high incidence of inadvertent phrenic nerve blockade, which results in temporary hemidiaphragmatic paralysis. Whilst this may go unnoticed in a healthy patient it may lead to respiratory failure in a patient with marginal lung function. Secondly, brachial plexus blockade (particularly supraclavicular) carries the risk of pneumothorax. The risk of both complications may be reduced by meticulous use of ultrasound guidance and thorough knowledge of the relevant sonoanatomy, as this will enable the precise placement of a smaller volume of drug and tracking of the needle tip position relative to the pleura. Pneumothorax can also occur following paravetebral or intercostal nerve blocks.

Other

These are rare and should be avoidable by good technique. They include:

- intravascular placement of an RA needle or catheter PNB in the neck. This is particularly hazardous and minute quantities of drug may lead to major central neurological system disturbance
- epidural block during paravertebral blockade
- intrathecal block during caudal block
- visceral perforation during abdominal wall blocks. This may occur during poorly performed transversus abdominus plane (TAP) blocks, ilioinguinal blocks and femoral nerve blocks. Injuries to bowel and liver have been reported
- globe puncture and dural puncture during ophthalmic RA (see below).

Wrong-site/side regional anaesthesia

Wrong-site and wrong-side PNBs can and do occur. The use of checklists such as the one promoted by the World Health Organization, pre-operative marking of the correct site of needle insertion and performing PNB in the awake patient may all reduce the incidence of wrong-site/side blockade. However, these systematic approaches to risk management do not absolve the clinician of the responsibility for the utmost personal vigilance when performing regional anaesthesia.

Complications of ophthalmic regional anaesthesia

Ophthalmic surgery can be performed under non-akinetic (topical) or akinetic regional anaesthesia. Akinetic regional anaesthesia is performed by placing local anaesthetic around the globe in a variety of positions, including in the intraconal space (retrobulbar block), extraconal space (peribulbar block) or the sub-Tenon's space (sub-Tenon's block). Although rare, there are some specific complications associated with orbital regional anaesthesia. These range from trivial to life-threatening. Complications are considerably less likely with sub-Tenon's blocks.

Chemosis

Chemosis or swelling of the conjunctiva due to anterior spread of local anaesthetic is a minor adverse event that responds well to gentle pressure over the eye, usually provided by a small weight or a Honan balloon.

Bruising

Visible bruising to the eye, usually in the subconjuctival space or the eyelids, is the result of damage to superficial blood vessels during placement of the needle, and is more common in the elderly and patients on steroids or aspirin. Spread may be limited by gentle oculocompression. Larger bleeds may require postponement of surgery but all resolve spontaneously.

Damage to the motor nerve of the inferior rectus and inferior oblique muscles

This can occur due to direct damage to the nerve during injection and can be avoided by placing the blocking needle as far laterally as possible in the inferotemporal quadrant.

Prolonged extraocular muscle malfunction

Unusually, clinically significant dysfunction of the extraocular muscles follows an intraorbital block. The mechanism is unclear, but may be related to direct injection of local anaesthetic into the intraocular muscles or damage to the motor nerve. In the latter situation, dysfunction may be permanent, but more frequently resolves spontaneously within three weeks.

Oculocardic reflex

The bradycardia that accompanies a rapid increase in intraorbital or intraocular pressure or traction on the ocular muscles can occasionally occur during ophthalmic regional anaesthesia. Slow and careful injection can mitigate the effects of this reflex and ECG monitoring enables prompt identification.

Globe ischaemia

The perfusion pressure of the globe is dependent on the local mean arterial blood pressure minus the intraocular pressure. When ocular compression devices are used to reduce intraocular pressure during surgery there is a risk that globe pressure can be increased above the local mean arterial pressure resulting in globe ischaemia. This risk increases with atherosclerotic disease, injection of large volumes of local anaesthetic into the orbit, in the elderly and in the presence of co-morbidities that reduce orbital compliance (e.g. scleroderma or glaucoma).

Retrobulbar haemorrhage

Retrobulbar haemorrhage is a more serious complication that results from damage to posterior blood vessels within the orbit. Arterial bleeding is more serious than venous bleeding and may lead to rapid (within minutes) proptosis of the globe accompanied by lid swelling and conjunctival injection. The intraocular pressure increases rapidly, and threatens the retinal circulation and ultimately the function of the eye. Oculocompression can limit the extent of the haemorrhage and an immediate ophthalmic opinion regarding further intervention (e.g. acetazolamide or surgical treatment, to reduce the intraocular pressure) must be sought. Retrobulbar hemorrhage may occur in up to 1 in 5,000 retrobulbar blocks. It is far rarer with peribulbar blockade and has not been reported with sub-Tenon's block.

Globe penetration and perforation

Globe penetration (passage of a needle into the globe) and perforation (passage of a needle through the globe) are emergencies, and require an urgent ophthalmological opinion to determine the need for surgical intervention. They occur most commonly during RA on myopic eyes with an axial length >26 mm, and in the uncooperative patient. They have been reported during retrobulbar and peribulbar blockade but not sub-Tenon's block. Globe penetration or perforation should be suspected when there is pain on injection, loss of vision, a loss of the red reflex or vitreous haemorrhage. If penetration is suspected no injection of fluid should take place as this increases the risk of visual loss.

Optic nerve damage

Optic nerve damage is the result of direct local anaesthetic injection into the nerve or nerve sheath leading to high intraneural pressures, or indirect damage from the use of adrenaline-containing local anaesthetic solutions in or around the optic nerve leading to vasoconstriction and optic nerve ischaemia. Optic nerve dysfunction may be delayed, and rarely optic atrophy can occur. Avoiding the use of long needles (>31 mm) and ensuring any injection is made with the eye in the neutral position will reduce the chance of the needle tip approximating the optic nerve and therefore reduce the incidence of this serious complication.

Brainstem anaesthesia

Inadvertent placement of the blocking needle into the optic nerve sheath risks spread of local anaesthetic into the subarachnoid space surrounding the brainstem. Rapid loss of consciousness and cardiovascular collapse may result, requiring ventilatory and cardiovascular support.

List of further reading

AAGBI. Safety guideline. Infection control in anaesthesia. October 2008. www.aagbi.org/publications/guidelines/docs/infection_control_08.pdf (accessed 15 April 2011).

AAGBI. Safety guideline. Regional anaesthesia and patients with coagulation abnormalities. Forthcoming 2011. www.aagbi.org/publications.

Auroy, Y., Benhamou, D., Bargues L. *et al.* Major complications of regional anesthesia in France: the SOS Regional Anesthesia Hotline Service. *Anesthesiology* 2002; **97**: 1274–80.

Cook, T. M., Mihai, R. & Wildsmith, J. A. W. A census of UK neuraxial blockage: results of the snapshot phase of the 3rd National Anaesthesia Project. *Anaesthesia* 2008; **63**: 143–6.

Cook, T. M., Counsell, D. & Wildsmith, J. A. W. Major complications of central neuraxial block: report on the Third National Audit of the Royal College of Anaesthetists. *Br J Anaesth* 2009; **102**: 179–90.

Cuvillon, P., Ripart, J., Lalourcey, L. *et al.* The continuous femoral nerve block catheter for postoperative analgesia: bacterial colonization, infectious rate and adverse effects. *Anesth Analg* 2001; **93**: 1045–9.

Hogan, Q. Pathophysiology of peripheral nerve injury during regional anesthesia. *Reg Anesth Pain Med* 2008; **33**: 435–41.

Kumar, C. & Dowd, T. Complications of ophthalmic regional blocks: their treatment and prevention. *Ophthalmologica* 2006; **220**: 73–82.

Lupu, C. M., Kiehl, T-R., Chan, V. W. S. *et al.* Nerve expansion seen on ultrasound predicts histologic but not functional nerve injury after intraneural injection in pigs. *Reg Anesth Pain Med* 2010; **35**: 132–9.

Mulroy, M. F. & Hejtmanek, M. R. Prevention of local anesthetic systemic toxicity. *Reg Anesth Pain Med* 2010; **35**: 177–80.

Royal College of Anaesthetists. Good practice in the management of continuous epidural analgesia in the hospital setting. November 2004. www.rcoa.ac.uk/docs/epid-analg.pdf (accessed 15 April 2011).

Szypula, K., Bogod, D., Ashpole, K. *et al.* Litigation associated with regional anaesthesia: an analysis of claims against the NHS in England 1995–2007. *Anaesthesia*; **65**: 443–52.

Wijeysundera, D. N., Beattie, W. S., Austin, P. C., Hux, J. E. & Laupacis A. Epidural anaesthesia and survival after intermediate- to high-risk non-cardiac surgery: a population-based cohort study. *Lancet* 2008; **372**: 562–9.

Chapter

Body temperature complications

John Andrzejowski and James Hoyle

Highlight of importance

Incidence

Core body temperature is one of the most tightly controlled parameters in humans. Behavioural changes and autonomic regulation maintain a preset value of approximately 37°C +/− 0.2°C. Induction of anaesthesia can result in quite marked changes in body temperature. The commonest change is a rapid drop in temperature of up to 2°C in the first 90 minutes. This is known as inadvertent perioperative hypothermia (IPH). Its incidence without measures to combat it would approach 100% due to the physiology described below. Clinicians have been aware of IPH for some time yet despite best efforts at prevention, the incidence remains >30%. The National Institute for Health and Clinical Excellence (NICE) published guidelines in 2008 in an attempt to increase awareness of IPH and decrease its impact on postoperative morbidity.

Hyperthermia as a complication of anaesthesia is addressed at the end of this chapter.

Physiology of thermoregulation

Peripheral afferent cold and warm thermal sensors feed back to the central thermoregulator located in the anterior hypothalamus. The peripheral sensors are located on the skin surface, in deep thoracic and abdominal tissues, in the spinal cord as well as in other portions of the brain and the hypothalamus itself.

The hypothalamus controls the efferent outputs of thermoregulation that are closely controlled around an 'interthreshold range' (ITR) of approximately 0.2°C in humans (Figure 13.1).

In awake patients, behavioural changes (such as adjusting clothing) are mediated largely by thermal discomfort. Autonomic changes are mediated by low body temperature and result firstly in peripheral thermoregulatory vasoconstriction of the arterio-venous shunts at the skin surface. This maintains core temperature at the expense of cutaneous blood flow. Flow can be changed by a factor of 100 through these shunts. This does not result in haemodynamic changes since they only account for <10% of cardiac output. Any further decrease in temperature results in shivering that can increase metabolic heat production by 200%. All thermoregulatory responses are diminished to some extent in elderly patients (e.g. less muscle mass).

During general anaesthesia, all behavioural thermoregulatory compensation is ablated leaving the maintenance of core temperature to autonomic protection. These defences are

Anaesthetic and Perioperative Complications, ed. Kamen Valchanov, Stephen T. Webb and Jane Sturgess. Published by Cambridge University Press. © Cambridge University Press 2011.

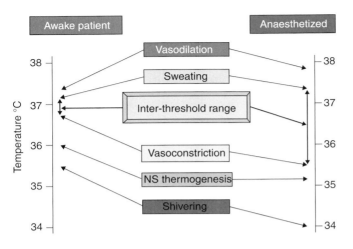

Figure 13.1 The large increase in the interthreshold range of autonomic control of body temperature homeostasis following induction of anaesthesia.

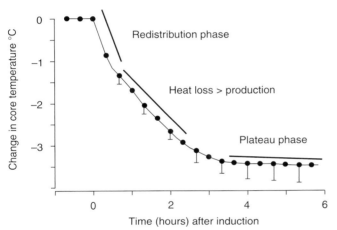

Figure 13.2 The triphasic drop in core temperature following induction of general anaesthesia.

greatly affected by anaesthesia, with the ITR being increased by a magnitude of up to 20. (Figure 13.1). The increase in range affects the response to cold more than the response to warmth (i.e. sweating and vasodilatation are better preserved). Patients become virtually poikilothermic over a temperature range of approximately 34 to 38°C. It is likely that these changes are due to central inhibition of thermoregulation although some peripheral inhibition may also occur. Any drug that acts as a peripheral vasodilator will have an added detrimental effect on thermoregulatory vasoconstriction.

Following induction of anaesthesia there is a triphasic drop in core temperature (Figure 13.2). Initially there is a rapid drop of up to 1.5°C, where inhibition of tonic thermoregulatory vasoconstriction results in a core to periphery redistribution of heat. Skin temperature may actually rise at this time. There follows a period of slower decrease in temperature where (radiative and convective) losses exceed heat production. A steady (plateau) state is then reached where heat loss equals heat production.

Regional anaesthesia results in ablation of tonic vasoconstriction below the level of any block and it is thought that some central inhibition may also occur, possibly as a result of a change in afferent input to the hypothalamus.

Causative and associated factors: why does perioperative hypothermia occur?

Lack of awareness

In a Europe-wide study published in 2007, it was found that only 25% of patients undergoing general anaesthesia and 6% of those having regional anaesthesia, routinely had temperature monitoring. In order to prevent IPH, clinicians need to know how widespread it is in their own practice. The National Institute for Health and Clinical Excellence has recommended recording core temperature every 30 minutes in all patients undergoing any type of anaesthesia.

Other factors affecting the incidence of IPH are as follows:

- ASA – Any grade greater than ASA I is a risk factor for IPH; the risk increases with ASA grade.
- Age – There is some evidence that the elderly are more at risk in terms of incidence of IPH and once cold they are at more risk of morbidity from the side effects and may take longer to rewarm. Children are at much higher risk of IPH due to their high surface area to weight ratio.
- Body morphology – Patients with a low BMI (less body fat) tend to have less heat insulation and thus more tonic thermoregulatory vasoconstriction. They may be at higher risk of IPH, especially if allowed to get cold pre-operatively. The opposite is true of patients with high BMI, where increased body weight may have a protective effect.
- Regional anaesthesia – Patients often feel warm due to vasodilatation, but they are at risk of IPH. Some central affect on thermoregulation is seen as well as direct peripheral vasodilatation. Warming should be used during regional anaesthesia. The patient can inform the clinician if they feel too hot so warming can be discontinued. Patients undergoing combined general and regional anaesthesia are at most risk of IPH.

Pre-operative core temperature

Some studies have shown that up to 10% of patients may have pre-induction temperatures less than 36°C. A low pre-operative temperature is a significant risk factor for IPH, since cold patients will have increased tonic vasoconstriction and subsequently more core heat redistribution as described above. Sedative premedication can affect patients' behavioural response to cold. If left in a cold environment pre-operatively they are more likely therefore to maintain their core temperature by further tonic vasoconstriction. Ideally, routine anaesthesia should not commence until the core temperature is >36°C. Pre-warming has been shown to be effective in such patients.

Type of surgery

Patients undergoing major or prolonged surgery with body cavities and major vessels exposed (e.g. major abdominal, thoracic, major vascular, hip arthroplasty) are at increased risk. These types of surgery are also more likely to need higher volumes of IV fluids and blood products, which if unwarmed can lead to a profound decrease in core temperature. Patients requiring urgent surgery are also at higher risk, as are those in whom large volumes of unwarmed irrigation fluid or intra-peritoneal gases are employed.

Theatre temperature

Low ambient temperatures predispose to IPH. Radiation losses are directly proportional to the fourth power of the patient-to-ambient temperature difference. This is of particularly significance in paediatric surgery and in short cases where other warming may not be used.

Complications of IPH

Prolonged drug action

All enzyme pathways in the body are temperature sensitive. The same is true of drug metabolism that relies on these enzymes.

Muscle relaxants

All relaxants are affected to some extent but vecuronium metabolism is affected the most. Duration of action is nearly doubled with mild (2°C) hypothermia.

Intravenous agents

Propofol concentration increases by 30% with a 3°C drop in temperature and plasma fentanyl concentration is increased by 5% for each degree drop.

Volatile anaesthetics

There is a 5% decrease in MAC for each degree drop in temperature. (Bispectral index drops by about 2 points for each °C drop in temperature.) Hypothermia also increases volatile solubility, so larger amounts need to be exhaled upon discontinuation.

Haematological disorders

Hypothermia results in a coagulopathy. Mild hypothermia (<1°C) significantly increases blood loss by 16% and increases the relative risk for transfusion by 22%. Platelet function is decreased due to structural changes and there is a reduction in the availability of platelet-activating factors such as thrombin. The coagulation cascade is delayed but this is not detected with standard tests since they are carried out at 37°C. Fibrinolysis appears to be unchanged, with clot formation alone being affected.

Cardiac complications

Postoperative hypothermia causes hypertension and tachycardia particularly in elderly patients. This is thought to be due to increases in norepinephrine levels, which lead to increased cardiac work and may augment cardiac irritability. The Perioperative Ischemia Randomized Anesthesia Trial Study Group in the United States has shown that patients with just 1.4°C of hypothermia have a three times higher risk of cardiac morbidity such as arrhythmias and ischaemia, especially in those patients with pre-existing coronary lesions.

Surgical site infections (SSI)

These are increased by up to 300% in patients with IPH. There is evidence that patients may also be at higher risk of decubitus ulcers. The mechanisms are thought to include tissue hypoxia secondary to thermoregulatory vasoconstriction. This is particularly important in the first few hours of bacterial contamination. It also leads to decreased collagen deposition.

Hypothermia also causes impaired immunity, mainly reflected by decreased neutrophil function.

Increased length of stay

Patients with IPH have been shown to stay longer in the recovery room and this is not simply because they take longer to achieve a core temperature of 36°C. They also stay longer in hospital, possibly as a result of an increase in SSIs and other postoperative complications.

Shivering

Shivering is an autonomic response that results in up to a two-fold increase in metabolic heat production. It can occur in normothermic patients. Patients sometimes complain that postoperative thermal discomfort is worse than surgical wound pain. Shivering also aggravates wound pain. Shivering interferes with monitoring (SpO_2, ECG and NIBP) and can result in a rise in intracranial and intraocular pressure. All cold patients (<36°C) must be warmed using forced air warming. Small doses of IV pethidine, alfentanyl, clonidine or doxapram can alleviate shivering.

Recognition: temperature measurement

In order to effectively detect and treat hypothermia, the clinician must understand body temperature homeostasis and correctly choose a device and site at which to measure it. Normal body temperature is best described as a range rather than an exact value for any one individual, and the site at which it is measured will affect the temperature recorded. Body temperature has a natural diurnal variation with an approximate 0.5°C higher reading in the afternoon. Temperature is also higher in women around the time of ovulation. Body temperature is also different at the extremes of age and tends to be lower in the elderly.

Site of measurement

The site of temperature measurement affects the accuracy of reading. The variation of core temperature at different sites is referred to as 'physiological offset'. Figure 13.3 summarizes the temperature variation at different body sites. Some thermometers automatically account for this offset by adding or subtracting a correction ('fudge factor') from the measured value when displaying the temperature measured. With any thermometer used it is essential that staff are trained in its use and understand any limitations the device may have.

For accurate perioperative temperature management it is important to record accurate and reliable core body temperature. This is most accurately measured using invasive methods but a number of non-invasive core temperature measuring devices also exist.

Invasive measurement

Core body temperature is most accurately measured using either a pulmonary artery catheter or a thermocouple placed on the tympanic membrane (direct tympanic measurement). Neither of these techniques is appropriate for routine intra-operative temperature measurement of all surgical patients. Acceptable alternatives closely reflecting core body temperature are: bladder temperature, distal oesophageal temperature and nasopharyngeal temperature (although this can be affected by airway gases).

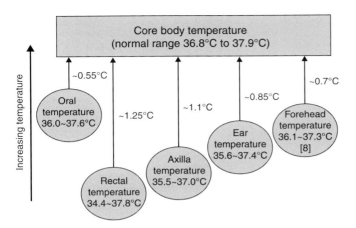

Figure 13.3 Temperature variation at different sites of measurement in healthy volunteers. (With permission from the Medicines and Healthcare Products Regulations Agency (MHRA) 04144, Thermometer Review: Evaluation, 2005).

Non-invasive measurement

A number of devices exist for non-invasive measurement of core body temperature at different anatomical sites.

One of the most commonly used devices is the infrared aural thermometer (indirect tympanic measurement). There are a number of limitations with this device. It is subject to incorrect use (inter-operator error) and misread if wax (or other matter) is present in the ear canal. One suggested way of improving the precision of this device is to measure the temperature in both ears, and record the higher of the two readings.

The most exact method for non-invasive core body temperature measurement is an electronic digital oral thermometer. The thermometer is placed in the sublingual pocket on either side of the mouth. Readings taken this way can be done in the intubated and ventilated patient.

The temporal artery thermometer is a more modern device, which in some studies has also been shown to correlate well with invasive core temperature measurements and is an alternative to oral measurement. Most published research with the device relates either to paediatrics or to patients in intensive care settings in whom sedatives might affect tonic thermoregulation. More research is therefore required before its accuracy and reliability for core temperature measurement can be confirmed in a more widespread population.

Frequency of measurement

Body temperature is a vital sign and should therefore be recorded. Current recommendations are that temperature should be recorded:

- prior to induction of anaesthesia
- continuously during the case (if this is not possible, then at a minimum of every 30 minutes throughout the case)
- every 15 minutes in the recovery room.

In our own practice we have found that patients who are maximally warmed rarely reach normothermia within the first hour of surgery. We therefore warm all patients according to the NICE guidelines but only routinely monitor those having operations lasting longer than one hour.

Pre-operative phase
- Assess each patient for their risk of inadvertent perioperative hypothermia (IPH).
- Commence forced air warming on all patients whose temperature is below 36°C.

Intra-operative phase
- The patient's temperature should be measured before induction of anaesthesia and then every 30 minutes until the end of surgery.
- Induction should not begin unless the patient's temperature is 36°C or above (unless urgent surgery).
- Intravenous fluids (500ml or more) and blood products should be warmed to 37°C using a fluid warming device.
- Patients at high risk of IPH and who are having anaesthesia for less than 30 minutes should be warmed intra-operatively from induction using a forced air warming device.
- All patients who are having anaesthesia for longer than 30 minutes should be warmed intra-operatively from induction using a forced air warming device.

Postoperative phase
- The patient's temperature should be measured on admission to the recovery room and then every 15 minutes. Warm if temperature < 36°C.

Figure 13.4 Summary of NICE guidelines from April 2008: prevention of inadvertent intra-operative hypothermia (IPH).

Prevention and treatment

Once the core temperature decreases it can take a considerable time to rewarm. To raise the core temperature from 35 to 36°C takes approximately two hours and a further one hour to reach 36.5°C. Undoubtedly perioperative maintenance of normothermia, prevention and treatment should be considered a high priority.The reduction in core body temperature associated with the induction of anaesthesia is due to:

- anaesthetic-induced inhibition of tonic thermoregulatory vasoconstriction
- redistribution of heat down the core-to-peripheral tissue temperature gradient.

Both of these mechanisms can be targeted pre-operatively to prevent inadvertent perioperative hypothermia (IPH) (Figure 13.4).

Pre-warming

Pre-warming the patient prior to anaesthesia with 30 to 60 minutes of forced air warming reduces the incidence of IPH. The technique works via two mechanisms:

- it decreases the normal core-to-peripheral temperature gradient
- the warm air provokes vasodilatation, and thus the induction of anaesthesia has relatively little effect since thermoregulatory vasoconstriction has already been defeated.

Pre-warming can be readily incorporated into pre-operative practice on the admission ward and a number of specifically designed forced warm-air devices are now available. Additional benefits are that venous cannulation is easier secondary to the induced vasodilatation and the same disposable warming blanket can be used for intra-operative warming in order to minimize extra costs.

Pharmacological methods

Administration of drugs abolishing normal thermoregulatory vasoconstriction well before the induction of anaesthesia, facilitates heat distribution from the core to the periphery. As the patient is not anaesthetized they are still able to mount a thermoregulatory response to generate and conserve sufficient heat to maintain their core temperature. This technique has been demonstrated with oral nifedipine given 12 and 1.5 hours prior to surgery.

A number of other pharmacological techniques have been tried in research trials looking to prevent IPH. These have included:

- amino acid and fructose infusions given in the perioperative period
- intra-operative administration of an alpha$_1$-adrenergic antagonist, urapidil.

There is currently insufficient evidence to routinely recommend either of the above two interventions.

General measures

There are a number of general measures that should be taken whenever possible for all patients in an effort to reduce the incidence of IPH:

- Pre-warm patients with a core temperature ≤36°C one hour before anaesthesia.
- Anaesthesia should not be commenced for elective surgery if the patient's core temperature is below 36°C.
- Ensure patients are kept comfortably warm whilst waiting for surgery. This includes encouraging them to wear additional warm clothing including dressing gowns and slippers. Patients should be encouraged to walk to the operating theatre when able.
- Ambient operating theatre temperature should be at least 21°C while the patient is exposed (it can be reduced once intra-operative warming is established to ensure staff comfort).
- The patient should be adequately covered throughout the intra-operative phase.
- All irrigation fluids used intra-operatively should be warmed to 38–40°C.

Intravenous fluid warming

A unit of refrigerated blood or one litre of crystalloid solution administered at room temperature decreases mean body temperature by approximately 0.25°C. Heat loss becomes significant even if small volumes of blood or fluid are being given. All IV fluid given should therefore be warmed to 37°C via one of the many available warming devices on the market. No one device shows any significant clinical advantage for routine clinical cases. Fluid taken from a warming cabinet at 41°C and administered within 30 minutes is equally effective. It should be noted that fluid warming alone does not keep patients normothermic and will not warm them to any important degree.

Passive insulation

A single layer of passive insulation reduces heat loss by about 30%. There is little difference in efficacy among insulators routinely available in the operating theatre (e.g. cotton or reflective blankets). There is little benefit in adding additional layers as it is the layer of still air under the first blanket that provides the majority of the insulation. Passive insulation at best can reduce cutaneous heat loss to zero but in practice rarely reduces heat loss by even 50%. It may be suitable for short cases lasting less than 30 minutes to limit the degree of IPH, but for longer cases or higher risk patients, active warming methods will be required.

Active warming

Current best practice evidence from NICE suggests that intra-operative forced air warming should be commenced for all patients whose expected duration of anaesthesia is greater than 30 minutes. It is worth noting here that not many operations last less than 30 minutes when anaesthetic time is included. Those patients at high risk of IPH should be actively warmed from induction even if their anaesthetic is of less than 30 minutes' duration. Patients should be managed as high risk if two or more of the following apply:

- ASA grade II to V (the higher the grade, the greater the risk)
- pre-operative temperature below 36°C
- undergoing combined general and regional anaesthesia
- undergoing major or intermediate surgery
- at risk of cardiovascular complications.

Comparison of active warming devices

The efficacy of surface warming devices depends on heat transfer per unit area and the total surface area used for rewarming. In clinical practice there is usually at least a 30-minute delay to the onset of core rewarming with any method chosen. This delay results from the time necessary to transfer heat from the skin surface to the body's core compartments. A number of different methods for active cutaneous warming are available for clinical use.

Forced air warming (FAW)

The active heating effects of forced air warming have been well proven over many years. It is relatively cheap and safe although it should not be applied to ischaemic tissues. The efficacy of all warming devices is proportional to the surface area available for heating. The use of surgical access blankets and under-body FAW may go some way to alleviating this problem. The warm air is distributed further than the extent of the actual warming blanket. To date this is the most widespread patient warming system. There have been some concerns relating to surgical wound contamination and infection as a result of FAW but these have been unfounded. Regular servicing of the air unit and changing the filters is required. Some units do not default to warm-air settings. When turning on FAW, a setting of 38°C or above should be selected. Blowing ambient temperature air onto patients leads to heat loss.

After surgery is finished, the same warming blanket can be taken to recovery for any further warming required.

Under-body circulating-water or electrical mattresses

These devices are placed under the patient on the operating table. Their efficacy is limited by a number of factors, which renders them less effective at preventing or treating hypothermia. The back is a relatively small fraction of the total skin surface area and approximately 90% of heat is lost from the anterior surface of the body. Blood flow is restricted in dependent capillaries, which limits the amount of heat that the body can absorb. The temperature of the mattress must be carefully regulated since they have been associated with increased risk of pressure-heat necrosis and burns. Newer pressure-relieving (resistive) mattresses are also available. They could help to decrease the incidence of IPH, but sufficient evidence for their use as a substitute for FAW is yet to emerge.

Overbody resistive heating

These devices are reusable and need careful disinfection between cases. They are linked to an electrically efficient (and silent) control box. Some are multipart devices. Heat exchange relies on close contact with the patient's skin so incorrect placement will lead to poor heat transfer. In some surgical procedures, many blankets can be linked to cover most exposed areas. This can, however, lead to an array of wires. The use of these devices has a mixed evidence base to date. Some trials have shown them to be as effective as FAW but others, in whom limited patient access is available, have found that they are less effective. Overall, despite the fact that their use would save on disposables and electrical running costs, these devices are less popular.

Hyperthermia

Intra-operative hyperthermia (>38°C) is a surprisingly rare yet potentially life-threatening complication. The low incidence of intra-operative fever occurs as a consequence of the impairment of thermoregulation by anaesthesia that has the potential to decrease core body temperature during surgery in febrile patients. It results in part from dose dependent inhibition of fever by volatile anaesthetics, opioids and neuromuscular blocking agents inhibiting shivering. Patients should be kept well hydrated.

Intra-operative hyperthermia can be caused by:

- malignant hyperthermia
- thyroid storm
- neuroleptic malignant syndrome
- drugs (ecstasy, cocaine)
- sepsis
- blood in 4th ventricle
- iatrogenic.

Iatrogenic (over-heating) occurs frequently in prolonged procedures with little blood loss. Warming should be temporarily switched off in such cases, when temperature is rising past approximately 36.4°C. Often it will continue to further increase.

Hyperthermia can be treated by blowing ambient air onto the patient from an FAW device. Other options include wet sheets, ice over the major vessels and more recent innovations such as cold-water garments and IV cooling.

Malignant hyperthermia

Malignant hyperthermia (MH) is a rare congenital disturbance of calcium regulation in skeletal muscle caused by volatile anaesthetics and the depolarizing agent suxamethonium. If left untreated, malignant hyperthermia is usually lethal. The earliest signs are tachycardia, hypercapnoea and muscle rigidity. The increased body temperature during malignant hyperthermia is caused by a huge increase in metabolic heat production resulting from uncontrolled calcium release in skeletal muscles.

Treatment must be instituted rapidly on clinical suspicion of the onset of malignant hyperthermia and includes:

- discontinuation of the trigger agent
- administration of intravenous Dantrolene
- supportive therapy directed at correcting hyperthermia, acidosis and organ dysfunction.

Thyroid storm

A thyroid storm, or thyrotoxic crisis, is an acute exacerbation of the hyperthyroid state caused by the sudden release of T3 or T4, or both, into the circulation. It is characterized by fever, tachycardia, agitation, shock and cardiac failure. Muscle rigidity as seen in MH is not a feature. It is most commonly seen in patients with thyrotoxicosis secondary to Graves' disease who are undergoing treatment, but can occur in newly diagnosed patients. It has an incidence of approximately 10% in patients hospitalized for thyrotoxicosis. The onset is usually 6 to 24 hours after surgery, but it can occur intra-operatively mimicking malignant hyperthermia.Treatment follows four principles:

- correction of precipitating events
- reducing the secretion and production of thyroid hormones, e.g. sodium iodide, propylthiouracil
- diminishing the metabolic effects of circulating thyroid hormones by beta-blockade
- general supportive care and resuscitation.

Neuroleptic malignant syndrome

Neuroleptic malignant syndrome is a rare idiosyncratic reaction to antipsychotic drugs. It is clinically similar to malignant hyperthermia and is characterized by fever, muscle rigidity and autonomic instability triggered by the use of phenothiazines, tricyclic antidepressants and monoamine oxidase inhibitors. Patients taking haloperidol and chlorpromazine are thought to be at greatest risk. It can also occur after sudden withdrawal of dopamine agonists. Rhabdomyolysis can lead to a raised plasma creatinine kinase (CK).

Hyperthermia should be aggressively treated. Any precipitating drugs should be stopped and close observation and support of renal function instigated.

List of further reading

Frank, S. M., Fleisher, L. A., Breslow, M. J. *et al.* Perioperative maintenance of normothermia reduces the incidence of morbid cardiac events. A randomized clinical trial. *JAMA* 1997, **277**(14): 1127–34.

Lenhardt, R., Grady, M. & Kurz, A. Hyperthermia during anaesthesia and intensive care unit stay. *Best Pract Res Clin Anaesthesiol* 2008; **22**: 669–94.

National Collaborating Centre for Nursing and Supportive Care commissioned by National Institute for Health and Clinical Excellence (NICE). Clinical practice guideline. The management of inadvertent perioperative hypothermia in adults. April 2008. www. nice.org.uk/nicemedia/pdf/CG65Guidance. pdf (accessed 15 April 2011).

Rajagopalan, S., Mascha, E., Na, J. & Sessler, D. I. The effects of mild perioperative hypothermia on blood loss and transfusion requirement: a meta-analysis. *Anesthesiology* 2008; **108**: 71–7.

Sessler, D. I. Complications and treatment of mild hypothermia. *Anesthesiology* 2001; **95**: 531–43.

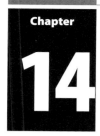

Chapter

14

Equipment malfunction

Rajinikanth Sundararajan and Peter Faber

Introduction

During the last five decades anaesthetic equipment has evolved from simple, manual devices to advanced, comprehensive workstations incorporating anaesthesia delivery and patient monitoring. Such technological advancement has followed the general medico-technical development of ever-more sophisticated equipment contributing to improvements in patient health and safety. However, notwithstanding the development and introduction of evermore technologically advanced equipment failure and malfunction of medical devices continue to occur. Hence improvements in patient safety, related to the interaction with medical equipment, may not have enjoyed a parallel, upward trajectory together with the technological advances of equipment. In England in 2009, approximately 9,000 medical device-related adverse events were reported to the Medicines and Healthcare Products Regulatory Agency (MHRA) – an almost 37% increase compared with a decade ago. Additionally, every year approximately 400 patient episodes are reported and investigated by the National Patient Safety Agency (NPSA) due to severe harm or death associated with failure of medical devices. Inherent equipment problems such as faults in manufacture, design, quality and packaging and human error have contributed equally towards two-thirds of the incidents. In the remaining one-third of cases no association was found between the critical incident and the equipment used during patient contact. These numbers emphasize the increasingly important link between the sophistication of medical devices and the ongoing need for comprehensive training preceding the clinical introduction of novel equipment.

Definitions

Most often critical incidents related to anaesthetic equipment cannot be solely ascribed to a single contributory factor and the majority of adverse events are a combination of human factors and equipment failure. The following two definitions assist in the apportioning of human error and equipment malfunction towards an adverse event:

- Equipment failure: The device is faulty and malfunctions in spite of proper use and maintenance.
  - Example: Ventilator suddenly fails to ventilate the lungs due to circuitry board failure.
- Equipment misuse: Medical device is working as per manufacturer's instructions, but malfunctioning is caused by human error, including improper preparation, maintenance and usage of the equipment.
  - Example: Ventilator malfunctions due to misassembled tubes and connections.

Anaesthetic and Perioperative Complications, ed. Kamen Valchanov, Stephen T. Webb and Jane Sturgess.
Published by Cambridge University Press. © Cambridge University Press 2011.

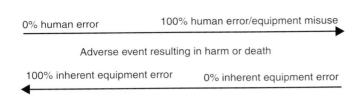

Figure 14.1 Relative contribution of human error and equipment malfunction to adverse events.

Because the above terms are inter-related the exact incidence of equipment malfunction in each category is difficult to assess and may be best illustrated by the diagram shown in Figure 14.1.

Anaesthetic equipment failure attributed to solely a technical breakdown is an uncommon event and unlikely to result in severe patient harm or death. A report, examining a five-year period, revealed the frequency of 'pure equipment problems' as 0.23% in general anaesthesia and 0.05% in regional anaesthesia. However, pure equipment failure still contributes up to 9% of the total anaesthetic adverse events as published in an Australian incident monitoring study. These numbers have been reproduced by a French safety database study reporting that 9% of device-related incidents resulted in severe harm defined as extended hospitalization, the requirement of (re)operation or causing permanent disability or death respectively. Anaesthetic equipment is increasingly complex but in the majority of cases remains reliable when maintained and used according to the manufacturer's instructions.

Operating theatres and critical care

The interface between operator and medical device remains the most frequent cause of critical incidents. For the years 2008 to 2010 approximately one-third of the total anaesthetic incidents reported to Safe Anaesthesia Liaison Group (SALG) were related to equipment – either as single primary cause or in combination with operator error. Most incidents occur in relation to the provision of general anaesthesia in the operating theatre. In the critical care setting equipment-related problems resulting in significant harm are uncommon. This may be due to either under-reporting or differences in operational procedures and policies between critical care and theatres. However, proportionally more patient safety incidents, namely 50% of all NPSA reports received from critical care, are related to equipment failure. Not surprisingly, equipment misuse was more likely to be associated with harm to patients compared with equipment failure due to other causes. Such statistics again emphasize the requirement for proper and maintained staff training in the operation of medical devices.

Considering the abundance and complexity of general and specific medical devices for anaesthesia and critical care it is unfeasible to describe all possible permutations of equipment malfunction. The following sections will provide an overview of commonly occurring equipment problems and how to address these to ensure continued patient safety.

The modern anaesthetic machine

The purpose of the modern anaesthetic machine is principally to:
1. provide and maintain adequate patient oxygenation and ventilation during anaesthesia
2. provide an accurate mixture of anaesthetic gases
3. provide patient monitoring.

Table 14.1 Medical gas supply pressures, size E cylinder.

Medical gas	Pressure in kPa
Oxygen	13,700
Nitrous oxide	4,400
Entonox	13,700
Air	13,700

Oxygenation and ventilation

Gas supply

Anaesthesia gas delivery systems form a pivotal component of the anaesthetic machine and constitute a complex design with a multitude of parts. Hence, the gas delivery system is associated with more critical incidents and severe patient injuries than any other component of the anaesthetic machine. Anaesthesia gas delivery systems were associated with 2% of the total claims reported to the American Society of Anesthesiologists (ASA). Most incidents were due to equipment misuse resulting in inadequate oxygen delivery causing irreversible brain damage and death in 3 to 5% of total anaesthesia claims.

High-pressure systems

Medical gas cylinders and central pipeline systems are the usual source of medical gas supplies. In most hospitals oxygen, air and nitrous oxide are supplied through a pipeline system. In the UK separate oxygen cylinders are mandatory backups in the theatre environment. Accessory cylinders should always be kept closed during normal pipeline supply because in the event of pipeline failure the cylinder source, if kept open, would be emptied before activation of the oxygen failure alarm. Subsequently, the oxygen failure alarm would be activated only after the accessory oxygen cylinders had been depleted.

The working gas supply pressures from the central pipeline and cylinder source should be displayed prominently on the anaesthetic machine or cylinder pressure gauges (Table 14.1).

The outlet pressure of all piped medical gas supply (O_2, N_2O and medical air) is approximately 400 kPa. Surgical air supply pressure is 700 kPa.

Gas supply failure and cross-connections of pipelines can cause severe permanent patient harm or death. Fortunately, cross-connections are very rare after the standard introduction of safety colour-coding, cylinder pin-index systems and non-interchangeable screw-thread (NIST) connections. Still, from 2000 to 2010 six deaths were reported due to accidental nitrous oxide contamination into oxygen gas delivery systems. Further away from operating theatres, misconnections of central hospital pipeline gas supply and failures can contribute to erroneous gas supply to the patient. Nitrogen purging of the central gas pipelines is carried out as a part of the regular servicing to remove the particulate debris collected on the walls of the pipeline system over a period of time. This type of pipeline servicing is known to have resulted in hypoxic brain injury to patients when nitrogen inadvertently has been purged into the central oxygen supplies.

In the case of pipeline misconnection the cylinder source would not be used unless the pipeline pressure is lower than the down-regulated cylinder pressure. The oxygen pressure failure alarm may not detect pipeline cross-connections as the alarm will be disengaged by the pressure of the erroneous gas supply. To circumvent such undetected failures in central oxygen supply an oxygen analyzer connected to an audible alarm has to be fitted at the common gas outlet on the anaesthetic machine. However, as such sensors are easily disconnected or concentration levels reset, the anaesthetic machines can still deliver a hypoxic gas mixture or contaminated oxygen without activating any oxygen failure alarm.

Low-pressure systems

The low-pressure system is from the second-stage pressure regulator on the anaesthetic machine to the common gas outlet. This includes the flow-meter system, vaporizers and in-between connections. Leaks can present anywhere along this line and result in low fresh gas flows. The most common causes for the bobbins to stick in the traditional flow-meters are dirt and static electricity. This may result in the delivery of inaccurate gas flows. Conventional anaesthetic machines have filters and antistatic material to overcome this problem. Cracks in flow-meters and trans-positioned flow-meter tubing are also known causes of equipment malfunction. To help overcome these problems newer generation anaesthetic machines have digital flow-meters. Though increasingly rare, gas flow-related equipment failures cannot be excluded even with modern anaesthetic machines where the complexity of the machines makes it increasingly difficult to trouble-shoot any unexpected faults.

Oxygen analyzers and oxygen failure alarms have greatly helped to prevent the delivery of hypoxic gas mixtures and both devices are mandatory parts of the anaesthetic machine. The Association of Anaesthetists of Great Britain and Ireland (AAGBI) insists the presence of alternative means of oxygenation and ventilation (self-inflating bag, oxygen cylinder, circuit) should at all times be readily available to manage accidental machine failure.

Breathing systems

Breathing systems contribute repeatedly to a high number of equipment-related events. Disconnections, leaks, misconnections and occlusions are common, pertaining to multiple interconnected disposable components like humidifiers, filters, catheter mounts and gas analyzers.

An analysis of 2,000 critical incidents in Australia revealed that 90% of events related to ventilation were due to either breathing-circuit disconnections or misconnections. Disconnection was the commonest cause for not being able to facilitate safe ventilation. In one-third of the cases, third-party interference was the reason for disconnection; mainly during surgery to the head or neck. A significant proportion of the disconnections were not detected by monitors alone. In two-thirds of disconnections, the low-pressure disconnect alarm was not triggered.

Within the circle breathing systems, malfunctions of unidirectional valves are the most frequently reported problems. During low-flow anaesthesia faulty unidirectional valves can result in hypoxaemic injury and hypercapnia due to rebreathing of carbon dioxide. Leaks within the circle breathing system are a common occurrence due to improperly fitted soda-lime canisters and the loss and wear of rubber seals.

Though disconnections are the predominant error associated with the breathing system, misconnections were equally common in the closed claim analysis of the ASA claims database. Misconnections can result in a sudden high airway pressure progressing rapidly to iatrogenic initiated tension pneumothorax. In contrast to disconnections, where the evolution of the outcome is slowly evolving, misconnections can progress very rapidly allowing less time for the clinicians to respond. For example breathing systems have mistakenly been connected to auxiliary gas outlets resulting in significant harm to patients. Even scavenging systems have been involved in misconnections with reports of the scavenging port (expiratory valve) of a Mapleson-D circuit mistakenly being connected to the common gas outlet resulting in no fresh gas flow.

The oxygen flush valve on the anaesthetic machine delivers oxygen at 35 to 75 litres per minute. With prolonged activation of the oxygen flush valve during mechanical ventilation, excessive airway pressure may cause lung injury. Protruding oxygen flush valves have accidentally been held open by anaesthetic staff. Although modern designs of anaesthetic machines incorporate a protective collar around the valve to avoid this user error, the accidental activation of oxygen flush valves in the fully or partially open position still happens and can result in patient awareness due to dilution of anaesthetic gases.

The standard oxygen reservoir bag will protect anaesthetized patients by limiting the pressure in the breathing system to rise beyond approximately 40 cmH$_2$0. The automated pressure limiting (APL) valve is another important part of the breathing system used to regulate the expired gas flows from the patient during spontaneous breathing and manually controlled ventilation. In modern anaesthetic machines the APL valve will open to the atmosphere if pressure inside the breathing system exceeds 60 cmH$_2$0. Failure of the APL valve allowing high-pressure build up can happen due to water condensation within the valve resulting in a permanently closed position. Additionally, the valve can fail due to breakage of the internal spring.

In 2004, the Department of Health published a guideline: *Protecting the Breathing Circuits in Anaesthesia* following 13 severe incidents related to breathing-system obstruction. Detailed analysis of the incidents revealed that foreign bodies in the breathing system were the most common cause of obstruction, predominantly in catheter mounts. The variety of foreign bodies identified were disposable protective caps from intravenous-giving sets, caps from arterial blood gas sampling syringes, breathing filter caps, small pieces of rubber or sticky tape. The guidelines emphasize the importance of keeping the package of the breathing system intact until use to avoid the accidental spillage of foreign bodies into any parts of the system. Co-axial breathing circuit obstructions due to kinking of internal tube and external pressure have been well documented. Defective electronic switch selectors between manual and automated ventilation have also been reported as a cause of critically low gas flows to the patient, as the fresh gas flow can leak to atmosphere from the breathing circuit while the patient is attached to an automated ventilator.

Breathing systems are continually revised and redesigned with additions like filters, sampling lines for anaesthetic gas monitoring, catheter mounts, angle pieces and tracheal tube connectors. All these supplements and extensions of the breathing system multiply the likelihood of adverse events occurring. For example, filters amplify the complexity of the breathing system and continue to be a common source for adverse events. Blocked heat and moist exchange filters have been associated with life-threatening complications including airway obstruction and high peak airway pressures resulting in tension pneumothorax.

Disconnections at the junction of an endotracheal tube and filters have also been reported to result in critical incidents. In general, leaks within the breathing systems occur more frequently at the distal patient end; between endotracheal or tracheostomy tube connections compared with proximal machine disconnections. Breathing systems completely integrated with the anaesthesia machine, would simplify the need for the user to configure the system before use and thus contribute to the elimination of human error in the failure of correctly connecting the breathing system. Acknowledging the potential for serious harm to patients, rigorous checks of the anaesthesia breathing system, such as those published by the AAGBI, include the following procedures:

- Inspect and manually check the configuration and assembly of connections.
- Check the functioning of all mechanical components of the breathing system (unidirectional valve, adjustable exhaust valve).
- Check all connectors, such as filter, angle piece and catheter mount, for leaks and ensure good flow.
- Prepare and confirm functioning of monitors (calibration, enabling alarms).
- Ensure the back-up ventilation mode is available.
- Specific tests including pressure leak tests are also recommended.
- Standard connectors of internal diameter 15 mm male and 22 mm female are used in breathing system and 30 mm connectors are mandatory for the scavenging system.

Ventilators

Mechanical ventilators are an integral component of modern anaesthetic machines although free-standing older style ventilators (e.g. Manley and Penlon) may still be found in many anaesthetic rooms. An integrated design of ventilator and anaesthetic machine provides fewer opportunities for the user to be involved in the configuration of the ventilator. This set-up should reduce human errors like mis- and disconnections. Contemporary anaesthetic ventilators with integrated alarms have the ability to measure flow, volume, pressure and analyze gas composition – all of which should promote patient safety. However, despite these advances, ventilators along with breathing systems remain a frequent source of severe harm and death to patients. Repeatedly, equipment misuse and human error are the most likely cause of these serious events compared with inherent device failure. Inappropriate alarm settings and silenced alarms on ventilators can additionally result in untoward consequences to the patient. It has been reported that a majority of anaesthetists incorrectly set the ventilator disconnection alarm limits, and hence the alarms would not have been activated during disconnections.

As previously discussed, the increased complexity and integration of a ventilator within the anaesthetic machine in order to eliminate the potential for human error can also make it more difficult to diagnose and correct equipment failure. For example, leaks from flow-sensors can be extremely difficult to identify as the sensors may be hidden within the anaesthetic machine. Poor preparation and inadequate machine checks prior to commencing anaesthesia have all been associated with failure to detect preventable incidents – e.g. power failure, non-functioning unidirectional valves and leaking ventilator bellows.

Similar to the APL valve of the anaesthetic breathing system, the incorporated pressure-relief valves within anaesthetic machines have been found to fail and result in high airway pressures. The anaesthetic gas scavenging system (AGSS) works in coordination with the ventilator pressure-relief valves ensuring the waste anaesthetic gas mixture is released to the atmosphere. Anaesthetic gas scavenging system transfer tubes incorporate a standard 30 mm female connector to be attached with either the breathing system APL or ventilator pressure-relief valve. The positive and negative pressure-release valves within the scavenging system protect against excessive alterations in pressure during ventilation. Failure of the positive pressure-relief valve can result in increased airway pressure. Anaesthetic gas scavenging system transfer tubing should be armoured to prevent any accidental obstruction.

Vaporizers

Over the past few decades, anaesthetic vaporizers have undergone regular design modifications to improve the safety profile along with other aspects of the anaesthetic machine. Control knob changes, agent-specific calibration, Selectatec interlocking system, colour-coded and geometric specific filling system are some of the changes aimed at reducing user errors. Temperature-sensitive bimetallic strips, wicks, bypass channels and copper-built vaporizers are all but few of the safety features included to ensure accurate delivery of anaesthetic vapour.

When not attached to the back bar of the anaesthetic machine vaporizers should be kept upright. If the vaporizer is tilted there is a risk of accidental spillage of anaesthetic liquid into the inspiratory limb or bypass channel of the vaporizer. When re-attached the vaporizer may accidentally deliver an erroneously high concentration of anaesthetic agent. Anti-spill systems present in some of the current vaporizers can prevent these accidents. If accidental tilting is suspected, it is recommended to purge the vaporizer with 5 litres/minute of fresh gas flow for about 30 minutes at dial settings of 5% vented to atmosphere.

The Selectatec interlocking system present on the back bar of anaesthetic machines physically prevents the use of more than one vaporizer at any one time. However, the interlocking system is not failsafe and failure may lock one vaporizer in an open position during the concomitant use of a second vaporizer. Inappropriately seated vaporizers on the back bar are another common source of leaks and may result in inadequate anaesthetic agent delivery with resultant patient awareness. Multiple safety features like colour-coding and specific geometric key patterns for both vaporizers and filling bottles have been developed to avoid filling the vaporizers with the wrong anaesthetic agent.

Intravenous infusion devices

Infusion systems are widely used in anaesthesia, pain and critical care. The Medicines and Healthcare Products Regulatory Agency categorizes infusion systems into three groups based on (i) drug therapeutics, (ii) patient group and (iii) clinical performance parameters, to help in choosing the appropriate infusion device. Although a common core of safety parameters apply across the groups, each group has specific requirements for use in clinical practice. Human error is consistently the major contributor to equipment failure of intravenous infusion devices. An analysis of the French anaesthesia safety database exposed approximately 50% of the device-related adverse events in anaesthesia and intensive care were related to infusion devices and almost one in three were due to inappropriate use. Such statistics are reproduced within the UK where infusion systems are the most common source of adverse events. Notably, the frequency of adverse events related to infusion systems is higher in the critical care setting as compared with perioperative use. If the design of the equipment is overly complex and not fit for purpose such circumstances may be defined as equipment failure – even if the device works according to the manufacturer's instructions (Table 14.2).

Monitoring equipment

An essential part of modern anaesthesia is the simple, yet comprehensive, display and continued monitoring of patient physiological parameters. Monitoring equipment

Table 14.2 Problems related to infusion devices.

Problem	Cause
Human errors	
Rate and concentration calculations	Lack of understanding
Setting up errors, e.g. multiple infusions, siphonage, air entrapment	Poor training, lack of support
Incorrect label/record	Poor communication
Technical errors	
Power failure, incorrect infusion rate	Design faults, poor maintenance
Failure of pressure limitation	–

enhances the senses of the anaesthetist by conveying objective clinical information. Thus, studies have repeatedly acknowledged the benefits to patient safety with reductions in morbidity and mortality by the application of modern monitoring equipment. However, although modern anaesthesia is reliant on monitoring equipment, it remains the task of the anaesthetist to interpret the abundance of information – hence the requirements for an anaesthetist to be present at all times during anaesthesia. Additionally, it is not uncommon for monitoring equipment to fail. Frequently reported problems are failure of non-invasive blood pressure equipment, gas analyzers, capnographs, pulse oximeters, oxygen analyzers, ECG and devices for temperature measurement. Those are the most frequently used types of patient monitoring equipment and the high failure rate is likely a reflection of their abundance in clinical practice, heavy use and insufficient maintenance and calibration.

Regional anaesthesia

Equipment failure has also been reported in cases relating to regional anaesthetic techniques. Most incidents relate to indwelling catheters used for the continuous delivery of local anaesthetics and opioids. Erroneous delivery of local anaesthetics into intravenous catheters when epidural delivery was intended, has been partly blamed on equipment design such as the lack of safeguards, e.g. Luer locks and safety locking devices, permitting the wrong attachments to be made between infusion pumps and catheters.

Reporting incidents associated with equipment failure

In the UK critical incidents associated with medical equipment should be reported to the following national organizations:

- National Patient Safety Agency (NPSA)
- Medicines and Healthcare Products Regulatory Agency (MHRA)
- Health and Safety Executive, Department of Health.

In addition a local reporting system may be in place facilitating a fast response and review of the equipment in question. Most reporting systems and organizations allow online reporting and regular safety guidelines, alerts and bulletins are published by the NPSA, MHRA, the Royal College of Anaesthetists and the Safe Anaesthesia Liaison Group (SALG).

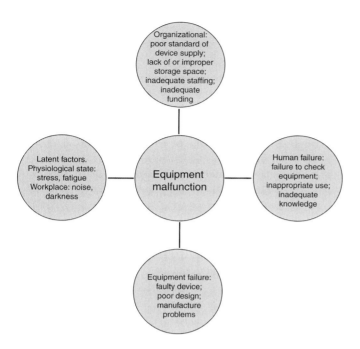

Figure 14.2 Contributory factors to equipment malfunction.

Prevention of equipment failure

It is widely acknowledged that the majority of equipment failures occur at the human–equipment interface. In order to reduce the risk of human error contributing to equipment failure, medical devices are all carefully designed. The evaluation of device usability and comparison of different types of equipment remains difficult to qualify. Recognizing these difficulties, the AAGBI has published guidelines on the safe management of anaesthesia-related equipment. These guidelines comprehensively encompass the procurement of medical equipment, maintenance, storage and replacement. The choice and introduction of new equipment should primarily be based on device safety, performance and quality. Protocols outlining the correct use of the equipment, staff training, device maintenance and safety testing should be produced prior to the introduction of new medical devices.

As with human errors and accidents, a device failure is most often caused by the alignment of several contributing factors. This is illustrated in Figure 14.2.

Only by recognizing the individual factors and their contribution to device failure is it possible to continue to improve patient safety and introduce evermore complex equipment into clinical care.

List of further reading

AAGBI. *Safe Management of Anaesthesia Related Equipment*. AAGBI, 2009.

Al-Shaikh, B. & Stacey, S. (eds) *Essentials of Anaesthetic Equipment*, 3rd edn. Churchill Livingston, 2007.

Beydon, L., Ledenmat, P. Y., Soltner, C. *et al.* Adverse events with medical devices in Anaesthesia and Intensive Care unit patients recorded in the French safety database in 2005–6.

Anaesthesiology 2010; **112**(2):
364–72.

Caplan, R. A., Vistica, M. F., Posner,
K. L. & Cheney, F. W. Adverse
anaesthetic outcomes arising from
gas delivery equipment: a closed
claims analysis. *Anesthesiology* 1997; **87**:
741–8.

MRHA. Safety warnings. www.mhra.gov.uk/
Publications/Safetywarnings/ (accessed 15
April 2011).

National Patient Safety Agency. Patient
safety alert 004A. Safer epidural,
spinal and regional devices, NPSA 2009.

National Patient Safety Agency. Patient safety
alert 004B. Safer epidural, spinal and
regional devices, NPSA 2009.

Thomas, A. N. & Galvin, I. Patient safety
incidents associated with equipment
in critical care: a review of reports to
the UK National Patient Safety Agency.
Anaesthesia 2008; **63**: 1193–7.

Webb, R. K., Russell, W. J., Klepper, I. &
Runciman, W. B. The Australian
Incident Monitoring Study. Equipment
failure: an analysis of 2000 incident
reports. *Anaesth Intens Care* 1993; **21**(5):
673–7.

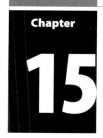

Chapter

Drug reactions

Alison Kavanagh and Martin Shields

Definition

An adverse drug reaction is defined as an unwanted or harmful reaction following the administration of a drug or combination of drugs under normal conditions of use, which is suspected to be related to the drug. Adverse drug reactions that occur during anaesthesia are a potential source of morbidity and mortality. Their incidence is difficult to determine due to under-recognition and under-reporting.

Classification

Adverse drug reactions have been classified in various ways. Rawlins and Thompson (1977) classified drug reactions as Type A or Type B. Type A reactions are an exaggerated response to a drug, the nature of which is predictable from the known pharmacology of the drug and is usually dose dependent. An example would include hypotension following the first dose of an angiotensin converting enzyme inhibitor. Type B reactions are not dose dependent, and are unpredictable given the known drug pharmacology. An example is anaphylaxis following penicillin administration.

The Rawlins and Thompson classification has been extended and modified to include Types C (dose and time dependent), D (delayed reactions), E (withdrawal reactions) and F (failure of treatment). Problems with this classification system are that some drug reactions can fall into one or more categories. Other adverse reactions can depend on both the dose and duration of treatment. Finally, some reactions do not occur in all patients, such as the exacerbation of asthma by NSAIDs. Aranson and Ferner (2003) have proposed a new classification, which takes into account the dose, timing and patient susceptibility to the drug reaction. This new classification aims to help drug development and management of adverse reactions.

Within anaesthesia adverse drug reactions are common, ranging from mild hypotension induced by hypnotics to life-threatening reactions such as anaphylaxis or malignant hyperpyrexia. The following sections aim to discuss the significant drug reactions encountered in anaesthetic practice.

Anaphylaxis

Anaphylaxis is a severe, life-threatening, generalized or systemic hypersensitivity reaction. It may be categorized as allergic or non-allergic, although the clinical features may be identical. Allergic anaphylaxis can be further subdivided into IgE-mediated and non-IgE-mediated.

Anaesthetic and Perioperative Complications, ed. Kamen Valchanov, Stephen T. Webb and Jane Sturgess. Published by Cambridge University Press. © Cambridge University Press 2011.

The incidence of perioperative allergic anaphylaxis is between 1:9,000 and 1:20,000, with a mortality rate between 3.5 and 4.7%. A further 2% of patients are left with permanent neurological deficits. Death or permanent disability can be prevented by early recognition and prompt treatment. The recognition and treatment of anaphylaxis is deemed to be of such high importance that protocols for the management of suspected anaphylaxis form an integral part of training for anaesthetists.

Pathogenesis

Exposure to an allergen in susceptible individuals results in sensitization. The exact mechanisms that induce sensitivity are unknown. Upon re-exposure the allergen then binds to IgE receptors on the surface of circulating basophils or mast cells in connective tissue. Anaphylaxis generally occurs on the second exposure to an allergen, but can also occur after the first exposure because of cross-reactivity between many drugs and other substances.

When two or more IgE receptors are cross-linked by allergen mast cells degranulation occurs releasing pre-formed inflammatory mediators including histamine, heparin and mast cell tryptase. This gives rise to the classical symptoms of anaphylaxis discussed later. Newly formed mediators are also synthesized and released following IgE-mediated mast cell activation including leukotrienes, prostaglandins, interleukins and platelet activating factor.

Females are more likely to develop anaesthesia-related allergic anaphylaxis than males, with a 3:1 ratio. Reactions tend to occur in those aged 20 to 50 years. Other groups with risk factors for allergic anaphylaxis include patients with spina bifida in whom there is an increased risk of latex sensitivity. Patients with food allergies may have an increased risk of perioperative anaphylaxis. Kiwi fruit allergy is associated with an increased risk of latex allergy and those with egg allergy have a higher incidence of reactions to propofol.

Causative agents

Neuromuscular blocking agents (NMBAs) are responsible for two-thirds of allergic anaphylactic reactions in anaesthesia, with succinylcholine and rocuronium being most commonly implicated. Neuromuscular blocking agents can, however, cause non-IgE-mediated histamine release from mast cells, which is dose dependent, but may mimic allergic anaphylaxis clinically. Non-IgE-mediated reactions occur more often with benzylisoquinoline NMBAs. Other common allergens that induce perioperative allergic anaphylaxis include latex (up to 20% of anaesthesia-related anaphylaxis), antibiotics (15%) and chlorhexidine.

Diagnosis

Recognition of anaphylaxis may be more difficult in an anaesthetized patient, as they will not be able to report symptoms and cutaneous signs may be obscured by surgical drapes. In addition the clinical features such as hypotension and bronchospasm are seen in everyday anaesthetic practice and are usually not related to anaphylaxis. The common clinical signs and the grading of the severity of allergic reactions are shown in Table 15.1. Most cases of anaesthesia-related anaphylaxis present as grade III or IV severity. Clinical signs usually appear within the first few minutes after exposure. However, with certain allergens such as latex, chlorhexidine and intravenous colloids, signs may be delayed. Haematological abnormalities due to release of heparin and platelet clumping are now known to occur early in allergic anaphylaxis but were not mentioned in the original Ring classification.

Table 15.1 Grading of the severity of symptoms and signs associated with anaphylaxis (Ring and Messmer, 1977).

Grade	Dermal	Abdominal	Respiratory	CVS
I	Pruritis			
	Flush			
	Urticaria			
	Angio-oedema			
II	Pruritis	Nausea	Rhinorrhoea	Tachycardia (>20 BPM*)
	Flush	Cramping	Hoarseness	Blood pressure change (>20 mmHg systolic)
	Urticaria		Dyspnoea	Arrhythmia
	Angio-oedema			
III	Pruritis	Vomiting	Laryngeal	Shock
	Flush	Defaecation		Oedema
	Urticaria	Diarrhoea		Bronchospasm
	Angio-oedema			Cyanosis
IV	Pruritis	Vomiting	Respiratory arrest	Cardiac arrest
	Flush	Defaecation		
	Urticaria	Diarrhoea		
	Angio-oedema			

Management

The management of patients with suspected anaphylaxis should follow a protocol such as that of the Association of Anaesthetists of Great Britain and Ireland in their publication *Suspected Anaphylactic Reactions Associated with Anaesthesia*. Their guideline is as follows.

Immediate management

- Use the ABC approach.
- Remove all potential causative agents and maintain anaesthesia, if necessary, with an inhalational agent.
- Call for help and note the time.
- Maintain the airway and administer 100% oxygen. Intubate the trachea if necessary and ventilate the lungs with oxygen.
- Elevate the patient's legs if there is hypotension.
- If appropriate, start cardiopulmonary resuscitation immediately according to advanced life support (ALS) guidelines.
- Administer adrenaline intravenously. An initial dose of 50 μg (0.5 ml of 1:10,000 solution) is appropriate (adult dose). Several doses may be required if there is severe hypotension or bronchospasm.
- If several doses of adrenaline are required, consider starting an intravenous infusion of adrenaline.

- Administer saline 0.9% or lactated Ringer's solution at a high rate via an intravenous cannula of an appropriate gauge (large volumes may be required).
- Administer chlorphenamine 10 mg IV (adult dose).
- Administer hydrocortisone 200 mg IV (adult dose).

Follow-up

There is no one test that can be used to diagnose with certainty that an allergic reaction has occurred. The follow-up of patients with suspected allergic anaphylaxis should take into consideration the clinical history including any temporal relationship between signs and symptoms and drug administration. As most anaesthetic drugs are administered intravenously, the onset of symptoms usually occurs within a matter of minutes. During induction of anaesthesia several drugs are administered in quick succession and it is therefore not possible to discern which of these may be the causal agent until later follow-up.

The response to treatment is important when determining which adverse events were allergic as these reactions tend to settle within a short time following treatment unless complicated by secondary events. The results of immediate blood tests and the results of skin testing, when examined in the context of the history, help to establish the overall likelihood that an allergic reaction occurred and what the offending drug was.

Serum mast cell tryptase is a useful test for the investigation of perioperative reactions that may have an allergic aetiology. The timing of mast cell tryptase sampling is variable between allergy centres. In the UK, the samples tend to be taken immediately and at one and 24 hours post-reaction. The 24-hour sample serves to provide a baseline value for individual patients. The degree of elevation of serum mast cell tryptase correlates with the severity of the reaction. The threshold for determining an elevated mast cell tryptase varies between centres commonly ranging from 14 to 25 µg/l.

Specific IgE immunoassays can help identify the causative agent in allergic anaphylaxis. They are only available for substances such as latex, chlorhexidine, penicillins, succinylcholine and rocuronium.

Skin testing forms the mainstay of allergy follow-up. Skin testing aims to identify the drug responsible for anaphylaxis. There are two tests available for type I hypersensitivity:

- **Skin prick testing (SPT)**: To perform skin prick testing, a droplet of solution is placed on the skin, and a lancet tip is used to prick the skin, allowing the potential allergen to come into contact with mast cells in the skin. A positive result is indicated by the presence of a wheal greater than 3 mm in size after 15 minutes, or 3 mm greater in size than a negative control. It is recommended to perform skin prick testing within four to six weeks following a reaction.
- **Intradermal dilutional testing (IDT)**: Intradermal testing involves injecting potential allergens into the dermis with a fine needle. A positive result is indicated by the presence of a wheal of 8 mm or greater after 15 minutes. Intradermal dilutional testing has a much higher risk of inducing allergic symptoms while the test is being performed, estimated at 1:1,000. Intradermal dilutional testing should be used only when SPT is borderline.

Prevention

Prevention of anaphylaxis involves identification of at-risk individuals and avoidance of known allergens. A careful history should be taken pre-operatively, including details of any allergies and previous allergic reactions. If the patient has a known allergy, this should be documented in the anaesthetic chart and on the drug prescription chart. It should also be flagged up by the WHO theatre checklist. The patient may also be wearing medical alert jewellery if they have had a previous severe reaction. The potential for cross-over reactions should also be noted. This is particularly important with neuromuscular blocker agents where an allergy to one means there is an increased risk of allergy to another.

Malignant hyperthermia

Malignant hyperthermia (MH) is a rare, life-threatening pharmacogenetic myopathy occurring between 1:10,000 and 1:15,000 of anaesthetics. The true incidence of MH susceptibility in the general population may be higher than expected, as many susceptible patients have never been anaesthetized. It affects men more often than women, and particularly affects children and young adults. All ethnic groups are at risk. The mortality has decreased dramatically to approximately 5% as a result of increased awareness and early recognition, improved standards of monitoring and the introduction of dantrolene.

Pathogenesis

Susceptibility to MH is inherited in an autosomal dominant pattern, with variable penetrance. There are at least six genetic loci of interest and around 60 to 70% of cases involve the coding for the ryanodine receptor, RYR1, on chromosome 19. Exposure to a trigger agent causes calcium release from the sarcoplasmic reticulum in an uncontrolled fashion, leading to prolonged and sustained muscle contraction. This is most likely due to an abnormality at the junction of the T-tubule (dipyridine receptor) and sarcoplasmic reticulum (ryanodine receptor). A hypermetabolic state results with increased glucose metabolism, oxygen consumption and heat production. The resulting hyperthermia and acidosis causes destruction of the sarcolemma, cell death and release of intracellular materials. This leads to electrolyte abnormalities, cardiac arrhythmias, disseminated intravascular coagulation (DIC), cerebral oedema, multi-organ dysfunction syndrome (MODS) and death.

Causative agents

Recognized trigger agents for malignant hyperthermia include succinylcholine and volatile anaesthetics. Other reported non-pharmacological triggers include intense physical activity, exercise-induced rhabdomyolysis and febrile illness. Malignant hyperthermia does not occur with every exposure to a trigger. Susceptible patients may undergo several uneventful anaesthetics before developing MH. Drugs that are safe to administer to MH-susceptible individuals include propofol, nitrous oxide, opioids, non-depolarizing muscle relaxants, benzodiazepines, local anaesthetics, barbiturates and ketamine.

Diagnosis

Malignant hyperthermia should be suspected in any patient who develops an unexplained, unexpected rise in end-tidal CO_2 and tachycardia, together with an increase in oxygen consumption. Patients who develop masseter muscle spasm after the administration of succinylcholine should be considered to have a high risk of MH susceptibility.

MH can be subdivided according to the clinical course:

- **Abortive MH** – Removal of the trigger agent may occasionally bring about resolution of symptoms with no systemic complications.

- **Acute MH** – Hyperthermia and acidosis will not resolve with removal of the trigger agents. Active treatment with dantrolene and cooling is necessary.
- **Fulminant MH** – Characterized by a rapid increase in the core temperature and development of cardiovascular collapse, DIC, cerebral oedema and MODS.

Given the inability to predict which of these categories an individual patient will fall into, withdrawal of the trigger agent and active treatment should be commenced immediately once there is clinical suspicion.

Management

Immediate management

- Stop administration of trigger agents.
- Use a new, clean non-rebreathing circuit, administer high-flow oxygen, hyperventilate.
- Maintain anaesthesia with intravenous anaesthesia (i.e. propofol) until completion of surgery.
- Give dantrolene 2 to 3 mg/kg as initial bolus then 1 mg/kg as needed according to response.
- Institute active cooling measures: cold IV fluid administration, cold gastric/peritoneal/bladder lavage, active forced air or water cooling devices, avoid peripheral vasoconstriction.

Treatment of specific complications

- Hypoxia: 100% inspired oxygen.
- Acidosis: hyperventilation and sodium bicarbonate.
- Hyperkalaemia: sodium bicarbonate, insulin and dextrose, calcium gluconate.
- DIC: fresh frozen plasma, cryoprecipitate, platelets.
- Myoglobinaemia: forced alkaline diuresis.
- Cardiac arrhythmias: magnesium, amiodarone, avoid calcium channel blockers.

Prevention

The avoidance of volatile anaesthetics and succinylcholine in MH-susceptible patients are the key elements for prevention of MH. The intra-operative management involves using a new breathing circuit and flushing it with 10 litres/minute of oxygen for at least 30 minutes pre-operatively, changing the CO_2 absorbent canister, removing the vaporizers from the anaesthetic machine and considering regional anaesthesia if appropriate.

Follow-up

Patients with suspected MH and their families should be screened to identify individuals at risk. Patients should be referred to a specialist centre for counselling and testing. In the UK this is carried out at the MH Investigation Unit at St James's University Hospital, Leeds.

In vitro contracture testing (IVCT) is the gold standard for diagnosis for MH. A muscle biopsy is taken from the vastus medialis muscle under femoral nerve block. The muscle tissue is exposed to caffeine and halothane in vitro, and the muscle tension at different concentrations is measured. Patients who are MH-susceptible will have increased muscle tension at a lower concentration of caffeine/halothane. The test has a high degree of sensitivity (99%) and specificity (94%). If MH-susceptibility is confirmed, the patient's family will also be offered testing, beginning with first-degree relatives.

DNA testing may be used in addition to IVCT. However, MH displays a high level of locus heterogeneity, therefore it is not possible to confirm or exclude MH-susceptibility on the basis of genetic testing alone. In particular a false negative result could have serious consequences.

Porphyria

The porphyrias are a group of rare, inherited diseases resulting from the overproduction and excretion of porphyrins. Porphyrins are intermediate compounds in the synthetic pathway of haem, which is involved in the biosynthesis of metallo-proteins such as haemoglobin, myoglobin and the cytochromes, including P450. A deficiency of one of the enzymes in the haem metabolic pathway results in accumulation of porphyrin, which is deposited in the tissues causing neurocutaneous manifestations. The incidence of porphyria is 1:20,000 in Europeans. Less than 10% of patients have any clinical signs, and are thought to have an enzyme deficiency rather than an absolute deficit. The prevalence of porphyria is higher in Afrikaners in South Africa, approximately 1:250 to 1:500. Porphyria may be inherited in an autosomal dominant pattern.

Pathogenesis

The first step in the haem metabolic pathway is the formation of d-aminolaevulinic acid (ALA) from glycine and succinyl CoA, catalyzed by the enzyme ALA synthetase. This is the most important rate-limiting step and is subject to negative feedback depending on the concentration of haem. In an acute attack of porphyria, there is increased haem production in response to a number of precipitating factors. Increased activity of the haem metabolic pathway leads to increased production of porphyrins, but because of enzyme deficiency, haem is not produced. There is therefore no negative feedback on ALA synthetase, and no control over the rate of porphyrin production.

An acute attack of porphyria can produce only mild symptoms or can be life-threatening by causing neuromuscular weakness leading to respiratory failure. The mortality from an acute attack of porphyria is around 3%. Clinical features include autonomic instability with tachycardia, blood pressure lability, electrolyte abnormalities (in particular hyponatraemia), abdominal pain, seizures and neuropsychiatric disturbances.

Precipitating agents

Acute porphyria can be precipitated by stress, fasting and dehydration, all of which can occur in the perioperative period. In addition, numerous drugs have been identified as porphyrogenic by causing hepatic enzyme induction, and should be avoided in order to reduce the risk of triggering an acute attack. Susceptible individuals can be safely anaesthetized with the knowledge of which agents are safe to use. The Porphyria Drug Safety Database held at the University of Cape Town applies recommendations to drugs depending on whether they can be safely used, used with caution, used with extreme caution only or avoided.

All barbiturates should be avoided as they can precipitate acute porphyria through induction of ALA synthetase. Etomidate has been shown to be porphyrogenic in animal models. It has been used safely in susceptible patients, although there is a single case report of an acute porphyric attack after its use. Propofol can be used safely as an induction agent, although it is unclear whether it is safe for continuous infusion. Nitrous oxide and halothane are both safe to use. Isoflurane appears safe and there is no data on sevoflurane or desflurane. Given their short duration of action it is presumed that they are safe. Most local anaesthetics can be used safely. Cocaine and mepivacaine should be used with caution and there is no data available for ropivacaine. Succinylcholine can be used safely. Atracurium and vecuronium are porphyrogenic in animal studies but have been used safely in patients. It is thought that rocuronium and mivacurium are safe to use. Opioids, paracetamol and aspirin are safe. Non-steroidal anti-inflammatory drugs should be avoided.

Prevention

Prevention of an acute attack relies on the identification of patients who have a personal or family history suggestive of porphyria along with appropriate laboratory testing. Patients with a history of recurrent acute attacks should be considered at particularly high risk. Pre-operative fasting should be limited to avoid dehydration. Carbohydrate intake should be maintained peri-operatively, aiming for at least 2,000 kCal/day. Solutions containing glucose alone should be avoided, as this increases the risk of hyponatraemia with an acute attack.

Diagnosis

During an attack of porphyria, the awake patient may complain of severe abdominal pain or display signs of neuropsychiatric disturbance. The anaesthetized patient may present with haemodynamic instability with tachycardia and hypotension or hypertension.

Management

Management of an acute attack is largely supportive. The suspected trigger agent should be immediately withdrawn if possible. Opioid analgesia should be given. Hypertension and tachycardia may be managed with beta-blockers. Phenothiazines can be used to treat nausea and vomiting and neuropsychiatric disturbances. Specific therapies include haematin and haem arginate, which both provide a supply of haem to inhibit ALA synthetase by negative feedback. Haematin is only available from specialist centres, is unstable and can cause thrombophlebitis, coagulopathy and acute renal failure. Haem arginate can be used as an alternative, at a dose of 3 to 4 mg/kg/day. The use of somatostatin in conjunction with plasmapheresis has also been described.

Succinylcholine apnoea

Succinylcholine apnoea is a rare condition that results in prolonged apnoea after the administration of succinylcholine and mivacurium. It results from a congenital or acquired deficiency of the enzyme pseudo-cholinesterase, also referred to as plasma cholinesterase or butyrylcholinesterase (BChE). Congenital succinylcholine apnoea results from a decreased level of pseudo-cholinesterase, whereas in acquired cases the level of the enzyme is normal but the activity is reduced. It is estimated that 1 in 3,500 people have genotypes that cause significant prolonged apnoea with succinylcholine and mivacurium.

Table 15.2 Relative frequencies of the different alleles and estimated duration of apnoea following administration of succinylcholine.

Genotype	Percentage of population (%)	Duration of apnoea
EU/EU	96	3 to 8 minutes
EU/EA	2.5	30 minutes
EU/EF or EU/ES	0.3	>3 hours
EA/EF	0.005	Apnoea only prolonged if acquired deficiency occurs concurrently
EA/EA	0.05	2 hours

Table 15.3 Causes of acquired changes in pseudo-cholinesterase levels.

Effect	Cause
Physiological decrease	Decreased in third trimester of pregnancy
	Decreased in elderly patients
Acquired decrease	Liver disease
	Malignancy
	Renal disease
	Malnutrition
Acquired increase	Obesity
	Alcoholism
	Hyperthyroidism

Pathogenesis

Pseudo-cholinesterase is a glycoprotein enzyme which is synthesized in the liver and found in plasma and tissues but not in red blood cells. It has a half life of 8 to 16 hours. The physiological function of pseudo-cholinesterase is not known. It is responsible for the metabolism of succinylcholine, first to succinylmonocholine and then to succinic acid. If the level or function of pseudo-cholinesterase is reduced the metabolism of succinylcholine will be prolonged with an increased duration of action.

Congenital succinylcholine apnoea has an autosomal inheritance. The allele for the normal pseudo-cholinesterase enzyme is EU. Approximately 96% of Caucasians are homozygous for this normal allele. Other variants include atypical (EA), fluoride (EF) and silent (ES), all of which result in altered affinity of the enzyme. The alleles EK, EJ and some silent variants result in a decreased quantity of the enzyme. Table 15.2 shows the relative frequencies of the different alleles in the population, as well as the estimated duration of apnoea following administration of succinylcholine.

Levels of pseudo-cholinesterase can also be altered in a number of acquired physiological and pathological conditions. Table 15.3 illustrates the various causes of increased and decreased levels.

Diagnosis

Succinylcholine apnoea is usually recognized at the end of surgery, with delayed emergence from anaesthesia accompanied by tachycardia, hypertension and sweating. Train-of-four stimulation may show absent twitches or reduced twitch height with succinylcholine or significant fade if mivacurium has been administered.

Management

Management of succinylcholine apnoea is supportive, and involves maintenance of anaesthesia and mechanical ventilation until adequate muscle tone has returned. Frequent assessment of the degree of neuromuscular blockade using a neuromuscular monitoring device should be performed. Fresh frozen plasma (FFP) has also been used in diagnosis and treatment of succinylcholine apnoea. In stored FFP, pseudo-cholinesterase activity does not decrease for seven weeks after being donated. Providing an exogenous source of pseudo-cholinesterase has been shown to shorten the duration of apnoea in several case reports. The risks associated with transfusion must be balanced against the risks of a period of mechanical ventilation and possible transfer to intensive care.

Follow-up

In the absence of a positive family history, there is no way to predict which patients will have prolonged apnoea with succinylcholine. Once an episode has occurred, the patient should be fully informed of the potential diagnosis and advised to alert the anaesthetist of the possible diagnosis until testing is completed.

To determine a patient's phenotype their dibucaine number can be determined. Dibucaine is an amide local anaesthetic, which reduces the activity of normal pseudo-cholinesterase. To perform the test, a sample of the patient's plasma is added to benzoylcholine. A chemical reaction occurs, which causes the emission of light. The wavelength of this light is then measured. Dibucaine is then added, which inhibits the reaction, and hence the amount of light emitted. This inhibition is given as a percentage and is referred to as the dibucaine number. Normal individuals have a dibucaine number of 77 to 83. In heterozygotes, it is reduced to 45 to 68, and in homozygotes is less than 30. Reduced pseudo-cholinesterase may also be used to diagnose this condition.

Once diagnosed, the patient should be advised to wear medical alert jewellery to prevent administration of succinylcholine or mivacurium in an emergency situation. The patient and their family should be offered testing to determine whether the condition is congenital or acquired and if any other family members are affected.

Idiosyncratic reactions specific to anaesthetic agents

Volatile anaesthetic agents

Hepatotoxicity may be caused by volatile anaesthetics. Mild self-limiting increases in transaminase and glutathione S-transferase are seen commonly following halothane administration. However, fulminant centrilobular liver necrosis related to halothane has an incidence of around 1:35,000. This condition presents with fever, jaundice and grossly elevated liver enzyme levels. The mortality associated with this drug-induced hepatitis is 50%. The risk with newer volatile agents is significantly lower as they rely less on oxidative metabolism.

Etomidate

Etomidate is an intravenous anaesthetic agent, which provides haemodynamic stability and may be useful for induction of anaesthesia in high-risk patients. However, etomidate also has a high affinity for 11-beta-hydroxylase, a cytochrome P450 enzyme, which is required for the synthesis of cortisol, corticosterone and aldosterone. Etomidate causes suppression of adrenocortical steroid production even at sub-anaesthetic doses. The effects of even a single dose can be prolonged, which is of concern in critically ill patients. Currently under development is carboetomidate, a pyrrole analogue of etomidate. It is designed to provide similar haemodynamic stability to etomidate but without adrenocortical suppression.

Opioids

Intravenous administration of large doses of opioids can cause life-threatening skeletal muscle rigidity. This occurs particularly when opioids are used as the sole or primary induction agent, and is more commonly associated with fentanyl, alfentanil and remifentanil. Chestwall rigidity leads to ineffective manual ventilation, hypoxia and hypercarbia. Management involves the immediate administration of a neuromuscular blocking drug, to enable manual ventilation and securement of the airway. Premedication with midazolam has been shown to reduce the risk of muscle rigidity.

Drug interactions

Drug interactions result when the effect of one drug is altered by the concurrent administration of another. In addition to the many drugs administered during an anaesthetic, the patient may be taking medication for their operative condition or concurrent medical problems. The risk of developing a drug interaction increases with each additional drug the patient receives.

Monoamine oxidase inhibitors

Monoamine oxidase (MAO) is an enzyme that catalyzes the oxidative de-amination of more than 15 monoamines, including adrenaline, noradrenaline, dopamine and serotonin. There are two subtypes: MAO-A and MAO-B, which differ in their substrate, specificity and tissue distribution. Newer monoamine oxidase inhibitors (MAOIs) are used as antidepressants. They are competitive inhibitors of MAO, and produce reversible inhibition of MAO-A. Because of the widespread inhibition of MAO and other enzymes, there is great potential for interactions with various drugs. Of particular concern to anaesthetists are interactions with indirectly-acting sympathomimetics and opioids.

Monoamine oxidase inhibitors lead to an increase in size of the noradrenaline pool stored within the brain and sympathetic nerve terminals. Administration of an indirectly acting sympathomimetic (such as ephedrine and metaraminol) will cause an exaggerated release of noradrenaline and a marked hypertensive response, which can be life-threatening. Directly acting sympathomimetics such as adrenaline, isoprenaline and phenylephrine are safe to use.

Pethidine can also cause life-threatening interactions with MAOIs. Two distinct reactions can occur: an excitatory form and a depressive form. In the excitatory form, intracerebral serotonin levels are increased due to inhibition of MAO. This is further potentiated by pethidine, which blocks neuronal uptake of serotonin. Clinical features include headache, delirium, agitation, hyperthermia, seizures and coma. The depressive form is characterized by cardiovascular and respiratory depression, and coma. It is caused by the reduced break-down and hence accumulation of pethidine, due to inhibition of hepatic N-demethylase by MAOIs.

List of further reading

Aronson, J. K. & Ferner, R. E. Joining the DoTS: new approach to classifying adverse drug reactions. *BMJ* 2003; **327**: 1222–5.

Rawlins, M. D. & Thompson, J. W. Pathogenesis of adverse drug reactions. In Davies, D. M. (ed) *Textbook of Adverse Drug Reactions.* Oxford: Oxford University Press, 1977.

Management of postoperative complications

Benias Mugabe and Saxon Ridley

Introduction

When dealing with patients who have immediate postoperative complications, using the relevant parts of life support protocols can ensure a standardized management approach and improved communication between personnel. Each patient presents a unique diagnostic and therapeutic challenge. Patient-tailored treatment can offer the best management.

Postoperative patients will generally follow one of three pathways.

Anaesthesia/surgery → recovery → postoperative care unit or return to general ward

In the recovery room, many complications such as incomplete reversal of neuromuscular blockade, pain, sickness and hypotension can be corrected quickly. Most patients can then be discharged to a general ward or postoperative care area and so follow the normal care pathway. However, once on the general ward further postoperative complications, such as new onset dysrhythmias, hypotension and oliguria, can develop. The response to these new complications requires both a systematic approach to identify the underlying pathophysiology and the essential skills of airway, breathing and cardiovascular support. Simple but timely measures may be all that is needed to prevent further deterioration and allow the patient to remain on the general ward.

Anaesthesia/surgery → recovery → return to theatre → recovery → ward/critical care unit

Patients who require immediate return to theatre will often declare themselves quickly, for example a rapid fall in the level of consciousness in a neurosurgical patient, or airway compromise in a patient following a thyroidectomy, bleeding after a tonsillectomy or vascular procedure. The anaesthetist's approach to such patients remains airway, breathing and circulation, with simultaneous resuscitation while the surgical management is undertaken.

Anaesthesia/surgery → (recovery) → critical care

Following either elective or emergency surgery, postoperative critical care may be necessary for control of the presenting condition (e.g. severe sepsis), support of limited premorbid physiological reverse (e.g. COPD, renal dysfunction), support after major surgery

Anaesthetic and Perioperative Complications, ed. Kamen Valchanov, Stephen T. Webb and Jane Sturgess.
Published by Cambridge University Press. © Cambridge University Press 2011.

(e.g. oesophageal resection, cardiac surgery) and unforeseen life-threatening intra-operative complications (e.g. massive haemorrhage, myocardial ischaemia). The management of these patients will be the focus of this chapter.

Admission to the critical care unit

Obtaining a complete history and undertaking a thorough clinical examination are essential at critical care admission. Although key facts will be presented by colleagues during hand-over of care, the patient's medical notes should be examined and the immediate family asked for further details, especially those pertaining to pre-morbid functional status, impact of co-morbid diseases on daily living and previous hospital admissions. Clinical examination and further investigations contribute to the identification of both the most relevant and serious pathophysiological disturbance and the principal underlying diagnosis.

The patient's response to treatment and the development of new complications are usually detected by close observation and monitoring. All patients in critical care will have basic level monitoring (i.e. ECG, SpO_2 and arterial pressure monitoring, and hourly urine output). Additional monitoring will be required as determined by the patient's clinical condition.

Critical care support may be broadly divided into general support and specific therapy aimed at the principal diagnosis; the general supportive measures (e.g. mechanical ventilation, renal replacement therapy) merely stabilize the patient allowing time for the specific measures (e.g. antibiotics) to work. General supportive measures on their own are unlikely to improve the patient's condition. As the patient's clinical condition evolves, changes in both the general supportive and specific measures may be required.

The following paragraphs outline the management of the commonest postoperative complications requiring critical care support.

Critical care for patients with respiratory complications

Postoperative respiratory support may be divided into basic or advanced support.

Basic support consists of controlled oxygen therapy, ideally provided by a fixed performance device, physiotherapy to encourage bronchial secretion clearance and a balance between effective analgesia and central (e.g. opiates) or peripheral (e.g. epidural) respiratory depression. The F_iO_2 is adjusted to achieve peripheral arterial oxygen saturation in the physiological range appropriate for the patient. This may be sufficient. If the patient develops signs of respiratory insufficiency (i.e. an increasing respiratory rate, use of accessory muscles, sweating, haemodynamic instability and confusion) basic support is inadequate and advanced techniques are indicated.

Advanced respiratory support includes continuous positive airway pressure (CPAP) and mechanical ventilation. Continuous positive airway pressure is usually delivered at levels between 5 and 15 cmH_2O via a tracheal tube and ventilator, or non-invasively via a tight-fitting facemask or hood. The F_iO_2 and CPAP levels are adjusted to achieve the appropriate age-compensated P_aO_2 (i.e. ((patient's age/2) – 100)/7.5 kPa); generally once the F_iO_2 falls below 0.5, the CPAP level can be gradually reduced.

Mechanical ventilation is required for hypoventilation and respiratory insufficiency, hypoxaemia (unresponsive to other forms of less invasive respiratory support). The aims of mechanical ventilation are to improve alveolar ventilation and oxygenation, prevent alveolar over-distension and minimize auto-positive end-expiratory pressure (auto-PEEP) while maintaining alveolar recruitment and patient–ventilator synchrony.

There are a variety of modes on modern ventilators but most can be classified into:

- continuous mandatory ventilation – where a minute volume is preset and consistently delivered
- continuous spontaneous ventilation (including pressure support, tube compensation, proportional assist and neurally adjusted ventilation) – where all breaths are triggered by the patient but no rate is set
- synchronized intermittent mandatory ventilation – where mandatory breaths are delivered and spontaneous breaths supported
- bilevel or airway pressure-release ventilation – where spontaneous breaths are supported at two different (i.e. inspiratory and expiratory) pressure levels.

More specialized modes include those that use closed-loop feedback (e.g. adaptive support ventilation) to provide combinations of pressure-limited, time-cycled ventilation allowing mandatory and spontaneous breaths and high-frequency ventilation (i.e. oscillatory, jet and percussive).

Ventilator settings depend upon the patient's respiratory system compliance and airway resistance. The main strategies of mechanical ventilation are to optimize gas exchange with minimal barotrauma and volutrauma. A simple guide for ventilatory settings is suggested below:

- The tidal volume should be set between 4 and 8 ml/kg based upon the patient's ideal body weight, calculated as $50 + (2.3 \times (\text{height in inches} - 60))$ for men and $45.5 + (2.3 \times (\text{height in inches} - 60))$ for women. If the plateau pressure exceeds 30 cmH$_2$O, reducing the tidal volume is necessary to avoid barotrauma and ventilator-associated lung injury; under these circumstances an increase in P$_a$CO$_2$ is acceptable.
- The respiratory rate should be set between 15 and 25 breaths per minute with a lower rate if there is evidence of excessive auto-PEEP and hyperinflation.
- The inspiratory:expiratory ratio should be set at 1:2 but longer expiratory times will be required if auto-PEEP is present and/or there is haemodynamic depression. Conversely if the patient is severely hypoxaemic, a longer inspiratory period will promote oxygen transfer from the alveolar gas to the pulmonary capillary.
- PEEP will increase the functional residual volume and lung compliance while decreasing intrapulmonary shunting. The appropriate level of PEEP can be set (1) by titrating the level of PEEP to allow the F$_i$O$_2$ to be reduced to 0.6; (2) according to a table resulting from a study of the acute respiratory distress syndrome; (3) slightly below the lower inflexion point; or (4) to optimize lung compliance or global oxygen delivery. However, there is no strong evidence suggesting that one method of selecting the PEEP level is better than another.

All mechanically ventilated patients should be nursed in a head-up position (between 30 and 45°) unless contraindicated as this reduces ventilator-associated pneumonia. However, if patients are critically oxygen dependent (e.g. F$_i$O$_2$ >0.9) or require potentially dangerous plateau pressures, they can be turned prone to temporarily improve gaseous exchange while other measures take effect.

The adverse effects of mechanical ventilation include over-distension, possibly through excessive or undetected auto-PEEP leading to alveolar rupture (i.e. barotrauma), de-recruitment predisposing to infection, oxygen toxicity and haemodynamic depression by decreases in venous return, increased pulmonary vascular resistance (if alveolar pressures exceed pulmonary venous pressures) and decreased left ventricular filling by reduced right ventricular output, leftward bowing of the interventricular septum and consequent decreases in left ventricular compliance.

Such adverse effects can generally be minimized by selection of the most appropriate ventilatory mode and minimizing the duration of ventilation. Patients will generally wean from mechanical ventilation when the pathophysiological problem precipitating the need for mechanical support has resolved. Gaseous exchange should be adequate (i.e. a P_aO_2 near the age-adjusted predicted value with the extrinsic PEEP level below 8 cmH$_2$O and a F_iO_2 <0.5) and all other organ systems (but principally the cardiovascular) stable without artificial support. Patients should have the muscle power to sustain a good inspiratory effort. While numerous weaning parameters have been tested to assess inspiratory effort or muscle power, generally patients who are able to raise their arms above their heads and have respiratory frequency/tidal volume (in litres) ratio of less than 105 are likely to successfully wean from mechanical ventilation.

Patients are likely to remain ventilator dependent if:

- the respiratory load remains high because of high airways' resistance (e.g. bronchoconstriction, secretions) combined with low lung compliance (e.g. increased lung water, consolidation, atelectasis or fibrosis)
- the patient's respiratory power remains inadequate due to poor nutrition (i.e. failing to reverse respiratory muscle catabolism), electrolyte imbalances (e.g. low phosphate and magnesium levels) and hormonal deficiencies (e.g. hypothyroidism)
- residual effects of sedative and analgesic drugs persist. This complication can be minimized by daily sedation breaks
- critical illness polyneuropathy or myopathy develops, especially with complicating sepsis, multiple organ failure, prolonged immobility and use of steroids and neuromuscular blockers particularly those with steroid-like ring (e.g. vecuronium)
- left ventricular failure persists and causes pulmonary congestion
- central neurological depression of respiratory drive (e.g. brainstem ischaemia, seizures) is present
- psychological dependence upon mechanical support has developed.

Weaning from mechanical ventilation largely depends upon its duration, with patients ventilated for short postoperative periods generally being promptly extubated following termination of sedation. With longer periods of mechanical ventilation, weaning may require a tracheostomy and several trials of spontaneous breathing supported initially with CPAP. If the patient suffers from chronic obstructive airways disease, non-invasive ventilation can be successfully used as a bridge to weaning.

Critical care for patients with cardiovascular complications

Although there is some overlap, the cardiovascular complications after anaesthesia may be broadly divided into shock (i.e. aberrations of the intravascular circulating volume) and primary cardiac dysfunction (i.e. decrease in cardiac output).

Management of shock depends on identifying and correcting its underlying cause, which may be:

- hypovolaemia secondary to depletion of the effective intravascular volume caused by excessive losses or inadequate intake or replacement

- cardiogenic shock due to impaired pump function in the presence of normal or elevated filling pressures caused commonly by acute myocardial ischaemia, left ventricular failure or less commonly cardiomyopathy, myocarditis or cardiac contusion
- obstructive due to impairment of flow to or from the heart caused by tension pneumothorax, abdominal compartment syndrome, pulmonary embolism or pericardial tamponade and less commonly by aortic stenosis, dissection or coarctation
- distributive caused by loss of systemic vascular resistance secondary to sepsis or systemic inflammation, anaphylaxis, spinal injuries, hepatic and adrenal insufficiency.

The initial stages of shock are usually compensated by sympathetic nervous system and rennin-angiotensin activation. Shock management aims to reverse this process before irreversible shock develops. When oxygen supply at the microvascular level becomes inadequate, cellular integrity disintegrates. General supportive measures start with optimizing inspired oxygen to maximize global oxygen delivery. Cellular oxygen delivery depends on appropriate circulating volume and cardiac output. Different types of shock can be treated by correcting the physiological derangement and are divided into the following groups: low circulatory volume, low cardiac output and low vascular tone.

Low circulatory volume

Low circulating volume (and hence poor venous return and consequent poor ventricular filling) should be treated by volume replenishment with crystalloids, colloids and blood products individually or in combination. The choice of fluid and the volume required depends upon the clinical situation. After surgery, additional volume over and above the patient's usual daily requirement may be required because of concealed but perhaps continuing haemorrhage, replacement of intra-operative blood and fluid losses, expansion of the vascular tree during rewarming and third-space losses. The most appropriate replacement fluid is determined by which blood component or fluid was primarily lost in theatre, the transfusion threshold appropriate for the patient, presence of ongoing losses and results of laboratory tests (i.e. coagulation parameters). The circulating volume must be restored but excessive fluid administration avoided as it may precipitate left ventricular failure, pulmonary and general tissue oedema. Fluid replacement should be guided by haemodynamic monitoring and regular clinical review of the patient assessing capillary re-fill, hourly urine output, core-periphery temperature difference, pulse pressure variability, central venous pressure measurement or jugular venous pressure assessment.

Low cardiac output

Low cardiac outputs caused by alterations in rate, rhythm and contractility. In the early postoperative period, cardiac contractility may be altered by displacement of the left ventricle from its usual position on the Frank Starling curve. Myocardial ischaemia, fluid shifts, depressant effects of anaesthetic agents, increased myocardial work caused by stressors such as pain, rewarming and surgical injury can all contribute to changes in cardiac output. Management plans to improve contractility and enhance cellular oxygen delivery often increase myocardial work. A balance between driving cardiac output and against present or potential myocardial ischaemia should be sought.

The commonest dysrhythmia post-operatively is atrial fibrillation. New atrial fibrillation is important because of decreased ventricular filling (i.e. loss of up to 30%). Atrial fibrillation may be treated pharmacologically by intravenous amiodarone (i.e. loading dose 5 mg/kg over 20 to 120 mins followed by infusion of up to 1.2 g in 24 hours), beta-blockers (e.g. metoprolol 2.5 to 10 mg six hourly). If the patient is sedated, direct current cardioversion can be used. Other dysrhythmias can occur and may be life-threatening (e.g. ventricular tachycardia) or stable (e.g. pre-existing heart block).

Primary pump failure requires inotropic support; dobutamine (2.5 to 10 µg/kg/min) is a suitable agent. It is a potent $beta_1$-agonist. Other agents such as dopexamine (0.5 to 6 µg/kg/min) or phosphodiesterase inhibitors (e.g. milrinone loading dose 0.5 µg/kg over ten minutes followed by infusion at 0.375 to 0.750 µg/kg/min) can be beneficial. When pharmacological treatment of depressed myocardial contractility is not sufficient, mechanical cardiovascular support with intra-aortic balloon counterpulsation, or other extracorporeal or intracorporeal devices, may be necessary.

The effectiveness of reversing reduced cardiac output and improved peripheral perfusion can be assessed by falling lactate levels (possibly after a transient increase due to a washout phenomenon) and return of mixed venous oxygen saturation toward normal levels (70% in the superior vena cava and 65% from the pulmonary artery).

Low vascular tone

Low vascular tone (afterload) can be due to inappropriate vasodilatation secondary to loss of usual control mechanisms (e.g. acetylcholine), unresponsiveness to usual neurohumoral control (e.g. loss of response to sympathetic activity) or release of pathologically induced vasodilators (e.g. induced nitric oxide). Improvements in vascular tone can be achieved by $alpha_1$ vasoconstriction with norepinephrine. Low-dose infusions of arginine vasopressin (0.01 to 0.04 IU/min) are commonly used and produce V_1 receptor-mediated restoration of the vascular tone.

Restoration of an adequate arterial blood pressure can most easily be judged by a urine output exceeding 0.5 ml/kg/hour in the absence of previously identified renal dysfunction.

Critical care for patients with renal complications

Acute renal dysfunction adversely affects outcome in critically ill patients. Intensive care unit severity scoring systems such as the APACHE III and the SOFA scoring systems use acute renal dysfunction in their calculation of mortality risk. The Risk, Injury, Failure, Loss and End-stage kidney (RIFLE) classification has improved the definition of acute renal dysfunction. RIFLE defines three grades of increasing severity of acute kidney injury according to serum creatinine changes or urine output. The system categorizes acute dysfunction as a risk (class R), injury (class I) and failure (class F) and two outcomes (Loss and End-stage kidney disease):

- Risk: Glomerular filtration rate (GFR) decrease of >25% but <50%
  urine output <0.5 ml/kg/hour for 6 hours.
- Injury: GFR decrease of >50% but <75%
  urine output <0.5ml/kg/hour >12 hours.
- Failure: GFR decrease >75%
  urine output <0.3 ml/kg/hour for 24 hours
  anuria for >12 hours.

Table 16.1 Potential causes of renal injury in the perioperative period.

Underlying medical disease

Nature of surgery

Nephrotoxin exposure

Hypovolaemia

Hypotension

Raised intra-abdominal pressure

Table 16.2 Perioperative measures to reduce renal injury.

Maintain hydration

Avoid nephrotoxins where possible

Maintain renal perfusion pressure – MAP within 25% baseline

Urine output >0.5ml/kg/hr

Avoid drugs that increase renal oxygen demand

Causes of postoperative renal dysfunction

As acute renal injury was poorly defined prior to the RIFLE classification, the incidence of postoperative renal failure has been reported as between 1 and 5% following elective surgery and 5 to 10% after emergency or vascular surgery. Postoperative renal failure occurs as either progression of pre-existing renal failure (i.e. acute on chronic) or as a new complication of anaesthesia and surgery (Table 16.1).

The aim of perioperative management should be to identify the patients at risk of postoperative renal failure and to employ a combination of strategies to prevent renal injury (Table 16.2).

The kidneys receive 25% of cardiac output but utilize only 10% of the total body oxygen uptake. As a result of the kidneys' ability to autoregulate, the GFR parallels the renal blood flow (RBF) over a wide range of perfusion pressures. The renal medulla is in a permanent state of near hypoxaemia (and is highly prone to ischaemia) due to the differences in regional blood flow within the kidney and because 90% of renal oxygen extraction occurs in the medulla. Glomerular ultra-filtration is the result of the difference between afferent and efferent arteriolar pressures, which in turn are influenced by intrinsic and extrinsic factors (e.g. catecholamines, renin, angiotensin, prostaglandins, nitric oxide and platelet activating factor). All anaesthetic drugs affect renal blood flow due to their vasodilatory effects and though they may reduce cerebral oxygen requirement, they have no effect on renal oxygen demand. Thus the pathogenesis of postoperative renal failure depends upon the nature of the surgery, pre-operative and intra-operative haemodynamics and intrinsic renal conditions.

Postoperative renal support may be divided into pharmacological intervention or renal replacement therapy. Pharmacological management involves the use of vasoactive drugs, diuretics and judicious fluid management to restore renal perfusion while waiting for the kidneys to recover. Renal replacement therapy involves a form of haemodialysis, haemofiltration or combinations of the two. In the postoperative period an important distinction needs to be made between pre-renal failure and acute tubular necrosis (ATN). The former can usually be reversed by a rapid restoration of renal perfusion and glomerular ultra-filtration pressure. Hence it is prudent to assume that patients who are oliguric in the postoperative period are hypovolaemic until proven otherwise.

Pharmacological management of postoperative renal failure

Diuretics

Loop diuretics such as furosemide, and other diuretics such as metalazone and bumetanide, induce a diuresis, which may convert oliguric to non-oliguric renal dysfunction. While not improving outcome, non-oliguric renal failure is generally easier to manage clinically. Loop diuretics decrease the metabolic demand of renal tubular cells and so may protect against ischaemia. Furosemide (unlike other drugs whose effects are mediated by the unbound fraction) needs to be bound to albumin in the renal tubules to have any effect. Correction of hypoalbuminaemia will help furosemide's efficacy. The presence of a highly protein-bound drug (e.g. warfarin, phenytoin) and hypoalbuminaemia can both contribute to resistance to the diuretic effect of furosemide.

Dopamine has historically been used as renal prophylaxis or as a treatment for oliguria in doses of 1 to 4 µg/kg/min. However, its effect on dopaminergic receptors diminishes with prolonged use. More importantly as dopamine increases GFR, increased solute load presented to the medullary thick ascending limb of the loop of Henle will increase its oxygen demand and may cause further ischaemia.

Fenoldopam mesylate is a dopamine analogue, which increases renal blood flow, natriuresis and urine output, and is many times more potent than dopamine. It has been used to treat postoperative renal failure. It exerts its effects via dopaminergic and beta-adrenergic receptors at the proximal tubule. Its effects can occur in the absence of vasodilatation. Importantly fenoldopam can be infused through a peripheral vein unlike dopamine, which requires central venous access.

Non-pharmacological management of postoperative renal failure

Renal replacement therapy

Post-operatively renal replacement therapy (RRT) is indicated for fluid overload, electrolyte imbalance (particularly hyperkalaemia) and acidosis (Table 16.3). Renal replacement therapy may be intermittent (dialysis) or continuous (haemofiltration). Although neither form of RRT has been shown to improve long-term outcome, in critical care units continuous RRT is usually employed. Patients with haemodynamic instability better tolerate it.

Continuous renal replacement therapy can be provided by a number of methods:

- SCUF (Slow Continuous Ultra-Filtration) removes ultra-filtrate at low rates without administration of a substitution solution. Ultra-filtration is the extracorporeal removal of plasma water by application of a transmembrane pressure. No dialysate or substitution solutions are used. The aim is to prevent or treat volume overload when waste product removal or correction of acid–base balance is not necessary.
- CVVHF (Continuous Veno-Venous HaemoFiltration) uses continuous convective removal of waste products (of various molecular sizes). Haemofiltration

Table 16.3 Renal replacement therapy treatment goals.

Removal of waste products (e.g. hypercatabolic states, trauma with rhabdomyolysis)

Restoration of acid–base balance

Correction of electrolytes abnormalities

Haemodynamic stabilization

Fluid balance in diuretic-resistant fluid overload

Generation of vascular space for nutritional support or blood products

Removal of drugs

Removal and/or modulation of septic and immune mediators

involves the simultaneous removal of plasma water by ultra-filtration and its replacement with a buffered electrolyte solution to maintain the acid–base balance.

- CVVHD (Continuous Veno-Venous HaemoDialysis) employs continuous diffusive removal of waste products; this is driven primarily by the transmembrane concentration gradients. Such gradients are maintained by a dialysis solution provided by a countercurrent mechanism.
- CVVHDF (Continuous Veno-Venous HaemoDiaFiltration) combines both continuous diffusion and convective removal of waste products using both dialysis and substitution solution.

Haemodialysis is based on diffusion along concentration gradients across a dialysis membrane, while haemofiltration depends upon convective solute removal through sieving by a membrane and formation of ultra-filtrate. If a solute can pass through a membrane, this solute can be swept or 'dragged' across the membrane by the plasma water. The rate of solute drag can be modified either by altering the rate of solvent (i.e. plasma water) passage or the effective mean pore size in the membrane.

The function of ultra-filtration membranes is affected by secondary membrane formation (caused by a proteinaceous layer on the inside of the membrane on exposure to blood) and concentration polarization (i.e. the build up of non-permeable proteins on the blood side of the filter). Substitution/replacement fluid can be added either before (pre-dilution) or after (post-dilution) the filter chamber. Post-dilution achieves a higher rate of solute clearance but pre-dilution is associated with longer membrane life and hence less frequent filter interruptions.

Anticoagulation

Renal replacement therapy requires the priming of the extracorporeal circuit with anti-coagulant to prevent the blood clotting usually with fractionated or unfractionated heparin. Heparin is delivered before the filter as either low dose at 5 to 10 IU/kg/hr or at 8 to 10 IU/kg/hr if excessive clotting is a problem. Heparin reaches the systemic circulation and so can trigger heparin-induced thrombocytopaenia (HIT). The patient's platelet count should be monitored daily while on heparin. Alternative anticoagulation strategies have been used for patients who cannot have heparin (e.g. allergies), those who are already coagulopathic (e.g. septic patients) and those who develop HIT whilst requiring continued treatment with

CRRT. The alternatives include prostacyclin, direct thrombin inhibitors (e.g. lepirudin, argatroban) and heparinoids (e.g. danaparoid).

Postoperative sepsis

The potential for developing sepsis in the early postoperative period is considerable, particularly after perforation or manipulation of the digestive tract or surgery on infected sites and abscesses, especially those within the renal or gynaecological tracts. Ideally the management of septic patients should follow the updated 2008 *Surviving Sepsis* guidelines. However, as the patients will be returning from theatre, they will be well resuscitated and the source of sepsis (and hence likely pathogen) usually recognized.

The *Surviving Sepsis* guidelines breaks down the management of septic patients into the following eight categories.

1. Initial resuscitation (first six hours)

Ideally the patient will be returned from theatre with the following goals achieved:

- central venous pressure 8 to 12 mmHg although a higher target of 12 to 15 mmHg may be required if the patient is ventilated and/or there is reduced left ventricular compliance
- mean arterial pressure over 65 mmHg
- urine output ≥ 0.5 ml/kg/hr
- superior vena cava oxygen saturation $\geq 70\%$, or mixed venous saturations $\geq 65\%$.

If these targets are not achieved, then further fluid loading, transfusion to a haematocrit $\geq 30\%$ and/or dobutamine (infused to a maximum 20 µg/kg/min) may be required.

2. Diagnosis and source identification

Following surgery, the source of sepsis will usually have been eradicated and the most appropriate antibiotics started. However, occasionally and unexpectedly the patient may display the signs of sepsis in the early postoperative period. In these circumstances it is vital to obtain relevant cultures (i.e. two percutaneous blood cultures, blood cultures from each vascular access device in place >48 hours and samples from other sites as indicated) before starting antibiotics.

3. Antibiotic therapy

If antibiotics were started in theatre, these should be continued; otherwise they should be administered as early as possible, and always within the first hour of recognizing severe sepsis and septic shock. Broad-spectrum agents active against likely bacterial/fungal pathogens and with good penetration into the presumed source are required. They can be stopped once pathogen susceptibilities are known, and appropriate anti-infective agents started. The duration of therapy should typically be limited to seven to ten days; longer therapy may be required if the response is slow, there is inaccessible foci of infection or immunologic deficiencies.

4. Fluid therapy

Fluid resuscitation may use crystalloids or colloids aiming for a target CVP ≥ 8 mmHg (≥ 12 mmHg if mechanically ventilated) using a fluid challenge technique (e.g. 1,000 ml challenges of crystalloids or 300 to 500 ml of colloids over 30 minutes). More rapid and larger volumes may be required in sepsis-induced tissue hypoperfusion.

5. Vasopressors

The target MAP is $\geq$65 mmHg. If fluid resuscitation does not restore MAP, then centrally administered norepinephrine or dopamine are the initial vasopressors of choice. If MAP remains unresponsive to increasing doses of norepinephrine or dopamine, vasopressin 0.03 IU/min may be added or epinephrine used as an alternative.

6. Inotropic therapy

Dobutamine may be used in patients with myocardial dysfunction as indicated by elevated cardiac filling pressures and low cardiac output, but predetermined supranormal levels of cardiac index should not be aimed for.

7. Steroids

Intravenous hydrocortisone (<300 mg/day) may be useful for adult septic shock when hypotension persists despite adequate fluid resuscitation and vasopressors. An ACTH stimulation test is not recommended to identify the subset of adults with septic shock who should receive hydrocortisone. Fludrocortisone is not essential if hydrocortisone is used but may be required if another glucocorticoid with less mineralocorticoid property is used. Steroid therapy may be weaned once vasopressors are no longer required.

8. Blood product administration

If the patient was previously fit and/or not requiring continued resuscitation, red blood cells transfusion may be deferred until haemoglobin decreases to <7.0 g/dl. However, a higher haemoglobin level may be required if myocardial ischaemia, severe hypoxaemia, acute haemorrhage, cyanotic heart disease or lactic acidosis are present. Platelets should be transfused when counts are <5,000/mm^3 regardless of bleeding and between 5,000 to 30,000/mm^3 when there is significant bleeding risk. Higher platelet counts ($\geq$50,000/mm^3) are required for only surgery or invasive procedures.

Mechanical ventilation of sepsis-induced acute lung injury (ALI)/ARDS

Patients who develop sepsis-induced acute lung injury will often require mechanical ventilation.

Sedation, analgesia and neuromuscular blockade in sepsis

Sedation protocols specifying the level of sedation required and incorporating a daily interruption/lightening to produce awakening shortens the duration of mechanical ventilation. Neuromuscular blocking drugs should be avoided where possible.

Glucose control

Insulin should be used to control hyperglycaemia in patients with severe sepsis; following stabilization in the ICU, the target glucose range is between 6.0 and 8.3 mmol/l.

Sodium bicarbonate therapy

Bicarbonate therapy does not improve the haemodynamics or reduce vasopressor requirements when treating hypoperfusion-induced lactic acidaemia with pH $\geq$7.15 and so should not be used.

Deep vein thrombosis (DVT) prophylaxis

Ideally low-dose unfractionated heparin (UFH) or low molecular weight heparin (LMWH) should be used unless contraindicated, in which case mechanical prophylactic devices (e.g. compression stockings or intermittent compression device) should be used.

Stress ulcer prophylaxis

Stress ulcer prophylaxis using H_2 blocker or proton pump inhibitor can be used but the benefits of prevention of upper gastrointestinal bleed must be weighed against the potential for development of ventilator-associated pneumonia.

Nutritional complications

Postoperative patients should be resuscitated and stabilized before considering nutritional support. Enteral feeding is the best route to supply nutrients and, in general, enteral feeding should be started within the first 24 to 48 hours and advanced towards full feeding within 48 to 72 hours. For a critically ill postoperative patient, a total of 25 kcal/kg is required of which about 20% (or 1.3 g/kg) are provided by nitrogen, 50% (or 5 to 7 g/kg) by carbohydrates and 30% (2.5 g/kg) by lipids. Critically ill patients may not be able to metabolize 2.5g/kg/day of lipid after major surgery, burns or severe trauma. In such cases the nitrogen intake will need to be increased. If gastric residual volumes are likely to be high, a jejunal feeding tube placed at the time of surgery can be helpful.

Patients unable to be fed via a nasogastric or small bowel feeding tube may require parenteral nutrition. Total parenteral nutrition (TPN) may be required for patients in whom calorie-protein malnutrition was present prior to surgery and in whom extensive upper gastrointestinal surgery prohibits enteral feeding.

Immune-modulating enteral feeds are now commercially available and contain supplements such as arginine, glutamine, nucleic acid, omega-3 fatty acids and antioxidants. However, these should probably be reserved for patients following major elective surgery, trauma, burns, head and neck cancer, and those on mechanical ventilation.

Concluding remark

In the UK, many patients require critical care support after surgery. Between 1999 and 2004 in 94 NHS hospitals, just over 4 million surgical procedures were performed (70% elective) of which 12.5% were identified as high risk. These high-risk patients had a prolonged hospital stay, particularly if they were admitted to the ICU, and a high mortality (19%). Improvements in the recognition and management of postoperative complications by the provision of high-quality consistently applied critical care will benefit such high-risk patients.

List of further reading

Albert, R. K., Slutsky, A., Ranieri, M., Takala, J. & Torres, A. *Clinical Critical Care Medicine*. Philadelphia: Moseby-Elsevier, 2006.

Berstein, A. D. & Soni, N. *Oh's Intensive Care Manual*, 5th edn. Edinburgh: Butterworth-Heinemann, 2003.

Dellinger, R. P., Levy, M. M., Carlet, J. M. *et al.* Surviving Sepsis Campaign: international guidelines for management of severe sepsis and septic shock: 2008. *Crit Care Med* 2008; **36**: 296–327.

Hall, J. B., Schmidt, G. A. & Wood, L. D. H. *Principles of Critical Care*, 3rd edn. New York: McGraw-Hill, 2005.

Powell-Tuck, J., Gosling, P., Lobo, D. N. *et al.* British Consensus Guidelines on Intravenous Fluid Therapy for Adult Surgical Patients, GIFTASUP. www.bapen. org.uk/pdfs/bapen_pubs/giftasup.pdf (accessed 15 April 2011).

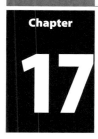

Before complications occur

Assessing, balancing and explaining risk;
Consent

Derek Duane

Introduction

Before agreeing to any medical intervention, a patient must be in possession of all of the relevant information to allow a reasoned appraisal prior to deciding what to do. The information that is given must include an assessment of the risks that a particular procedure may present. By explaining to the patient the nature and extent of the possible complications, the doctor fulfils a moral and legal duty that enables the process of consent. In general, to limit the harm to a patient as a result of a medical procedure, the starting point must be a well informed participant who has made an autonomous decision free from undue influence and accepts the risks involved.

The foundation of the doctor–patient relationship is trust. This is necessary to permit actions related to diagnosis and treatment to be carried out on a patient. Establishing this trust requires both parties to recognize the necessity of communicating freely and honestly thereby facilitating a mutually beneficial pact. This pact is formalized in the requirement for an individual's consent, which, to be valid, must be given voluntarily by a competent and well informed patient. The purpose of this consent is firstly to provide a legal justification for a doctor's duty of care towards the patient, thereby allowing touching of another person in a therapeutic context. This legal construct avoids committing the tort of battery and needing to defend this criminal charge. Secondly, obtaining consent upholds the ethical principle of autonomy and a doctor's legal duty to inform, thus avoiding a charge of negligence by the patient from lack of appropriate information. In *Sidaway v Board of Governors of the Bethlem Royal Hospital and the Maudsley* ([1985] AC 871), Lord Diplock pointed out that a doctor's general duty of care incorporated in addition to diagnosis and treatment, the requirement for advice on the side effects, risks and implications of any proposed treatment.

Legal issues and consent

The extent to which a patient needs to be informed of risks, complications and implications of any proposed intervention is at the heart of much of the legal controversy surrounding the issue of consent. The idea of *informed consent*, a term that has its medico-legal origin in the United States, was defined by Justice Bray (*Salgo v Leland Stanford Junior University Board of Trustees*, 317 P 2d 170 Cal 1957) as 'any facts which are necessary to form the basis of an intelligent consent by the patient to the proposed treatment'. Although grounded in the principles of self-determination as endorsed by Justice Cardozo in *Schloendorff v Society of*

Anaesthetic and Perioperative Complications, ed. Kamen Valchanov, Stephen T. Webb and Jane Sturgess.
Published by Cambridge University Press. © Cambridge University Press 2011.

New York Hospital (105 NE 92 NY 1914) that 'every human being of adult years and sound mind has a right to determine what shall be done with his own body' and with its legal validity confirmed in the United States Court of Appeals case of *Canterbury v Spence* (464 F 2d 772 DC 1972), informed consent, in the American sense, forms no part of English law. Therefore, the juristic basis of consent would appear to differ between continents with the UK law taking a unique stance. English law simply extends a doctor's duty of care and obligation to act in the patient's best interest, entered into by establishing a therapeutic relationship, and this it translates into a duty to inform such that a valid consent can be obtained from a patient.

Having established that a duty to inform exists to validate consent, what parameters define the extent of this disclosure and who should set the standard? Decisions at first instance had begun to explore this issue, particularly the cases of *Chatterton v Gerson* ([1981] QB 432) and *Hills v Potter* ([1983] 3 All ER 716). In the first of these cases, Miss Chatterton underwent on two occasions, an intrathecal injection of phenol to treat a neuropathic pain condition but she did not derive any great pain relief and suffered a weak leg as a result. She claimed against the doctor and hospital based on battery and negligence. Justice Bristow dismissed the claim in battery stating that 'the cause of the action on which to base a claim for failure to go into risks and implications is negligence, not trespass'. This particular decision underlined the reluctance of the judiciary to bring a charge of battery against a doctor who invalidated a patient's consent by failing to give sufficient information about particular complications. As long as a patient consented to the basic nature and character of a medical intervention, there could be no charge of intentional invasion of his or her person. On the negligence issue, the judge took his lead from *Bolam v Friern Hospital Management Committee* ([1957] 2 All ER 118) and paraphrased Justice McNair by declaring that 'the duty of the doctor is to explain what he intends to do and its implications, in the way a careful and responsible doctor in similar circumstances would have done'. He therefore imposed the *Bolam* standard to settle cases in negligence arising from failure to disclose sufficient information.

In *Hills v Potter* ([1983] 3 All ER 716), a case where the plaintiff was left paralyzed after an operation for spasmodic torticollis, a claim was brought in battery and negligence against the neurosurgeon. Justice Hirst presiding over the case dismissed the claim in battery and concluded, 'in my judgment McNair J. in *Bolam's* case applied the medical standard to advice prior to an operation, as well as to diagnosis and to treatment'. Justice Hirst rejected the arguments that he should apply the standard laid down in North American jurisdictions, i.e. the doctrine of informed consent and was only willing to allow this to be incorporated into English law as a result of a decision of an appellate court. He therefore upheld the *Bolam* principle as appropriate for deciding cases in negligence when it related to a doctor's duty to inform.

It would be up to the House of Lords to rigorously defend this stance and to consider the position of the doctrine of informed consent, which it had occasion to do in *Sidaway v Board of Governors of the Bethlem Royal Hospital and the Maudsley* ([1985] AC 871). In this case, the plaintiff Mrs. Sidaway claimed she was not warned of the risk of spinal cord damage suffered by her following a cervical laminectomy operation performed by a neurosurgeon Mr. Falconer. The risk of damage to the spinal cord was much less than nerve root injury but the consequences were much more serious. What the House of Lords had to determine was whether a patient's right to information including risks of a medical intervention was a legal duty of the doctor to disclose. They also gave consideration to further matters namely: (1) the nature, extent and standard by which to judge disclosure; (2) if medical opinion or a rule of law should guide a court's decision; and (3) whether full disclosure embracing the American doctrine of informed consent was appropriate. Of the four judgments handed down by the Law Lords, each one gave different reasons why the case should be rejected and to this date, no one speech is seen as defining this area of the law. The *Bolam* principle was at the heart of this case and Lord Diplock declared it as the legal standard when it came to disclosing risks related to medical procedures.

Should the nature and extent of the information disclosed be judged by a professional standard, i.e. from the viewpoint of the 'prudent doctor' or should the standard be patient centred, i.e. from a 'prudent patient' standpoint? At the end of the day it seemed that the 'prudent doctor' test was more consistent with English law and Lord Templeman ([1985] AC 871, at p898) affirmed this by stating 'the doctor…must decide what information should be given to the patient. The court will award damages against the doctor if the court is satisfied that the doctor blundered and that the patient was deprived of information'. Subject to certain caveats, the *Bolam* test was not to be seen as giving the medical profession carte blanche when it came to information disclosure. Lord Templeman emphasized that he did not subscribe to the theory that the patient was entitled to know everything or that the doctor was entitled to decide everything. Lord Bridge ([1985] AC 871, at p893) also echoed these sentiments when he claimed that a judge might find, despite medical opinion to the contrary, that 'disclosure of a particular risk was so obviously necessary to an informed choice…that no reasonably prudent medical man would fail to make it'.

The judgment of Lord Scarman ([1985] AC 871, at p882) is seen as the dissenting view. He accepted the 'prudent patient' test acknowledging a preference for the patient's right to self-determination. Drawing upon the judgment in *Canterbury v Spence*, Lord Scarman favoured the approach of the American courts, which expects the doctor to disclose all material risks which are those 'a reasonable person…would be likely to attach significance to…in deciding whether or not to forego the proposed therapy'. He proposed that medical evidence would be required and great importance would be attached to it when attempting to answer the questions of the probable occurrence of a risk, the seriousness of its consequences and the justification of withholding information on the grounds of 'therapeutic privilege'.

In the final analysis Lord Scarman ruled in favour of the neurosurgeon despite applying the substituted principles of the doctrine of informed consent. By astute reasoning, he showed that the plaintiff had not proved the risk was sufficiently significant to her, although the defendant had informed her of the broad nature and intention of the proposed surgery thereby fulfilling the *Bolam* principle. Lord Scarman had certainly attempted to make prominent the concept of informed consent but was mindful that if it became the new legal standard there was the possibility of a rise in litigation and the practice of defensive medicine.

If nothing else, *Sidaway* confirmed that a duty of disclosure existed but issues regarding the nature and extent of this disclosure were somewhat blurred. Was the *Bolam* standard to be adhered to? Was the transatlantic doctrine of the 'prudent patient' to become the norm or was there to be some hybrid legal formula adopted? Following the *Sidaway* case and despite Lord Scarman's non-conformist views, rulings from other cases did not see judges embracing anything but the *Bolam* standard. In *Gold v Haringey Health Authority* ([1988] QB 481), a case that involved a lack of warning of the failure rate of female sterilization and that of vasectomy, the Court of Appeal followed the *Bolam* approach as per Lord Diplock in *Sidaway* and rejected that there was a difference in a doctor's duty in the context of non-therapeutic treatment. Similarly, in *Moyes v Lothian Health Authority* ([1990] SLT 444), Lord Caplan was in no doubt how he saw the direction given in the *Sidaway* ruling when he said 'I can read nothing in the majority view in *Sidaway* which suggests that the extent and quality of warning to be given by a doctor to his patient should not in the last resort be governed by medical criteria'. In *Blyth v Bloomsbury Health Authority* ([1993] 4 Med LR 151), the Court of Appeal overturned a trial judge's decision in a case that involved a failure to answer the plaintiff's enquiries concerning Depo-Provera. Neill LJ supported the *Bolam* principle when he said 'the amount of information to be given must depend upon the circumstances, and as a general proposition it is governed by what is called the *Bolam* test'.

It appeared therefore that in the UK at least the status quo remained regarding the legal test required to determine negligence in relation to non-disclosure of medical information in the context of consent. However, other non-UK common law jurisdictions were not so bound to *Sidaway*. In *Rogers v Whitaker* ([1993] 4 Med LR 79), the Australian High Court considered a case involving a plaintiff who suffered blindness in her one good eye after developing sympathetic ophthalmia, a risk that was not disclosed to her. Here the court rejected the *Bolam* principle stating that it would not be appropriate to apply it to a situation where a patient asked direct questions about a risk only to be subject to what medical opinion thought useful to impart. Therefore, they adopted the 'prudent patient' approach while taking into consideration the specific circumstances of the patient.

Internationally, there seemed to be no allegiance to *Bolam*. America had its doctrine of informed consent, the Australian courts had a prudent patient test with a subjective component and Canadian law had set its precedent as far back as 1980 in the case of *Reibl v Hughes* ([1980] 114 DLR 3d 1) – a case where the patient, uninformed of the complications, suffered a stroke post carotid endarterectomy. However, over time *Bolam's* grip weakened in the face of these opposing views. In *Smith v Tunbridge Wells Health Authority* ([1994] 5 Med LR 334), the risk of impotence and bladder dysfunction was not revealed to the patient being treated for rectal prolapse and Morland J. held the doctor negligent despite supporting medical opinion. He had indeed felt that these risks were obviously necessary to an informed choice and ruled accordingly.

The case of *Bolitho v City and Hackney Health Authority* ([1997] 4 All ER 771) certainly impacted on the supremacy of the *Bolam* standard used to decide cases of failure to inform. This case involved a negligent claim against medical staff who failed to attend a child who later suffered a cardiorespiratory arrest and was left brain damaged. However, the plaintiff's legal action did not involve the issue of information disclosure per se but the case did influence significantly the Court's approach to professional negligence as laid down in *Bolam v Friern Hospital Management*. Following the ruling in this case, UK courts were now able to demand that the opinion of the reasonable and responsible body of medical opinion be subject to 'logical analysis'. The Court of Appeal in *Pearce v United Bristol Healthcare NHS Trust* (48 BMLR 118) delivered its ruling in the post-*Bolitho* era. This case involved a claim against a doctor who was alleged to have failed to advise the plaintiff of the increased risk of a stillbirth beyond term delivery. Lord Woolf in his judgment stated that it was the responsibility of a doctor to inform a patient of any significant risk that would affect the judgement of a reasonable patient. Both *Sidaway* and *Bolitho* seemed to have been used to produce a hybrid standard of disclosure with a significant risk made reliant on more than just percentages but all the relevant considerations. It would seem that this case had injected the courts with a stimulant of healthy scrutiny of the reasoning behind expert evidence and had taken the UK's legal framework on non-disclosure of relevant risks and complications of medical procedures closer to the 'prudent patient' standard.

Ethical issues and consent

The ethical basis of informed consent is the absolute commitment to the ethos of self-determination as enshrined in the ethical principle of autonomy. In addition, we aspire to uphold and respect all the rights of a patient enshrined in the articles of the European Convention on Human Rights. These moral values, which form one of the cornerstones of UK law, were emphasized by the House of Lords judgment in *S v S; W v Official Solicitor* ([1970] 3 All ER 107), when Lord Reid said 'English law goes to great lengths to protect a person of full age and capacity from interference with his personal liberty'. Medical paternalism no longer justifies a doctor's actions especially if it contravenes the autonomy of the competent patient. This view of the law was stated clearly in the speech of Lord Keith of Kinkel in *Airedale NHS Trust v Bland* ([1993] AC 789), when he stated that '[even]…the principle of the sanctity of life…is not an absolute one. It does not compel a medical practitioner on pain of criminal sanctions to treat a patient'.

Disclosing information to a patient to obtain a valid consent respects that patient's right to self-determination. It diminishes the 'doctor knows best' perspective and in theory should encourage and foster a more collaborative approach to medical decision making. Undue deference to unquestionable medical judgement is now a phenomenon of the past. The recent rise in the pre-eminence of autonomy in medical ethics is partly due to a growing mistrust in medical expertise, a demand by patients to judge their own best interests and a desire to endorse a moral code to promote the right to individuality and control of one's destiny. When a person is the dominant agent choosing which decisions to impact their lives, they derive fulfilment and purpose from existence. It is repellent to most people to have external forces dictate the progress of their lives. In this environment, and given the ongoing technological advances in all aspects of communications, patients armed with greater information than ever before are keen to be the final arbitrator of possible medical intervention. Doctors should be willing to promote this autonomy by providing expert information to facilitate independent and informed decision making.

What is meant by an autonomous decision? Is its promotion always in a patient's best interests and must it always be respected? Autonomy can be viewed simply as self-determination with or without rationality. It may be referenced to some objective or universal moral standard or subject to one's immediate inclinations. Some hold that not all autonomous decisions demand respect and that autonomy should not be the sole guiding ethical principle supplanting all others in consent issues. Autonomy is regarded by others as valid only if it is exercised to promote human wellbeing, is unharmful to others and based on a framework of sound moral values. Acting out autonomous wishes without moral restraint may not promote wellbeing and one must ensure all facets of the issue are balanced. An overemphasis on the ideal of self-determination in healthcare matters may overlook the symbiotic perspective many hold with their community and interpersonal relationships. Obligations to these other agents may need to be fulfilled thus involving restrictions on one's choice. This idea of 'relational autonomy' can have a significant impact when consent issues are discussed with patients. Many may take a broad view of the implications of their decisions on others despite the individual nature of the consent process and this may appear not to reflect a true choice by them. There is always the danger with this approach that an individual's wishes may be displaced to accommodate the needs of others, thus shifting the balance too far away from traditional liberal autonomy.

By obtaining a patient's consent, do we really uphold the principle of autonomy in its authentic form incorporating a desire to promote a person's wellbeing or does it just become a ritual of information exchange? Patient's decision making often depends on a host of factors separate from the probability of perceived benefits over risks. Obtaining the required consent to treatment does not equate with respect for autonomy if it fails to: (1) appreciate the complexity of the decision-making process; (2) diminishes a patient's trust in their doctor; and (3) ignores a patient's capacity to comprehend what is involved. Difficulties can be encountered when putting the principle of autonomy in relation to consent into practice. Among these are concerns relating to the explanation of complex medical procedures. Here patients with limited understanding may simply accept to have the procedure performed or their inappropriate focus on a trivial risk may invite indecision and thereby warrant undue persuasion by the doctor to get them to accept treatment. Often there are limitations in the time permitted to allow sufficient assimilation of the facts and not all details can be explained to everyone's satisfaction. Sometimes patients may have contradictory wishes. While both choices may be autonomous, one may not be compatible with the patient's best interests or sense of identity thereby forcing a doctor to choose the treatment option. Not infrequently doctors meet patients who do not want to make their own decisions about treatment intervention. In some circumstances they surrender their autonomous choice allowing the doctor to decide for them. At times, patients may make use of their right to place a relative in charge of their medical care, which is an acceptable exercise of autonomy and requires equal respect. While respecting a patient's autonomy is central to the consent process, the information relating to the balance of risks and benefits must be imparted with prudence. Too much information will encourage confusion and impair effective decision making while too little places a limit on a patient's ability to judge the correct course of action. Either error of information disclosure when consenting a patient undermines autonomy as the ethical foundation in this fundamental interaction between doctor and patient.

Consent in practice

The law protects an individual's right to self-determination. This legal principle was clarified by Lord Donaldson in *Re T* (Adult: Refusal of Treatment [1992] 3 WLR 782) when he stated that decision making regarding medical interventions for the competent adult patient is an absolute right. Personal autonomy and the right to bodily integrity is safeguarded by giving patients control through the legal instrument of consent and providing sanctions when a breach occurs through a tortious or negligence remedy. All aspects of healthcare involve medical decisions and patients and doctors must work in partnership to ensure that the best care is given so as to avoid conflict. This process involves listening, discussing and sharing information with patients, about their diagnosis and treatment thus helping them to decide on the available options thereby facilitating a meaningful consent. Implicit in a patient's right to bodily integrity is their entitlement to refuse treatment and in the absence of capacity issues, a patient's decisions must be respected.

For the patient with capacity, the information that should be provided about a particular intervention as part of the consent process should include a discussion of the potential benefits, risks, side effects, burdens and the possibility of other available treatment options. Weighing up all of these factors as well as some relevant non-clinical ones allows the patient to exercise their autonomous choice. Information must be imparted in a way that takes account of a patient's level of knowledge and understanding of what is being proposed. Patients should be encouraged to ask questions to gauge their level of understanding and any reply needs to be honest and comprehensive as dictated by the wishes of the patient. In general, there are few reasons for not sharing information about a medical procedure with a patient. Some may not want as much detail and while their wishes need to be respected they must still get a broad outline of the intended intervention. Withholding information is only justified on the basis of needing to avoid serious harm to a patient's wellbeing and this must be documented in the medical notes. All doctors must be prepared to explain their decision for non-disclosure, which should uphold logical reasoning.

As part of the consent process, all information should be presented in a balanced way without undue pressure to accept one opinion over another. Patients need to be given time to consider their decision especially if the medical treatment is complex and involves significant risks. All necessary communication needs must be catered for to allow the information to be understood even if this requires an interpreter or a written and audio record of the discussion. It may be desirable, should the patient want, to have relatives or advocates present when discussions about benefits and risks of a procedure are being explained.

When consent for a medical intervention is being sought, it is the responsibility of the doctor performing the procedure to have the discussion with the patient. However, if this is not possible, this responsibility can be delegated to another who is suitably qualified and has sufficient knowledge and understanding of the complications that may arise from a particular intervention. This information in relation to risks must be communicated in such a way that the patient can have a clear comprehension of what they are consenting to. The amount of information imparted will depend on the individual patient and their unique medical and non-medical circumstances. Clarification of the risks involved will need to cover side effects both minor and serious, complications either expected or unexpected and the probability of failure of the procedure. It must be remembered that patients may prioritize differently and attach a distinct significance to particular adverse outcomes not considered as important to the doctor explaining the procedure. Most patients do not understand completely what they are told in their first interview with the doctor and as a consequence little of this information can be recalled later. A more structured format and the provision of written details about the risks of the procedure can often improve understanding and recall.

Clear and simple language should be used when describing the probability of a risk. In general, patients prefer risk conveyed numerically rather than verbally and referencing these numbers to something familiar to the patient may improve their understanding and awareness of the problem. When making decisions about treatment, patients must be informed of the possibility of changes to the plan as investigations or alternative treatment options dictate. They must consent to all or part of the interventions planned and the doctor must not exceed any limitations imposed by the patient. Only if an emergency arises can a doctor go beyond the authority given by the patient and perform interventions based on the common law principle of necessity when the treatment undertaken must allow immediate survival, be essential and not just convenient.

When consent is obtained from a patient it must be voluntary and free from any undue bias or pressure from external agencies. Patients must consent or not to a treatment by making an autonomously informed choice. They have a right to refuse all treatment, which must be respected by a doctor 'notwithstanding that the reasons for making the choice [were] rational, irrational, unknown or even non-existent (per Lord Donaldson in *Re T. (adult: refusal of treatment*) [1993] Fam 95). Challenging a decision is only allowed if there is doubt about that patient's capacity in the circumstances prevailing. In this situation, the assessment of capacity must follow the advice and practice as stated in the Mental Capacity Act 2005.

Adult patients can give their consent in writing or in verbal form. It may also be implied by their cooperation with a procedure. What is essential is that the patient has received sufficient information that allows them to come to an informed decision as to whether they should proceed and accept the risks outlined. It is also imperative that some attempt is made to assess how well the patient understands the detail and implications of what is proposed. For minor treatment interventions, a verbal consent is usually sufficient, but when greater risks are involved, a written consent is considered more appropriate. In the absence of a formal consent form that can provide a record of what was discussed, it is good practice to document the detail in the patient's medical notes. When consent has been obtained far in advance of treatment, it is important to check again, prior to the intervention, that the patient is satisfied with the situation and is willing to proceed. If new information has come to light, then it becomes necessary to review all of the decisions again.

Consent involving children and young people is a specialized area and should be undertaken by experienced doctors. In general: (1) young people and children need to be involved in discussions about their care; and (2) at 16 years it is legally presumed that young people have the ability to make decisions about their own care and some young people under 16 may be considered to have this capacity. The foregoing principles relating to consent in adults will in broad outline be the same when taking consent from children and young people for medical procedures. However, the guidelines issued by the General Medical Council (*0–18 Years: Guidance for All Doctors*) must be followed when dealing with this age group.

Conclusion

No medical intervention is without risk, and complications occur despite the best efforts of the doctors involved. The majority of patients who undergo medical treatment do so with an expectation that a good outcome will prevail. They also accept that, within reason, they may be subject to a less favourable result. The burden of any complication that befalls a patient is carried with greater acceptance if they believe that all of the relevant adverse eventualities were explained to them sufficiently and that they were not denied any information that would have altered their decision-making process. The law will endeavour to redress any wrongdoing with regard to the information disclosed during the consent procedure by an action in negligence based on the *Bolam* standard subjected to logical analysis. However, a legal instrument that helps doctors adhere to certain professional standards is secondary to the overriding ethical principle of respect for patient autonomy. The interaction between doctor and patient is founded on this fundamental principle and its application in practice while challenging can inevitably strengthen this relationship. Guidelines on the day-to-day management of the consent process is clearly outlined in a recent publication by the General Medical Council. This aims to promote a partnership between doctor and patient that advances the principles of overall benefit, best practice and best outcome.

List of further reading

Foster, C. *Choosing Life, Choosing Death. The Tyranny of Autonomy in Medical Ethics and Law*. Oxford: Hart Publishing Ltd, 2009.

General Medical Council. Guidance for doctors. Consent: patients and doctors making decisions together, GMC Publications 2008.

Herring, J. Consent to treatment. In *Medical Law and Ethics*, 3rd edn. Oxford: Oxford University Press, 2010, p. 193.

Maclean, A. The legal regulation of consent. In *Autonomy, Informed Consent and Medical Law*. Cambridge: Cambridge University Press, 2009.

Moppett, I. K. Conveying risks and benefits. In Hardman, J. G., Moppett, I. K. & Atikenhead, A. R. (eds) *Consent, Benefit and Risk in Anaesthetic Practice*. Oxford: Oxford University Press, 2009.

Chapter

18

After complications occur

Explaining complications and outcome;
Allocating blame; Implications for the
hospital and the anaesthetist

Aoibhin Hutchinson and Clare Bates

Introduction

An anaesthetic complication is an unfavourable outcome that arises following the provision of anaesthesia, or following a procedure or treatment undertaken by an anaesthetist. Anaesthetists are trained with the intention of providing them with the skills required to assess and balance risk for those in their care and to respond to unanticipated hazards to reduce harm to their patients. Dealing with the aftermath of an unforeseen complication is also a necessary skill.

Safety is at the core of anaesthetic practice. An anaesthetic complication has implications primarily for the patient but also for the anaesthetist. Complications are a source of stress to both patients and healthcare staff and can lead to complaints and litigation. The subsequent management of complications can greatly influence the outcome for patients, in terms of satisfaction or dissatisfaction, and the likelihood of legal action.

Medical ethics

Medical ethics is the study of the moral values and judgements applied to good medical care. There are six basic concepts (Table 18.1). These principles do not tell us how to manage a patient's particular condition, but they form the skeleton for a balanced approach to providing good medical care.

Clinicians have an ethical obligation to respect patients' autonomy, i.e. their right to be involved in decisions that affect them. Guaranteeing a patient's autonomy implies due consideration of beneficence and non-maleficence, ideally resulting in an informed patient, aware of the risks and potential benefits, making a choice to consent to or decline treatment. This concept is intrinsic in the contemporary process of gaining consent and is in fact the first step in managing a potential complication. Ensuring the patient is adequately and effectively informed in advance has positive effects if something goes wrong. If a patient has been appropriately involved in discussion about their care then the potential complications will have been conveyed.

Anaesthetic and Perioperative Complications, ed. Kamen Valchanov, Stephen T. Webb and Jane Sturgess.
Published by Cambridge University Press. © Cambridge University Press 2011.

Table 18.1 Principles of medical ethics.

Ethical concept	Definition
Autonomy	Preserving the patient's right to choose
Beneficence	Acting in the patient's best interest
Non-maleficence	Doing no harm to the patient
Justice	Distribution of available resources to individuals and populations
Truth	Honesty in providing information, including when seeking consent
Dignity	Acting with propriety and treating the patient with respect

Pre-complication preparation

Pre-operative visit

The process of consent involves ensuring the patient understands the nature and purpose of the procedure, the intended benefits and risks, the alternative treatments and the likely outcome of doing nothing. Patients should be informed of common risks, even those unlikely to cause significant harm, as well as rare risks with serious consequences. All discussions relating to consent should occur in an appropriate environment in a timely fashion and contemporaneous notes should be made. The anaesthetist's pre-operative visit is essential for establishing rapport with the patient, building trust and allaying fears.

Postoperative visit

Likewise a postoperative visit demonstrates the anaesthetist's commitment to seeing a patient safely through the immediate perioperative period. The postoperative visit may be the first opportunity that an anaesthetist has to inform a patient of a complication. Alternatively it may be the first time that the anaesthetist is made aware of a complication by the patient or by other staff.

After the complication

The first priority

The first priority after a complication is to provide effective treatment to prevent further harm and if possible to reverse any harm incurred. Some complications will result in little or no harm, others will require longer term intervention. A patient may need immediate intervention to manage a complication. The first duty of the anaesthetist is to the care of their patient and this should not be compromised. Anaesthetists are trained to work in stressful situations and to deal with critical events. Calling colleagues for help in emergency situations should be encouraged.

General considerations

Complications and harm cannot be totally eliminated. Healthcare staff will cause some degree of harm at some stage in their careers, but it is how staff deal with error, failings and complications that is important with respect to outcome. The outcome includes the physical

- Talk to the patient at the earliest opportunity that allows the conversation to be undertaken with adequate time, in an appropriate location and with sufficient information available

- Give an honest, factual account of the events in language the patient can clearly understand

- Allow the patient time to consider what has happened and to ask questions

- Answer all questions honestly

- Keep to the facts and avoid opinions or blame

- Explain what happens next in terms of follow-up and treatment

- Explain what steps will be taken to investigate what has happened

- Finish with a willingness to be contacted again for further discussion or make arrangement for a follow-up meeting

- Clearly and concisely document the details of the discussion in the medical records

Figure 18.1 Informing a patient after a complication.

and psychological effects on the patient and also how the patient perceives the event has been handled by the anaesthetist. The aftermath of a complication is a vulnerable period when appropriate management can positively influence the patient's experience, the doctor–patient relationship and the likelihood of litigation. If handled correctly, damage may be limited. Patients can suffer in two ways: firstly, from the complication itself; and, secondly, from the way the complication is handled.

Informing the patient

The patient has a right to be informed about any complication related to their care (Figure 18.1). Doing so early and honestly is likely to assist in resolving any subsequent difficulties. The anaesthetist providing the patient's care should inform the patient of the complication. If this is an anaesthetist in training then it is advisable that a consultant should be present in addition.

Two overriding principles prevail in communicating with the patient after a complication: firstly, be open and honest; and, secondly, believe the patient. The patient may provide information about additional symptoms they have experienced. Apologizing for an event does not mean that you are accepting that you are at fault, but does demonstrate empathy. It is difficult to confront our potential failings or deal with complex situations that did not end as intended, but evading patients following a complication is likely to result in a much more difficult encounter in the future in terms of complaints and litigation.

Documentation

It is paramount that contemporaneous legible records are made after a complication. These should be accurate and clear, with the appropriate date, time, signature, printed name and designation in place. If a note can only be made retrospectively then this should done with the actual time of writing noted, and the accurate time of the incident referred to in the description of the events. Pre-operative discussions should have already been documented. However, if this is not the case any retrospective documentation of pre-operative discussions should clearly acknowledge this as a retrospective note.

Medical notes are a source of information for medical staff and for the patient. It may be several years later that a specific incident or case is examined as a formal complaint or in the form of litigation. Such a significant passage of time would make it unlikely for a doctor to recall details unless of course the situation was particularly stressful. Therefore, the notes form the doctor's record of what happened and how they managed it. The notes should include details of postoperative discussions, explanations offered and planned management and follow-up. It is also recommended to note in the patient records the reference number of any incident report forms completed at the time, for cross-referencing purposes.

Patient follow-up

The follow-up required for a patient following a complication is guided by the severity of the event. A complication resulting in minimal harm may not require any further action. Complications leading to significant harm may need arrangements for specific inter-specialty referral. The anaesthetist, in association with the patient's admitting consultant, should arrange appropriate and timely referral.

The anaesthetist

The majority of anaesthetists will be involved in an anaesthetic complication during their careers. The attitude of anaesthetists in relation to risk and potential harm is an important consideration. Anaesthetists strive to provide safe care but a doctor who cannot accept the potential to cause harm would be ineffective in their daily practice. Practice should be guided by the best evidence to support decision making but should acknowledge the possibility of untoward outcomes, and deal with such adverse events appropriately. The psychological effect of more serious complications on the anaesthetist should not be underestimated, and the individual should be supported by a senior colleague or mentor. Depending on the severity of the complication the anaesthetist's clinical commitment may need to be reviewed, both in terms of consideration for the anaesthetist's wellbeing or if there are concerns regarding fitness to practice.

Incident investigation

All UK NHS Trusts have clinical governance and risk management systems in place to record and investigate incidents of harm arising in patient care. As a result of a complication harm may or may not have occurred, the event may or may not have involved error on the part of the operator and the situation may have been preventable or not. However, such events may need further exploration to identify potential areas for improvement, to reduce future events and to improve safety. Incident reporting allows staff to report the details of complications so that they can be followed up by risk management to identify the degree of harm incurred, the likelihood of future recurrence and to decide if formal root cause analysis is required. Most risk management departments use risk matrices to grade events depending on likelihood of recurrence and severity of outcome. A risk assessment is carried out by risk management departments to determine the level of investigation required for a given event.

Despite the potential for local critical incident reporting systems to enhance the safety profile of healthcare there have been problems encountered during its evolution. Firstly, the concept of '*first do no harm*' may make it difficult for staff to accept that they can and will cause harm to their patients. Secondly, the worry that 'someone must be to blame' may leave staff feeling vulnerable and concerned about potential litigation. Lack of feedback to staff can result in a corrosive belief that reporting makes no difference. Confusion can arise about what to report, how to report it and how to deal with it. However, the profile of patient safety and incident reporting has risen significantly in the past decade on a global and national level.

In the UK hospitals use local risk management structures to handle and analyze all incidents reported across all specialties using a generic form. However, in addition to this local management the NPSA developed the National Reporting and Learning System (NRLS) in 2003 to collate reports from local risk management departments to pool learning at a national level. The advent of the NRLS in England and Wales was the first time data moved to an independent body for further collective analysis with the intention of improving pattern detection and learning. From 2003 to 2008, 2.8 million incidents in England were reported to the NRLS. Reporting has increased year on year suggesting effective reinforcement of the importance of reporting. Through the NRLS valuable lessons have been disseminated.

Sources of information

Medicine has a long history of trying to learn from its mistakes. There are multiple methods of identifying and analyzing safety deficits in healthcare (Figure 18.2).

Medico-legal implications

Blame allocation

Blame refers to how a complication is perceived by others and where responsibility lies for the complication and adverse outcome. Healthcare staff are trained with an expectation to get things right and error can be seen as being fallible. Blame directed at the anaesthetist can arise from several sources: from the patient or relatives, from colleagues, from the hospital, from lawyers and from the media. When dealing with blame allocation, there can be a conflict, perceived or real, between the hospital and the anaesthetist. Should the focus be on organizational systems or the individual professional? The reality is that both the hospital and the anaesthetist need to identify the underlying cause of what went wrong and identify opportunities for change. Fear of blame and of the consequences of being held responsible

- Critical incident monitoring
- Morbidity and mortality meetings
- Internal enquiries
- External enquiries
- Case reports/series
- Indemnity organisations' publications
- National Confidential Enquiries

Figure 18.2 Sources of information available to healthcare staff in relation to patient safety incidents.

Table 18.2 Implications for the hospital and anaesthetist.

Hospital	Anaesthetist
No future implications	No future implications
Complaint and review of care	Involvement in complaint and review of care
Involvement of Care Quality Commission or similar external regulatory body	Investigation under *Maintaining High Professional Standards in the NHS* and referral to National Clinical Assessment Service (NCAS)
Referral of anaesthetist to the GMC	Referral to the GMC leading to a professional conduct hearing
Serious untoward incident investigation	Involvement in serious untoward incident investigation
Coroner's inquest	Witness at coroner's inquest
Media coverage	Involvement in media coverage
Clinical negligence claim	Witness in clinical negligence claim (if NHS care), or defendant in clinical negligence claim (if private care)
Public inquiry	Witness at public inquiry
Corporate manslaughter charges	Defendant for manslaughter charges

can inhibit this process. Conflict between hospital and anaesthetist can also prevent an open consideration of events. Blame allocation is a difficult process but one that is necessary when litigation ensues following a complication.

Implications for the hospital and anaesthetist

The potential implications for the hospital and anaesthetist are far ranging and depend on the nature of the complication, the harm incurred, the response of the patient or relatives and the risk of future harm to other patients (Table 18.2).

The following examples have been provided to illustrate how each of these factors can affect both the hospital and the anaesthetist.

No future implications

Example: A patient regurgitated gastric contents during induction of anaesthesia and developed pulmonary aspiration pneumonitis. Gastric aspiration is a potential risk in any operation performed under general anaesthesia. The patient brought a clinical negligence claim for compensation but there was no evidence that the anaesthetist had been negligent and the claim failed.

Impact: The hospital was not required to make any changes to practice or procedure and the anaesthetist was found to have provided an appropriate level of care. There were no long-term implications for either party.

Complaint

Example: A patient was admitted to hospital complaining of vomiting and abdominal pain. She was admitted to the surgical ward where she was treated with intravenous fluids, intravenous antibiotics and analgesia. The next day her condition deteriorated. The patient was assessed by the consultant intensivist who agreed that ICU admission was necessary. Admission to ICU was delayed due to lack of available beds. The patient suffered a stroke and died several days later. Her husband raised concerns about the lack of ICU beds. The complaint was investigated through the hospital's complaints procedure. The hospital acknowledged the delay and advised the patient's relatives that it was in the process of increasing the number of ICU beds and that a regional network for ICU beds would be established.

Impact: The complaints process can provide a useful forum to assess the care provided to a patient. In this case it was not thought that the delay in admission to ICU contributed to the patient's death but it did give the hospital the opportunity to learn lessons and make organizational changes. No specific allegations were raised against the intensivist.

Involvement of an external statutory authority

Example: Following a series of high-profile critical incidents, the Regulatory and Quality Improvement Authority (RQIA) in Northern Ireland (the equivalent of the Care Quality Care Commission in England) carried out a review of intrapartum care in maternity units. The report recommended that one hospital review the level of anaesthetic cover available and that two other hospitals identify a lead obstetric anaesthetist.

Impact: Hospitals must meet the recommendations of external regulatory bodies. For an individual anaesthetist, the role of external regulatory bodies means that one adverse outcome may lead to a full investigation of care throughout the entire hospital. The anaesthetist may be referred to the National Clinical Assessment Service (NCAS), which provides assistance with the management of poorly performing doctors. Assistance may be provided to manage concerns locally or there may be a more formal assessment by NCAS. Less than 5% of referrals to NCAS are related to anaesthetists. Concerns about an anaesthetist may be so serious that the individual is suspended from work. Through NCAS steps may be taken to ensure that there is a prompt return to work or, alternatively, disciplinary action. The process of investigation under *Maintaining High Professional Standards in the NHS* is stressful and if there is a prolonged period of time out of the workplace, the risk of deskilling becomes a valid concern.

General Medical Council referral

Example: An anaesthetist had worked at a specialist unit for patients who required conscious sedation for dental treatment. Complaints were made by the parents of five children who had received sedation from the anaesthetist. A GMC Fitness to Practice panel found that there was:

- failure to obtain informed consent
- failure to comply with drug protocols and guidelines
- failure to ensure that the children had recovered before they were discharged
- excessive sedative dosing in four of the five cases
- the technique used was novel and had not been the subject of any audit
- the side effects and risks were not sufficiently explained to the parents of the children.

The panel held that the care provided to these five children fell below the standard expected of a medical practitioner. The anaesthetist was found guilty of serious professional misconduct and registration made subject to conditions for a period of 12 months.

Impact: The implications of a GMC hearing for any anaesthetist are significant. If a complaint is made to the GMC and a Fitness to Practice hearing takes place, the available sanctions are no action, undertakings, conditional registration (maximum of three years), suspension or erasure.

Serious untoward incident investigation

Example: Mrs. Elaine Bromiley was a 37-year-old mother who presented for elective nasal surgery. Due to anaesthetic complications, she sustained irreversible brain damage and subsequently died. Following her death, an independent review of the care provided was commissioned by the hospital. The relatives of the patient have made an anonymous copy of this report freely available on the internet for learning purposes. The review found that the management of the emergency 'can't intubate, can't ventilate' situation was unsatisfactory. The review made a number of recommendations including obtaining an Aintree catheter for difficult intubation, training in the Difficult Airway Society (DAS) airway management protocols, ensuring that timings are recorded and that staff are aware of the passage of time during an emergency situation, improved anaesthetic record keeping, improved arrangements for transfer of care from anaesthetist to recovery staff and enforcing a break for all staff after a major incident before continuing with an operating list.

Impact: The independent review of this incident gave both the hospital and the anaesthetist the opportunity to learn from the tragic outcome in this case and improve practice for the future.

Coroner's inquest

Example: The coroner's inquest into the death of Elaine Bromiley is available on the internet. The coroner gave a narrative verdict, which stated that:
'The management of the "can't intubate, can't ventilate" emergency did not follow the current or any recognized guidance. Too much time was taken trying to intubate the trachea rather than concentrating on ensuring adequate oxygenation. The clinicians became oblivious to the passing of time and thus lost opportunities to limit the extent of damage caused by the prolonged period of hypoxia. Not all the clinicians were aware that there was a problem with ventilating Mrs. Bromiley. Surgical airway access by either tracheotomy or cricothyroidotomy should have been considered and carried out. Given the prolonged period of hypoxia, Mrs. Bromiley should have been admitted to an intensive care unit rather than to the recovery room. To send her to recovery in an unconscious state and breathing spontaneously was inappropriate. Subsequently transferring Mrs. Bromiley to (the NHS) hospital without a secure airway was an unnecessary risk.'

Impact: A coroner's inquest is an investigative process, not an adversarial one. In England, Wales and Northern Ireland the coroner must first determine whether or not an inquest is necessary. Where a coroner proceeds to hold an inquest, his or her role is to ascertain who the deceased was, when they died and what the cause of death was. The system is different in Scotland where the prosecutor fiscal may hold a fatal accidents enquiry. Although the process is not adversarial, the competing interests of the interested parties often lead to a degree of cross-examination. The hospital will want to establish that appropriate systems were in place to provide the required level of care. The anaesthetist will want to establish that the care that he or she provided was acceptable. The relatives will want to establish if either the hospital or the anaesthetist were responsible for the death and if the death was avoidable. It is likely that the various parties will have separate legal representation. The hospital will provide legal representation but if a conflict of interest exists between the hospital and the anaesthetist, then separate representation will be required from a medical indemnity organization. The coroner will not explicitly allocate blame but will come to a verdict that may imply fault.

Media coverage

Example: A six-week-old boy was being treated for pyloric stenosis. A volume of air was accidently administered into the boy's blood supply instead of his nasogastric tube. The anaesthetist was referred to the GMC and received a period of suspension. The anaesthetist was also tried for manslaughter and acquitted. Significant interest in the case was generated in the media. An apology was issued to the relatives by the hospital.

Impact: The media have developed a great interest in reporting medical errors. What had previously been a private professional issue has now become of public and political interest. Dealing with the media often presents an anaesthetist with a difficult dilemma. The anaesthetist has a desire to defend their own reputation but must realize that they are constrained by their duty of confidentiality. The impact of media coverage is likely to be stressful. The positive effects of media coverage include raising the awareness of medical errors and resultant changes in practice to prevent recurrence.

Clinical negligence claims

Example: A patient underwent hip replacement surgery under combined spinal–epidural anaesthesia at a private hospital. The patient subsequently complained of loss of power and sensation in her legs. The anaesthetist advised that her symptoms were residual effects of the anaesthesia. She was subsequently diagnosed as suffering from a vertebral canal haematoma. A claim for damages for the permanent neurological deficit affecting her legs was brought against the anaesthetist. The patient suffered loss, which was avoidable, and she received an award of damages.

Impact: If care is provided in an NHS hospital, the hospital will be the defendant. In a private hospital, the anaesthetist will be the defendant. The impact on the hospital will include the time and resources spent investigating the claim, the effect on staff morale and the ability to learn lessons for the future. In financial terms there is the potential to be held responsible for the claimant's legal costs and an award for damages. The impact is more personal for the individual anaesthetist. Dealing with allegations of negligence is stressful, time-consuming and frustrating. An individual anaesthetist may struggle with the decision by the NHS hospital to settle a claim for financial reasons even if they believe that the care provided was defensible.

Public inquiry

Example: On 9 June 2010 the Secretary of State for Health, Andrew Lansley MP, announced a full public inquiry into the role of the commissioning, supervisory and regulatory bodies in the monitoring of Mid Staffordshire NHS Foundation Trust. The inquiry is established under the Inquiries Act 2005 (which means that the inquiry will have the authority to compel witnesses to attend and to give evidence under oath) and is chaired by Robert Francis QC, who will make recommendations to the Secretary of State based on the lessons learned from Mid Staffordshire. The public inquiry will build on the work of his earlier independent inquiry into the care provided by Mid Staffordshire NHS Foundation Trust between January 2005 and March 2009. The 800-page report of the independent inquiry was published in February 2010. Whilst the alleged failures in patient care do not arise from specific anaesthetic issues, this inquiry is a prime example of the far-reaching consequences of a public inquiry.

Impact: The hospital has already taken steps to address concerns and improve services. They have been the subject of ongoing assessment from the Care Quality Commission (CQC). Despite the best efforts of the inquiry to minimize interference with the work of the hospital, the inquiry will undoubtedly place pressure on the hospital in terms of resources, staff morale and adverse publicity. For the clinicians involved, they will be required to attend the inquiry, give evidence and face questioning and cross-examination. The inquiry will attract a high level of media interest, placing the clinicians under additional pressure.

Manslaughter charges

Example: Systematic problems with anaesthetic equipment may result in death and the failure to act in response to earlier concerns may lead to a prosecution for corporate manslaughter. An anaesthetist was convicted of manslaughter when the oxygen supply to a patient undergoing an eye operation was cut off. The anaesthetist failed to check the connection until after resuscitation had been commenced.

Impact – corporate manslaughter: The Corporate Manslaughter and Homicide Act 2007 creates the criminal offence of corporate manslaughter. An organization will be guilty of corporate manslaughter if the way in which its activities are managed or organized causes a death and amounts to a gross breach of duty of care to the deceased. The Sentencing Guidelines Council recently published a Definitive Guideline that must be considered by every court in England and Wales when sentencing organizations for corporate manslaughter. The effects of this new guideline include scope for the imposition of punitive fines and publication of conviction details. If a hospital is convicted of corporate manslaughter the consequences can be direct and indirect. Direct consequences include:

- imposition of unlimited fines
- remedial orders – that is the requirement for the organization to improve risk monitoring or to ensure that a similar problem will not occur again in the future
- publicity orders – requiring the organization to publicize details of its conviction and fine.

Indirect consequences could include:

- loss of reputation
- further prosecution for breach of health and safety, which may lead to the disqualification of directors
- poor staff morale.

    Impact – individual manslaughter: Whilst the consequences are serious, the impact on an individual of a prosecution for gross negligence manslaughter is much greater. The offence of gross negligence manslaughter is tantamount to a civil test in a criminal setting. In the case above, the House of Lords set out the key elements of the offence. The first question is whether the defendant is in breach of a duty of care to the victim. The second question is whether the breach of duty caused the death. The final hurdle is whether the breach of duty could be considered so serious as to constitute gross negligence and a criminal offence. If a criminal offence is established, a custodial sentence is likely. The implications for an anaesthetist facing criminal charges cannot be underestimated.

List of further reading

AAGBI. *The Anaesthesia Team*. AAGBI, 2005.

AAGBI. *Consent for Anaesthesia*. AAGBI, 2006.

AAGBI. *Pre-operative Assessment and Patient Preparation: The Role of the Anaesthetist*. AAGBI, 2010.

Clinical Human Factors Group. www.chfg.org (accessed 15 April 2011).

Department of Health. Inquiry into the Operation of the Commissioning, Supervisory and Regulatory Bodies in Relation to their Monitoring Role at Mid Staffordshire NHS Foundation Trust. Terms of reference. www.dh.gov.uk/prod_consum_dh/groups/dh_digitalassets/@dh/@en/@ps/documents/digitalasset/dh_116651.pdf (accessed 15 April 2011).

General Medical Council. Indicative sanctions guidance for the fitness to practice panel, GMC 2005.

House of Commons. Hansard Debates for 9 June 2010: column 333. Mid Staffordshire NHS Foundation Trust. www.publications.parliament.uk/pa/cm201011/cmhansrd/cm100609/debtext/100609-0004.htm#10060953000002 (accessed 15 April 2011).

National Clinical Assessment Service. *NCA Handbook: Resolving Concerns about Professional Practice*, 6th edn. National Patient Safety Agency, 2011.

National Health and Medical Research Council. *General Guidelines for Medical Practitioners on Providing Information to Patients*. Canberra: Australian Government Publishing Service, 1993.

Reason, J. Human error: models and management. *BMJ* 2000; **320**(7237): 768–70.

Vincent, C. *Patient Safety*. Elsevier Churchill Livingstone, 2006, pp.123–38.

Risk factors for litigation

19

Dominic Bell

Introduction

Despite the content of this textbook emphasizing the extensive range and severity of complications, litigation only arises from an exceptionally small percentage of finished patient episodes, including those cases where complications have materialized. This observation does not, however, neutralize the ill-defined threat hanging over practitioners, given the number of interventions over a professional lifetime, changing demographics towards the morbidly obese or increasingly elderly population with associated co-morbidity, more heroic surgery and logistical barriers to optimal practice such as admission on the day of surgery. Within such a system, complications, some potentially serious, appear inevitable and whilst all practitioners would aspire to or indeed claim the highest standards of patient care, it is unrealistic to consider that such complications would always be viewed as inherent to the anaesthetic process and therefore defensible.

The goal of the following chapter is to set out the circumstances in which litigation is likely to arise and to tease out those outcomes, actions, omissions and overall standard of professional delivery, which individually or cumulatively will meet the criteria for the 'breach of duty', which is fundamental to litigation success. It is hoped that both practitioners and anaesthetic departments will approach this subject constructively by reflection on their responsibilities to the population we serve at an exceptionally vulnerable phase in their lives, and promote a standard of care that minimizes adverse outcomes, rather than simplistically adopting strategies that limit liability in the event of an adverse outcome.

Triggering factors for the litigation process

There can be no doubt that society has moved away from gratitude for healthcare with naïve acceptance of complications, and become more litigious, fuelled by explicit advertizing of the legal sector specializing in this market and the offer of 'no win, no fee' arrangements. Despite such accessibility, additional factors are usually required before patient or next-of-kin are driven to legal advice, some of which are beyond the practitioner's control, but others reflecting the response of the clinician, healthcare team or broader institution to adverse incidents.

Whilst persistent pain, disfigurement or disability are always likely to trigger consideration of litigation, it is not necessarily the severity of the adverse outcome, but the impact on employment and other responsibilities over the longer term, that determines whether proceedings will be initiated.

Anaesthetic and Perioperative Complications, ed. Kamen Valchanov, Stephen T. Webb and Jane Sturgess.
Published by Cambridge University Press. © Cambridge University Press 2011.

The category of shortcoming may also be relevant at this primary stage, with the public particularly intolerant of what is perceived to be a failure to deliver on fundamental responsibilities, with reference to awareness under general anaesthesia or pain and discomfort under regional techniques when there are no obvious extenuating circumstances.

It can be noted that these complications are obvious to the patient from the outset, whilst others require communication from the practitioner, a scenario demanding a high level of skill and integrity. Doctors have a primary professional responsibility to inform patients or their next-of-kin of complications and to answer any subsequent questions fully and truthfully. They are not, however, under any obligation to indict themselves from a civil or criminal perspective by relating how the complication might have been avoided by the availability of additional equipment, an alternative technique or the attendance of practitioners with a higher level of experience or expertise.

Complications triggering this primary interface between patient and practitioner will inevitably be on a spectrum of 'culpability'. At one end will be patients carrying a significant level of risk through co-morbidity such as ischaemic heart disease, being aware pre-operatively of those risks but hoping for the greater benefit of the surgical intervention and accepting that those risks have materialized despite all precautions. At the other end of the spectrum lie the predictably avoidable complications in the patient with no relevant risk factors identified pre-operatively, who could reasonably expect answers on how the complication occurred and actions taken to avoid recurrence.

The nature of this primary interaction is a key determinant of the subsequent course of action on the part of patient or their next-of-kin. It is often stated by defence societies and patient action groups that first and foremost patients wish for an honest explanation of the event, an apology if this was avoidable and reassurance that action will be taken to avoid recurrence of a similar class of complication or error. Whilst competent handling of this scenario may avoid escalation of a grievance to destructive complaints to the regulatory bodies, it is unrealistic to anticipate that where identifiable harm has occurred, that a full explanation of the event, the implications, the prognosis and possible remedial treatment, will be enough to abort contact with legal advisers. It is predictable, however, that where there has been even a perception of an unsatisfactory or evasive response to questions or a formal complaint, there is a high likelihood of litigation being initiated.

Legal evaluation of a potential claim

The handling of a medical negligence claim requires specialized expertise, but this should be accessible to every member of the public, since solicitors must comply with professional expectations defined by their regulatory authorities and refer clients to firms and individuals accredited under the Clinical Negligence Accreditation Scheme if they themselves do not have this affiliation. Alternatively, agencies such as AvMA (Action against Medical Accidents) provide initial advice for individuals facing uncertainty, including referral to appropriate legal representation.

Whilst legal aid is still available for medical negligence cases, the criteria for eligibility as defined by the Legal Services Commission render this a limited option, leaving most cases to be managed on a 'no win, no fee' or conditional fee agreement (CFA). It might be considered in these circumstances that only claims with a high likelihood of success will be pursued, but the possibility of syndicating the costs of failure with an insurance company and the significantly higher level of fee chargeable with success, are responsible for increasing activity in this field.

Given the burgeoning costs of defending litigation, an additional driver is the likelihood of a healthcare provider settling a relatively low-level claim, such that even when the 'balance of probability' criteria for negligence are unlikely to be met, solicitors knowledgeable in the field and confident in their brinkmanship will initiate a claim.

The primary criteria to be examined will be whether or not the adverse event would normally happen given the circumstances of the case. If on such crude primary analysis the answer to this question is no, it is likely that there will be some initial investment in accessing the clinical records and reviewing these, potentially with in-house ex-healthcare professionals, usually nursing staff. Secondary analysis, still all potentially in-house, would focus on why the event occurred and whether there was any deviation from accepted standards, seeking disclosure of any relevant documentation such as departmental guidelines or serious untoward incident investigation reports.

Despite extensive reforms to the civil justice system in 1999 to minimize unnecessary cost, delay and inconsistency where possible, there still remains significant variation in how legal firms then proceed. The *Pre-Action Protocol for the Resolution of Clinical Disputes* is intended to avoid the high initial costs of litigation by incorporating strategies such as alternative dispute resolution (ADR). If a robust case can be established without resorting to formal expert opinion, a request for settlement either directly or through mediation will usually be contained in the first correspondence following request for the medical records, as exampled below:

> It is our view that in litigation of this nature there is a need for cooperation and openness on both sides. An unnecessarily adversarial approach will cause detriment to both our clients and in our view it is important that this should be avoided. We must make it clear to you that this are prepared to meet with you or your client at anytime on a without prejudice basis to discuss this case, the future conduct of the litigation, selection of experts or a possible settlement and would urge you to consider the matter being referred for mediation.

Despite this promotion of a non-adversarial system, apart from very low-order claims, the combination of professional unwillingness to self-define as negligent and institutional reluctance to be perceived as a soft target usually triggers a defensive response, placing the onus on the claimant to define precisely why causation and breach of duty can be proven on the civil burden of proof, and preparing a rebuttal on at least one point in the chain of breach of duty and causation. The process of litigation is thereby triggered, and predictably remains both adversarial and expensive until the claim is abandoned, settled or adjudicated on within the civil courts.

Defining negligence

With the majority of cases placed somewhere on the spectrum between unequivocal negligence and defensible care, the initial construction of the claim is critically dependent on the expertise of the legal team and instructed medical experts. A competent law firm will usually derive the key areas for further scrutiny, consider any relevant clinical standards or guidelines and request further information from the 'culpable' practitioner or institution on the course of events, internal protocols and any critical incident investigations. It is increasingly likely therefore that a medical expert will be presented not only with the relevant facts but with a series of very specific questions on 'breach of duty' given that causation is usually a less contentious issue.

It could reasonably be expected therefore that a practitioner professing expertise in the area could address these questions in a comprehensive and unambiguous manner, and secondarily identify any other aspects of care relevant to the litigation, in line with that expertise.

The reality is that the key issues might not be so identified, the points of reference for defining 'breach of duty' may be unclear or non-existent and the expertise of the expert witness variable. Whilst the rules for the conduct of expert witnesses have been increasingly refined over the last decade, with explicit responsibility to the court rather than any instructing party, there is at least a perception that more senior figures within the profession are likely to be instructed by institutions, defence societies or the NHS Litigation Authority. With such seniority and experience there is inevitable acquisition of 'court craft' and robustness in joint discussion that would predictably disadvantage a less experienced claimant's expert when there is near equipoise on a case. Given that the claimant's case may succeed or fail on the slimmest balance of probability, these issues are clearly relevant to whether litigation is initiated, maintained or ultimately successful. This is also the primary reason for barristers preferring to conduct a conference with the experts directly in attendance, prior to formalizing and thereby investing in Particulars of Claim, to determine whether an expert will maintain their position even under hostile cross-examination and seemingly authoritative counter-opinion.

Establishing 'breach of duty'

Defining 'breach of duty' is not only difficult for the above reasons when the case falls in the amorphous and debatable middle area, but also because society and indeed the regulatory bodies recognize that not every practitioner will possess all relevant knowledge, achieve the highest level of competence for technical interventions or be able to consistently perform at an optimal level, particularly when care is compromised by personal or environmental challenges or institutional shortcomings. There is indeed implicit recognition of these factors in the arbitrary pass mark for undergraduate and postgraduate medical examinations, when members of the public may take the view that in relation to healthcare, knowledge should be mandatory and absolute rather than relative. The evolving use of high-fidelity simulation for critical incident training also demonstrates how many practitioners may lack situational awareness and be unable to maximize efficient use of all available resources including personnel at times of crisis. Whilst there is an expectation that anaesthetists should competently handle a range of problems, limited access to training in this field or adverse outcomes despite such training, may be construed as a professional norm, thereby increasing the hurdle to proving negligence.

The law itself remains unhelpfully ill-defined on the issue of *Bolam* reasonableness versus *Bolitho* obligations to incorporate new knowledge and technology to minimize the risk of patient harms. Although there is an expectation under *Bolitho* to subject any defence argument to the test of 'intrinsic logic', there is no apparent barrier to the declaration by the defence expert: 'it is not what I would have done, and does not represent the highest standard of care, but that does not make it unreasonable or negligent'. There remains therefore a significant impediment to successful litigation unless the claimant's expert can ultimately persuade a judge that either the clinical judgement of the relevant doctor, his undertakings or his omissions, placed that individual beyond the expectations on his colleagues collectively, i.e. he did what no reasonable colleague would have done in the circumstances. There is unfortunately no unequivocal point of reference for this task, since the specialty has no 'code of conduct, competence and performance' that defines the limits of defensibility for the range of undertakings of any anaesthetist from pre-operative assessment to postoperative care.

Observations on professional standards

One of the key roles of the professional bodies is, however, to promote patient safety, and standards have been established on basic responsibilities such as monitoring, through to the management of significant complications such as anaphylaxis. If therefore patient harm were to arise from delayed recognition of endotracheal tube displacement in the absence of functional capnography, even with extenuating circumstances such as emergency life- or limb-saving surgery, it is unlikely that there would be any significant financial investment in defending the claim. Similarly, if mortality or morbidity followed clear deviation from the protocol for management of anaphylaxis, including secondary reactions due to a failure to appropriately investigate an initial incident, it would be difficult to defend a 'breach of duty' claim even if causation were more contentious.

It can be seen, however, that the professional standards are neither comprehensive in defining every safety precaution or the management of every complication, and are not pre-scriptive as to how these aspects of care should be delivered. There are multiple reasons why this situation pertains, including the conflict between effectiveness and efficiency if, for example, an exhaustive machine checklist with a third party was undertaken and docu-mented before every case on a list. There is also a concern that converting the anaesthetic process into a series of rigid protocols will not only alienate intelligent professionals, but introduce different categories of human error as clinical scenarios are approached by the best-fit algorithm, which is then slavishly followed to an untoward outcome that may not have occurred if the practitioner had utilized more generic principles for problem solving.

There is in addition, however, conflict between specifying the highest attainable stand-ard to support investment in departments looking for such support, and creating jeopardy for individual practitioners or departments if these standards are not met for whatever rea-son. The adoption of ultrasound scanning for central venous access demonstrates this con-sideration, with recognition that despite the technology reducing the incidence of major complications such as carotid artery puncture, not every unit had immediate access to the equipment, training in its use or the resources to achieve ongoing education. There was also a less defensible parallel recognition that certain practitioners refused to accept the possi-bility of complications of a landmark-based technique in their hands and the profession had neither the willingness nor the mandate to veto this practice. The end result is that almost a decade after national guidance, there is still ambiguity as to whether ultrasound guid-ance means initial review of the anatomy or continuous visualization during placement, and whether training in the landmark technique is justified for the occasional circumstances when access to ultrasound devices is problematical.

It can be seen therefore that defining negligence by reference to unequivocal professional standards is relatively rare, and the process of claiming negligence is predominantly arbi-trary and individual opinion-based, with the predictability of counter-argument and there-fore robust defence.

Generic responsibilities of a doctor

Given that 'breach of duty' equates with deviating from reasonable conduct, competence or performance, and there is no primary specialty-specific definition of 'reasonableness', an alternative point of reference is the generic duty of a doctor as defined by the General Medical Council as regulatory body. If therefore adverse events occurred from the point of induction onwards, which were foreseeable and avoidable by undertaking a competent history, examination and review of the medical records, this would unequivocally equate with negligence since the practitioner would have deviated from the standards that are mandated as a condition of registration, namely that good clinical care must include adequately assessing the patient's condition. These principles would apply if primary medical conditions with the potential to destabilize such as asthma or ischaemic heart disease, therapy relevant to anaesthesia and surgery such as steroids, the likely problematical airway or a history of adverse drug reaction to anaesthetic agents, were not identified at pre-operative assessment. If the patient died as a consequence of these omissions, given a fundamental failure of care in circumstances where the serious consequences of such an omission should have been recognized, it is predictable that the question would not be whether negligence occurred, but whether the criteria for gross negligence manslaughter and unlawful killing could be met.

The second stage after acquisition of all relevant patient information is making defensible decisions on the basis of that information. A fundamental professional responsibility of a doctor is to recognize limits of competence, and within anaesthesia there is an assumption that on entry to the specialty any practitioner would acknowledge the non-therapeutic nature of anaesthesia, the inherent risks and the primary responsibility during provision of anaesthesia to maintain near normal physiological status, particularly with regards to ventilation and cardiovascular performance. Any failure to act upon relevant information, such as severe bronchospasm during a previous anaesthetic, and follow this with evaluation of the relevant records, to consider the nature of the reaction and identify or eliminate certain agents as causal, thereby facilitating a rational choice for the proposed procedure, would in the event of a subsequent severe reaction, be interpreted as going beyond incompetence and the standard for civil negligence, and raise questions of recklessness.

This principle, that any competent anaesthetist should recognize the inherent risks of what is proposed and undertaken, and correspondingly take all effort to minimize the likelihood of such risk materializing, including seeking assistance, becomes therefore a defining standard when assessing negligence. It is a principle furthermore which is intrinsic to concepts of informed consent, whereby the generic risks of anaesthesia are explained to the patient, any additional specific risk associated with co-morbidity is also identified and the plan for anaesthesia to maximize benefit and reduce risk is set out as the basis of informed consent. If therefore the documentation and available evidence does not demonstrate a comprehensive pre-operative assessment for anything other than life-saving surgery in a patient lacking capacity, with engagement of the patient on both excess risk and strategies to minimize such risk, in circumstances where adverse consequences then arise, it is inevitable that questions will be raised not only over competence, but also conduct, and defence of any claim for negligence will be correspondingly problematical.

The above basic principles in relation to practitioner competence and patient consent permeate any analysis of anaesthetic care in the context of litigation, where competence equates with understanding the risks associated with any anaesthetic undertaking, and having the expertise to avoid, identify and appropriately manage any such complication, or recognizing the need to ensure supervision or the direct provision of care by practitioners with such expertise. It is accepted that certain scenarios may be unpredictable and beyond the experience of even senior anaesthetists, such as metabolic derangement during protracted prone surgery, which raises questions of pressure-induced hypoxic hepatic injury, drug toxicity or malignant hyperpyrexia. In these circumstances it would not be negligent not to reach the definitive diagnosis, but it would be negligent if the patient came to avoidable harm because anaesthetic or critical care assistance was not considered at an early stage.

Core responsibilities of an anaesthetist

Pursuing these principles, the nature of certain complications rather than the actions of the anaesthetist constitute negligence until proven otherwise, because it is considered to be the fundamental role of an anaesthetist to maintain oxygenation and ventilation and optimize cardiovascular status. This expectation goes beyond the avoidance of an adverse outcome in the context of a problematical airway, with every anaesthetist expected to ensure the availability of and be familiar with the extensive range of equipment currently provided for such an event. There is a fundamental expectation that any equipment intended for patient use would have been tested and passed as 'fit for purpose' prior to application to a patient. The public could reasonably expect an anaesthetic circuit to be demonstrably functional prior to induction of anaesthesia, i.e. be free from obstruction or leakage, and if difficulty with ventilation is encountered following induction, that the practitioner take logical steps to determine whether the problem lies with the patient, the airway or the breathing circuit, within the time frame necessary to prevent secondary sequelae. It has been argued previously that a blocked angle piece was beyond the expectation of an anaesthetist and that professional body recommendations on checking of anaesthetic equipment did not unambiguously specify that the angle piece should be included when assessing the patency of a breathing circuit. Whilst current UK guidelines do not stipulate a single reproducible functional test of the breathing circuit prior to induction, such as the 'double-bag' technique endorsed by ANZCA, there is an inevitability that in the aftermath of previous incidents and surrounding publicity, an adverse outcome attributable to equipment blockage would be investigated in the first instance for gross negligence manslaughter rather than for negligence, with the latter predictably unable to be defended.

It can similarly be expected that a competent anaesthetist would be able to differentiate between acute bronchospasm, whether occurring in isolation or as part of a more generalized reaction, endotracheal tube misplacement, equipment blockage and other induced conditions such as tension pneumothorax, before any significant secondary sequelae arise.

The other area in which there is reasonable anticipation of expertise relates to cardiovascular optimization, which incorporates rational use of invasive monitoring, and defining an acceptable degree of hypotension based on an individual's age and co-morbidity that would predictably avoid neurological, renal or cardiac injury. The logical use of inotropes and vasopressors, and defensible transfusion of blood and other products are other aspects where expertise can be expected. Unless therefore protracted hypotension is due to a scenario such as uncontrolled major haemorrhage despite all attempts to maximize transfusion in, for example, aortic aneurysm rupture, unanticipated and unresponsive anaphylaxis or cardiac decompensation in a patient with established severe primary myocardial disease, it is likely that hypoxic-ischaemic brain or spinal cord injury will be viewed as predictable, avoidable and thereby negligent.

Paralleling this core responsibility to maintain physiological homeostasis during the conduct of anaesthesia, and sometimes creating conflict with these goals, is the accompanying principal duty or raison d'etre of an anaesthetist to prevent awareness during general anaesthesia and discomfort and distress when relying on regional techniques. Unless there are extenuating circumstances in a case of awareness, such as life-saving surgery for major haemorrhage in a patient with profound hypotension, or for discomfort in the awake patient, such as the urgency due to fetal compromise in a caesarean section under epidural block-ade, and contraindication to any anaesthetic or analgesic adjuncts, it can be predicted that most institutions or defence organizations would not invest heavily in attempting to defend a claim for negligence.

Complications of invasive interventions

As set out above, anaesthetists also carry out invasive interventions in the form of vascular monitoring and regional analgesia, which carry significant additional risks for the patient and are likely to trigger litigation if such complications materialize. In the light of rec-ommendations regarding ultrasound guidance, complications of carotid artery puncture following a landmark-based technique or failing to use continuous scanning, are increas-ingly difficult to defend, particularly if deviation from optimal practice occurs at multiple stages.

If therefore a patient with anatomical hurdles such as obesity or limited neck movements, has undergone previous access at the same site, or there is intention to use a large device such as a dialysis catheter with predictably greater morbidity if misplaced within the artery, there is little justification for not using an ultrasound-based technique. There would simi-larly be little defence to adopting a blind technique in a hypotensive hypovolaemic patient, in whom cannulation of the vein would be predictably difficult and in whom aspiration from the artery would in a low-pressure state not necessarily suggest arterial puncture, thereby encouraging secondary dilatation and increased risk of significant morbidity. The debate regarding initial visualization versus continuous scanning outside the above scenarios has been alluded to previously and most experts would acknowledge that a primary technique of using the ultrasound machine to confirm normal neck anatomy, followed by a blind attempt at cannulation, is not in itself unreasonable, but only if the internal jugular vein was large, relatively superficial, full and unlikely to collapse on needle pressure and confirmed on ultrasound to be in the specific place predicted by a landmark-based technique and remote from the carotid artery.

If, however, an attempt at cannulation on this basis was unsuccessful, it would be unrea-sonable to persist with a blind technique because of the known hazards of perforating the carotid artery with just a seeker needle. If, furthermore, recognition of cannulation of the artery with a wide-bore catheter simply triggers immediate removal and local pressure with-out acknowledging the risk of stroke with this manoeuvre, as opposed to vascular surgery or radiology review, a picture of sequential and cumulative deviation from best practice becomes established with little merit in attempting to defend a civil claim. Interesting debate arises when successful cannulation of the carotid artery follows continuous ultrasound scan-ning, but this does not undermine the validity of the above arguments, and invariably dem-onstrates limited competence in the use of ultrasound.

Similar principles can be derived in relation to regional techniques, namely that even if most practitioners would agree that a procedure was indicated to avoid morbidity, a com-plication will not be viewed as intrinsic to the procedure, simply because it is a recognized and described complication. The questions that will be asked of the practitioner will relate to whether or not they had the appropriate training and expertise to minimize the risk of such complications arising, whether they conducted the technique in a way to minimize the risk and whether the procedures were put in place to identify the complication early and manage this appropriately. Whilst a dural puncture may in certain circumstances be defensible therefore, even if the epidural is conducted in the anaesthetized as opposed to awake patient, using loss of resistance to air as opposed to saline, it is likely that a case would succeed if the patient was not informed of the additional risks of this approach and offered the option of the procedure being carried out awake in the sitting position, particularly if factors such as obesity were present, which would increase the technical difficulty in the lying position.

Litigation is, however, more common for serious complications such as epidural haematoma or abscess, and in these circumstances there will be scrutiny not only of the primary technique, but of the process of postoperative supervision. This can reasonably be expected to include neurological assessment of the lower limbs, early identification of markers such as severe back pain and neurological deficit disproportionate to the volumes and concentration of local anaesthetic infusions and the early triggering of MRI imaging and expeditious liaison with neurosurgical services. Infection is becoming less acceptable as a complication of healthcare interventions in today's climate, and in the absence of an obvious primary source and secondary seeding, an isolated epidural abscess is likely to be interpreted as inadequate aseptic precautions until proven otherwise, and even secondary seeding is likely to raise questions over the advisability of siting an epidural in the presence of infection.

Late complications of dural puncture, such as intracranial subdural haematoma, still occur, and although interesting debate as to the optimal timing of a blood patch will take place in these circumstances, if it is apparent that standards of postoperative supervision have not ensured basic components of care such as a positive fluid balance, and there has not been discussion with the patient as to the condition, prognosis and benefits and risks of more invasive interventions such as a blood patch, with full documentation of the same, litigation is likely to be successful.

Broader considerations in the evaluation of negligence

The above considerations highlight the scrutiny that the overall process of care will be subjected to, looking for markers that suggest a shortfall in broader professional responsibilities including assessment, consent, documentation, handover of care and involvement of the patient in decision making, which ultimately may influence judicial opinion on the defensibility or otherwise of a specific complication.

The written explanation of events leading to a complication is also of critical importance, and whilst it is understandable that a practitioner may wish to present their actions in the most favourable light, any incompatibility between written documentation and the anaesthetic record, or a diagnosis that is not likely on a balance of probability, not supported by the available evidence or not subsequently pursued, for example anaphylaxis, is likely to colour the opinion of any instructed expert as to whether the complication or its consequences were avoidable with due care and attention.

Summary conclusions

Given the absence of definitive templates against which to evaluate anaesthetic care, it is inevitable that practitioners will be vulnerable to the vagaries of patient attitude, legal process and expert opinion in the aftermath of complications. This situation serves neither the patient, the practitioner, the profession nor the institution and remains refractory to the proposed amendments to civil procedure. It is possible, however, to derive what can reasonably be expected of an anaesthetist with regards to clinical competence and performance and the broader discharge of professional responsibilities.

The primary goals of anaesthesia are to keep the patient asleep or pain-free during regional techniques, facilitate the intended surgery and avoid longer term harms from the physiological derangement associated with this process. Such protection involves diligent identification of any excess risk, modification of anaesthetic procedure to minimize such risk, continuous optimization of gas exchange and cardiovascular performance, normalization of other physiological variables such as temperature, biochemical profile and coagulation status, and the early identification, correct diagnosis and appropriate management of complications of either surgery or anaesthesia.

Competence is anticipated in all technical anaesthetic interventions as is compliance with the broader professional responsibilities of involving the patient in decision making, achieving informed consent where feasible, maintaining vigilance at all stages of the anaesthetic journey, completing legible and comprehensive documentation that would allow another practitioner to maintain care and ensuring a high standard of patient handover whether to another anaesthetist, recovery staff, the acute pain team or a critical care facility.

At a time when the majority of consultants are losing an educational role as the combination of senior expansion and working time directives limit exposure to trainees, and the appraisal process has not embraced direct supervision of clinical practice, it is predictable that professional standards in the above fields may drift for certain individuals, leaving them vulnerable to both complications and subsequent litigation. Whilst initiatives such as *Safe Surgery Saves Lives* from the World Health Organization are providing useful reminders on issues such as machine checks, thromboprophylaxis, antibiotics and blood availability, safe anaesthesia is a broader concept than a simple checklist, and the challenge for individual practitioners, departments and the profession, is how competence and performance can be maintained in an increasingly isolated pattern of working. Attaining and maintaining the highest standards of care goes beyond this intellectual exercise, however, given the fundamental importance for both patient safety and accompanying professional fulfilment, reputation and sustainability. Avoiding risk factors for litigation should be a natural consequence of this aspiration towards the highest standards of care, rather than the primary driver.

List of further reading

Action against Medical Accidents. www.avma.org.uk (accessed 15 April 2011).

Australian and New Zealand College of Anaesthetists. Recommendations on checking anaesthesia delivery systems – 2003. www.anzca.edu.au/resources/professional-documents/ps31.html (accessed 15 April 2011).

Bell, M. D. D. Avoiding adverse outcomes when faced with 'difficulty with ventilation'. (Editorial) *Anaesthesia* 2003; **58**(10): 945–8.

Bell, M. D. D. & Bodenham, A. R. Problems and pitfalls of practical procedures: a medico-legal perspective. *Curr Anaesth Crit Care* 1998; **9**(6): 278–89.

Civil Justice Council. Alternative dispute resolution answerbank. www.adr.civiljusticecouncil.gov.uk/Home.go;jsessionid=baa5jU1d3m3C3_ (accessed 15 April 2011).

General Medical Council. Guidance on good practice. www.gmc-uk.org/guidance/index.asp (accessed 15 April 2011).

House of Lords. Judgments – *Bolitho v City and Hackney Health Authority*. www.publications.parliament.uk/pa/ld199798/ldjudgmt/jd971113/boli01.htm (accessed 15 April 2011).

Law Society. Accreditation schemes. www.lawsociety.org.uk/productsandservices/accreditation.page (accessed 15 April 2011).

National Institute for Health and Clinical Excellence. Guidance on the use of ultrasound locating devices for placing central venous catheters. *Technology Appraisal Guidance – No. 49*, September 2002.

Reuber, M., Dunkley, L. A., Turton, E. P., Bell, M. D. D. & Bamford, J. M. Stroke after internal jugular venous cannulation. *Acta Neurol Scand* 2002; **105**(3): 235–9.

World Health Organization. Safe surgery saves lives: the second global patient safety challenge 2009. www.who.int/patientsafety/safesurgery/en/ (accessed 15 April 2011).

Management of complaints and litigation in the UK

Jane Sturgess and Sam Bass

Introduction

Much of anaesthetic and perioperative practice could result in unfavourable or undesirable outcomes. These have been discussed earlier in this book. They can result from a fault of the healthcare professionals who may have neglected their role or simply made a human error. Failure of the anaesthetic machine, equipment, systems errors or a myriad of other causes can also be culpable. Often there is an array of factors leading to harm.

Modern society has become more aware, risk adverse and keener to apportion blame. Patients and their families expect compensation when errors occur. The result of this is an increase in litigation. Fortunately, anaesthesia is relatively safe and litigation is infrequent. Still, relatively minor, non-life-threatening problems such as dislodged teeth, sore throat or poor analgesia are common and are more likely to be the cause of a complaint.

The cases that have led to serious harm in anaesthetic practice are rare and are available in the medical law reviews. The case of *R v Adomako* ([1990] 1 AC 1) is a typical example. In this case, the level of negligence was so 'gross' that it amounted to criminal negligence. The defendant, the anaesthetist during an eye operation, had failed to notice the disconnection of the tracheal tube from the ventilator. The patient suffered a cardiac arrest and died. Cases of this kind are likely to lead to litigation.

The increase in prosecutions for medical manslaughter is due to changes in social attitudes. Modern-day intolerance of medical mistakes has turned medical errors resulting in death into tragedies calling for criminal investigation. Death is a serious and unusual end to the anaesthetic or perioperative process. Further, there are numerous complications of the perioperative practice, which may result in complaints and deserve compensation. This chapter will discuss the management of such complaints.

Proportion of anaesthetic complaints

In the UK it is almost impossible to assess the exact magnitude of complaints. Patients and relatives complain to different bodies and no organization has compiled a full set of data. The number of written complaints received also differs across the Strategic Health Authorities in England (Figure 20.1).

The Health and Social Care Information Centre compiles figures for written complaints (England) but this may only be the tip of the iceberg and does not make reference to serious

Anaesthetic and Perioperative Complications, ed. Kamen Valchanov, Stephen T. Webb and Jane Sturgess. Published by Cambridge University Press. © Cambridge University Press 2011.

Percentage of written complaints by Strategic Health Authority 2008–9

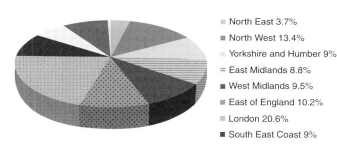

- North East 3.7%
- North West 13.4%
- Yorkshire and Humber 9%
- East Midlands 8.8%
- West Midlands 9.5%
- East of England 10.2%
- London 20.6%
- South East Coast 9%

Figure 20.1 Diagram to show the distribution of written complaints (total 89,139 received) in England according to Strategic Health Authority 2008–9 (from the Health and Social Care Information Centre).

untoward events. When trying to analyze the information available 39,981 complaints (of the 89,139 total) were made against doctors, and 908 against dentists. Another way of attempting to assess the size of the problem is to look at the number of complaints relating to hospital inpatient acute services. In this instance for 2008 to 2009 there were 29,033 complaints. Out of all service areas considered in this data set, acute hospital treatment had the largest number of complaints. The figures are actual numbers rather than percentage figures relating to patient episodes.

Complaints may arise from many different medical areas and can take any form. Some patients will complain to the doctor verbally, or in writing by letter or e-mail. These may not be reflected in reports compiled by the hospitals.

The National Health Service Litigation Authority (NHSLA) gives a broad overview of complaints but does not include information on direct complaints in its figures either. Private practice anaesthesia complaints fall outside the remit of the NHS indemnity scheme and are therefore dealt with by the relevant defence organizations. Again figures for the numbers of complaints are difficult to assess and it is hard to find exact details. Information from the Medical Defence Union (MDU) suggests that approximately 10% of all complaints are related to anaesthesia.

The distribution of medico-legal claims in English anaesthetic practice is unreported. Cook *et al.* studied NHSLA claims related to anaesthesia from 1995 to 2009. All claims were reviewed by three clinicians and variously categorized, including by type of incident, claimed outcome and cost. Anaesthesia-related claims account for 2.5% of all claims and 2.4% of the value of all claims. Of 841 relevant claims 366 (44%) were related to regional anaesthesia, 245 (29%) obstetric anaesthesia, 164 (20%) inadequate anaesthesia, 95 (11%) dental damage, 71 (8%) airway (excluding dental damage), 63 (7%) drug related (excluding allergy), 31 (4%) drug-allergy related, 31 (4%) positioning, 29 (3%) respiratory, 26 (3%) consent, 21 (2%) central venous cannulation and 18 (2%) peripheral venous cannulation.

Table 20.1 demonstrates the five commonest reasons for written complaints to the NHS in England for 2008 to 2009. The total number of written complaints received for all causes was 89,139. It is clear from the Cook paper that complaints in anaesthesia make up only a very small proportion of the total number of complaints recorded. In addition anaesthetic claims are often related to specific clinical events. Regardless of this we can learn that improved attitudes and communication with patients may protect us from a complaint.

Table 20.1 Table to show the five most frequent written complaints about hospital and community services in England, 2008–9 (from the Health and Social Care Information Centre).

	Subject of complaint England 2008–9	Number of complaints
1	All aspects of clinical treatment	37,149
2	Attitude of staff	11,332
3	Appointments, delay/cancellation (outpatient)	9,738
4	Communication/information to patients (written and oral)	8,970
5	Appointments, delay/cancellation (inpatient)	2,364

The NHS Litigation Authority

The number of written complaints (for hospital and community services in England) received year on year between 1997 and 2009 has remained reasonably constant at around the 90,000 mark. Yet the NHSLA reports an increase of 10% in the number of clinical cases dealt with up to 6,652 from 2008. In 2008 clinical negligence claims cost the NHS £650m: £385m of this was for damages but other costs amounted to £266m. This cost is increasing. The NHSLA was set up primarily to keep the costs of litigation low.

The payment of large sums in compensation for devastating complications appearing in the media is seldom the whole story. Large numbers of complaints do not ever become formal and warrant investigation. Most are dealt with at a local hospital level. Ward managers and doctors deal with a substantial number of incidents either by the standard incident reporting system or simply by answering queries on an informal basis. Many complaints are started because of the lack of information that a patient has, or are related to a lack of understanding combined with an unrealistic expectation of what is possible. Lack of communication is frequently the unifying theme in complaints.

Receipt of a complaint

Before 2009 the complaint process was felt to be complicated, cumbersome and unsatisfactory. There were strict time limits detailing the framework within which a claimant could complain (up to six months from the event occurring) and also within which the defendant should respond. The complainant had to receive written receipt of the complaint from the organization within two working days. This letter had to detail the expected time when a full response to the complaint would be made. A response from the chief executive officer (CEO) was expected within 20 days. If the complainant was not satisfied the complaint could be sent for independent review. A referral to review had to be made within the next 28 days and a response was expected within six months. If there was still no resolution further appeals could be dealt with by the Healthcare Commission, the ombudsman or a judicial review. A judicial review could only take place within three months of the incident occurring. Patients and carers felt disengaged from the process and it was time-consuming.

The *NHS Constitution* was published in January 2009 and stated a numbers of rights for every patient and carer (Table 20.2). It placed a great deal of importance on the 'customer experience' and this in part led to the need to reform the complaints procedure within healthcare (Table 20.3).

Table 20.2 The *NHS Constitution* (published January 2009) and patient/carer rights.

1. To have any complaint made about NHS services dealt with efficiently and investigated promptly
2. To know the outcome of the investigation
3. To take the complaint to an independent body if unsatisfied with the NHS resolution
4. To make a claim for judicial review if of the opinion that an unlawful act or decision has occurred by an NHS body
5. To claim compensation when harmed by negligent treatment

Table 20.3 Complainants wishes (from the *NHS Constitution* 2009).

Complainants wishes

To be treated with courtesy and receive support throughout the complaint process

To have mistakes acknowledged

An apology

An explanation of what went wrong

To put 'things' right quickly and effectively

To know the organization has learned from the mistake and put measures in place to prevent the same mistake from recurring

Table 20.4 Table to explain the difference between PALS and ICAS.

PALS	ICAS
Patient Advice and Liason Service (PALS) – usually on site	Independent Complaints Advisory Service (ICAS)
Provide advice and support for complainants trying to resolve their complaint informally	Free and confidential service to help patients and carers make formal complaints about NHS services
PALS do not take up the complaint	

Listen, Respond, Improve came into force from the 1 April 2009 as a shared complaints procedure for health and social care. Its aim was to make the process easier to access, more flexible and more responsive to patient and carer.

The main differences are as follows.

- Up to 12 months in which to make a complaint. This time period is either from the actual time of the event or the time the complainant became aware of the event or was able to complain about it (e.g. grieving, prolonged ITU stay or other trauma).
- Simple two-stage process to the complaint. Local resolution or recourse to Parliamentary and Health Service Ombudsman.
- Receipt of complaint should be acknowledged within three working days, and an appointment made to listen to the complainant. The complainant can choose how this is done – face to face, telephone or in writing.
- There should be an opportunity to have a meeting with all parties concerned.
- Advice given about the Patient Advice and Liaison Service (PALS) and the Independent Complaints Advocacy Service (ICAS) (Table 20.4).

- CEO made aware of serious complaints to ensure lessons are learned and policies put in place to prevent further similar episodes.
- Investigation report to be reviewed by complainant and staff concerned. This should increase patient involvement in resolution of the complaint.
- No more time constraint on CEO letter – but patient to be kept fully informed of the progress of the investigation. If a delay of more than six months is anticipated for a full review this (with reasons) must be communicated to the patient.
- An annual report should be produced detailing the lessons learned from complaints made in the preceding year.

NHS Trust services

Every NHS Trust and Primary Care Trust is required to have its own Patient Advice and Liaison Service (PALS) with staff available to listen to patients' and relatives' concerns and to offer information and support. They deal with any issue that may affect patients. The Patient Advice and Liaison Service liaise with other professionals to resolve complaints and issues before a formal complaint is made. Most complaints are dealt with in this way. Approximately 10% of the initial enquiries referred to the PALS department lead to a formal written complaint. Patients who require support or advocacy from an external source to the hospital can use the Independent Complaints Advocacy Service (ICAS) who will write letters and attend meetings at the hospital with the person involved. Some complaints may lead to a serious untoward incident inquiry depending on the nature of the complaint. Other agencies can be involved (from the coronial service to the police) at any time during the investigation. If criminal activity is thought to have occurred the police may make inquiries and prosecutions might follow. It is important to note that many patients or relatives are scared and upset with what they see as poor treatment or care. Complaints are not always justified – but patients have rights, which were started with the Patients' Charter in the 1980s and then formally incorporated in the recent *NHS Constitution*.

The General Medical Council

Patients may complain to the GMC directly about the treatment given by or the conduct of a doctor. The GMC publishes data on the number of complaints (www.gmc-uk.org/publications/7263.asp). Anaesthesia makes up a relatively small percentage of referrals to the GMC. The GMC investigates the complaint and decides whether it is necessary to investigate further. Actions taken may result in a hearing. Further information is available on the GMC website.

The coronial service

If a patient has died the relatives may complain to the coroner. If the coroner considers it appropriate and it is in his jurisdiction, then he may open an investigation into the death of the patient. Potentially the patient could complain before they die but this would be rather unlikely. The coroner has significant powers to examine the manner and circumstances that led to the death of the patient and can make recommendations under rule 43 of the Coroners Rules 1984 to improve or change practice. He is not allowed to apportion blame to any individual but can find that gross neglect of the organization had contributed to the death of a patient. He could also refer a case to the Crown Prosecution Service via the police. However, initially the coroner is likely to notify the medical director of the hospital in which the doctor worked. The coronial service can sometimes be used as a fact-finding mission to explore if a case for negligence could be brought and the service is funded by the tax payer. Legal aid is not normally available. Hospitals and Trusts are bound in law to comply with requests that the coroner makes and the coroner has wide powers to call witnesses to give evidence at an inquest. The questions can be wide ranging and the coroner determines the scope of the inquest. Thus complaints about services or the functioning of a hospital or organization can be examined and ultimately those services improved. Families who have lost a relative and are aggrieved by the care that has been received may want to know that it will not be repeated and any mistakes have been useful for effecting change.

Management of a complaint

If the patient or the complainants are not satisfied with the response to their complaint, the next stage is the local resolution of the complaint. The complaint should be dealt with quickly and efficiently. Formal responses are dealt with by the CEO of the Trust, who is responsible for answering complaints but can delegate this to the PALS department. Only 2% of complaints progress beyond the local resolution stage.

If there are still unanswered questions and the complainant is still not satisfied then the next route is to complain to the Health Service Ombudsman. This changed in April 2009 when the Healthcare Commission ceased to exist and the Quality Care Commission did not have a role in resolving complaints. The patient must bring the complaint within a year of becoming aware of the events and must show that they have suffered hardship or injustice. The ombudsman does not investigate cases where there is likelihood of a claim for negligence or if it appears that the patient is using the service as a fact-finding mission to see if litigation is possible without incurring any cost. The ombudsman can offer some financial payment if there is proven financial loss. The ombudsman received 4,257 complaints against the NHS in 2008. Most were premature as local resolution had not been exhausted and were referred back to hospital for resolution. Many hospitals employ lawyers who have the ability to settle low-value claims and reduce the need for expensive litigation. The costs of these claims may not be made public and therefore are related to the hospital alone. The vast majority of written complaints are resolved within 25 days, or outside 25 days but with complainant consent (Figure 20.2). Only a few are still being pursued after this time frame (1,935 out of a total of 89,139).

Written complaints about hospital and community services, England, 2008–9

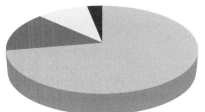

- Concluded within 25 working days (%)
- Concluded outside 25 working days with consent (%)
- Concluded outside 25 working days without consent (%)
- Still being pursued (%)

Figure 20.2 Chart to show the speed of complaint resolution in England 2008–9. Total number of written complaints received 89,139 (from the Health and Social Care Information Centre).

Resolution of a complaint

In most of the cases despite significant negative impact of healthcare system errors the complaints are resolved by an apology and explanation why a complication has occurred, as well as the organization taking action to preclude such complications from happening again in the future. However, a proportion of the complaints progress further and it is reasonable the case attracts financial compensation once the organization has admitted liability. A small proportion of complaints progress to a formal lawsuit. These on the whole represent serious medical negligence or a system blunder where individual or organization guilt is sought. Cases of this kind attract high costs as well as media publicity. The hospitals involved are represented by their solicitors, and healthcare professionals by their defence medical organizations. The modern society complaint procedures are designed to preclude such serious complaints from progressing to the law courts as this attracts undesirable negative publicity and expenses.

Complaint management systems

Although recently modernized there has been criticism of the existing complaints systems. It is viewed as complicated and not patient focused. The difficulty with any complaints system is to provide a sensitive and caring atmosphere and environment that puts patients first and takes any issues seriously. The PALS system is in place in every hospital and should deal with the complaints as they arise. The litigation system is expensive and difficult to access, especially as there is a reduction in the legal aid budget in the current economic climate. A discussion of the need to change the system to allow no-fault compensation is beyond the scope of this chapter. The aim of a perfect system is that patients who are entitled to compensation should receive it with minimum difficulty, but unsubstantiated complaints be dismissed fairly and promptly.

Simple measures taken by frontline staff helping those patients raising a complaint can not only ease the complaint procedure for the complainant but they may also help to resolve the issue at the first stage and prevent evolution of the complaint into litigation (Table 20.5).

Medical indemnity

Broadly speaking there are two types of medical indemnity: NHS indemnity and professional indemnity.

NHS indemnity covers anaesthetists for clinical negligence but not for any other liability. Clinical negligence may be a negligent act or an omission of an act. Before liability of negligence can be declared a number of prerequisites must be fulfilled:

- the person treated must be owed a duty of care by the relevant professional
- there must be a failure to reach an appropriate standard of care by action or omission, or consent – the duty is breached
- this breach must have injured or harmed the complainant in the way alleged
- the courts must be able to recognize and compensate for the loss the complainant has suffered
- the loss or injury should be seen as a possible consequence of the breach of duty.

NHS indemnity applies where the negligent person was under contract of employment and the act occurred during the period of employment. This stands regardless of whether or not the person remains under contract when the claim is brought. It also applies to individuals

Table 20.5 Advice in dealing with patients/carers with complaints (from *Listen, Respond, Improve* April 2009 – shared complaints procedure for health and social care).

Advice for frontline staff when dealing with a complaint (from *Respond, Listen, Improve*)
Ask the complainant how they would like to be addressed
If you have been phoned, offer to call back, and a chance to meet face to face to discuss the issue
Ask how the complainant would like to be informed about the investigation (e-mail, post, phone) and make sure contact details are correct
Ask when it is a convenient time to phone
Ensure the complainant knows they can request an advocate to support them
Systematically go through the reasons for the complaint to clarify why they are unhappy
Ask what outcome the complainant would like from the investigation. Let them know if this is realistic or not
Agree a plan of action – to include when the complainant will hear from the organization
Resolve the complaint yourself if possible and no risk to other patients
Check whether consent is required to access patient notes

contracted to the NHS body who owed the claimant a duty of care, who are not necessarily under a contract of employment (i.e. contracted for services). Locums, doctors in training, medical academics with honorary contracts, military doctors and medical students are all covered. There are times when it is worthwhile checking on special circumstances, e.g. medical students when the medical school may provide indemnity, or during a clinical trial when the university or sponsoring pharmaceutical company may provide indemnity.

The NHS body will cover the legal and administrative costs of defending the claim, damages and, where appropriate, plaintiff costs.

It is wise to check whether the main hospital NHS indemnity covers an individual when the contract of employment is with one hospital but the individual provides services to a second hospital.

Former NHS employees are covered so long as they were under contract at the time of the alleged incident.

There are a number of areas not covered:

- Treatment by consultants of private patients within the NHS hospital. However, the junior medical and nursing staff that assist in the patient's care would be covered.
- Category 2 work (e.g. reports for insurance companies).
- Defence of staff reported to their regulatory bodies (e.g. GMC).
- Local Research and Ethics Committees – these are covered by the Health Authority.
- 'Good Samaritan' acts.
- NHS staff working for other agencies, e.g. the prison service.

There have been difficulties in clarifying the indemnity of NHS employees providing services to NHS patients in the private sector. This has become more prevalent with the pressures of 'choose and book', and some hospitals are outsourcing their case loads to the private sector. The document *NHS Indemnity – Arrangements for Clinical Negligence Claims in the NHS* states, in Annex A item 2, that 'A consultant undertaking contracted NHS work in a private hospital would also be covered.' Nonetheless it is worth checking this cover before proceeding.

Professional indemnity comes in many guises but is considered essential by most professionals. Although not a legal requirement, the GMC recommends professional indemnity. It can be used in addition to NHS indemnity for NHS patients, but will also cover the individual for cases brought by private patients or the areas mentioned above that are not covered by NHS indemnity. On the whole medical defence can be provided as insured, discretionary or occurrence-based.

Insured protection provides a contractual agreement of assistance 'under the terms of the policy'. As with any insurance it is essential to read the small print to ensure this policy provides the cover required.

Discretionary cover allows the doctor to ask for help, advice and assistance but does not guarantee the doctor has the right to receive it.

Occurrence-based indemnity provides cover to the doctor if they had a policy at the time the event occurred, regardless of the policy cover at the time of the claim, i.e. a retired doctor not currently subscribing to an insurance policy, with a claim being brought about events in the past when the policy was in place.

The premiums are based on the areas of clinical practice and the likelihood of a claim being brought, and also the amount of work performed. The higher the risk, the bigger the practice, the higher the cost.

List of further reading

Cook, T. M., Bland, L., Mihai, R. & Scott, S. Litigation related to anaesthesia: an analysis of claims against the NHS in England 1995–2007. *Anaesthesia* 2009; **64**: 706–18.

Dorries, C. *Coroners Courts: A Guide to Law and Practice*, 2nd edn. Oxford: Oxford University Press, 2004.

General Medical Council. After registration. www.gmc-uk.org/doctors/information_for_doctors/after_registration.asp (accessed 15 April 2011).

General Medical Council. Good practice. www.gmc-uk.org/ (accessed 15 April 2011).

Independent Complaints and Advocacy Service. www.pohwer.net (accessed 15 April 2011).

Jackson, E. *Medical Law, Text, Cases and Materials*, 2nd edn. Oxford: Oxford University Press, 2009.

NHS. Consitution. www.nhs.uk/NHSConstitution (accessed 15 April 2011).

NHS Litigation Authority. www.nhsla.com/home.htm (accessed 15 April 2011).

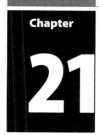

The role of the expert witness

Jurgens Nortje

Introduction

Modern healthcare has become increasingly patient centred. In fact, the National Institute for Health and Clinical Excellence (NICE) has a patient and public involvement policy aimed at being patient centred, with the public's needs as its focus. This ensures patient and public involvement in decision making and production of NICE guidance.

Greater patient engagement and knowledge, coupled with better access to information through media such as the internet, has meant high numbers of complaints that require arbitration, often in the courts. The latest NHS figures for hospital and community services for 2008 to 2009 reveal 89,139 complaints of which 45% are medical. Lawyers and judges usually lack detailed medical knowledge, and rely on expert witnesses to clarify medical issues and determine the standards of care.

What is an expert witness?

An expert witness is a person, from any walk of life, whom the court recognizes as being an authority on a topic through having greater knowledge about the topic than the average person by virtue of qualifications and experience. It should be noted that the role of the expert witness is to provide impartial factual information and analysis of circumstances and not to testify on legal matters. This chapter refers to medical expert witnesses.

In medicine, expert witnesses are medical practitioners who by virtue of their standing, experience and knowledge, are able to provide information to the court, including plaintiffs and defendants, to indicate best practice. This information may be used to secure or avoid criminal convictions.

A professional witness, on the other hand, is a medical practitioner who only provides the direct facts. Unlike an expert witness, he does not provide an expert medical opinion.

Several high-profile cases in the UK in the past few years in cases of suspected infanticide where initial expert witness evidence was subsequently cast into doubt, have highlighted the importance of strict adherence to impartiality and remaining within expert witness's area of expertise. It has also focused attention on the expert witness process, caused public debate and driven changes.

Expert witness regulation and advice

Both the government and medical organizations provide guidance on the principles of best practice for professionals acting as expert witnesses.

Anaesthetic and Perioperative Complications, ed. Kamen Valchanov, Stephen T. Webb and Jane Sturgess. Published by Cambridge University Press. © Cambridge University Press 2011.

The Ministry of Justice

The UK Ministry of Justice provides Civil Procedure Rules (CPR), part 35 of which relates to experts and assessors. A protocol, drafted by the Civil Justice Council, initially prepared in June 2005 and amended in October 2009, has been produced for the guidance of experts and those instructing them on giving evidence in civil proceedings.

Noteworthy excerpts from the duties of experts include:

Experts always owe a duty to **exercise reasonable skill** and care to those instructing them, and to **comply with** any relevant professional code of **ethics**. However, when they are instructed to give or prepare evidence for the purpose of civil proceedings in England and Wales they have an overriding duty to help the court on **matters within their expertise** (CPR 35.3). This duty overrides any obligation to the person instructing or paying them. Experts must not serve the exclusive interest of those who retain them.

Experts should be aware of the overriding objective that courts deal with cases justly. This includes dealing with cases **proportionately, expeditiously and fairly** (CPR 1.1). Experts are under an obligation to assist the court so as to enable them to deal with cases in accordance with the overriding objective. However, the overriding objective does not impose on experts any duty to act as mediators between the parties or require them to trespass on the role of the court in deciding facts.

Experts should provide opinions which are **independent**, regardless of the pressures of litigation. In this context, a useful test of 'independence' is that the expert would express the same opinion if given the same instructions by an opposing party. Experts should not take it upon themselves to promote the point of view of the party instructing them or engage in the role of advocates.

Experts should confine their opinions to matters which are material to the disputes between the parties and **provide opinions only in relation to matters which lie within their expertise**. Experts should indicate without delay where particular questions or issues fall outside their expertise.

Experts should take into account all material facts before them at the time that they give their opinion. Their **reports should set out those facts and any literature or any other material on which they have relied in forming their opinions**. They should indicate if an opinion is provisional, or qualified, or where they consider that further information is required or if, for any other reason, they are not satisfied that an opinion can be expressed finally and without qualification.

The protocol also addresses matters relating to the conduct of experts, whether experts are needed, how experts are appointed and remunerated, how experts are instructed, how experts accept or withdraw from assigned tasks and how experts should prepare their reports. It also addresses the use of single joint experts, i.e. where the expert, through his obligation to the court primarily, is used to state unbiased facts for the benefit of both the plaintiff and defendant as opposed to acting on behalf of either party alone.

The Ministry of Justice also provides Criminal Procedure Rules (2010), part 33 of which relates to requirements around providing expert evidence in criminal proceedings.

The Crown Prosecution Service (CPS)

The CPS is the government department responsible for prosecuting criminal cases investigated by the police in England and Wales. It provides guidance for expert witnesses in the form of a *Guidance Booklet for Experts Disclosure: Experts' Evidence, Case Management and Unused Material* (May 2010).

Complying with the requirements of the Ministry of Justice, this guidance is described as a 'practical guide to preparing expert evidence and the disclosure obligations for expert witnesses instructed by the Prosecution Team. When properly applied, these instructions will assist expert witnesses, investigators and prosecutors to perform their disclosure duties effectively, fairly and justly, which is vitally important to the integrity of the criminal justice system.'

The General Medical Council (GMC)

Good Medical Practice (2006)

Through documents like *Good Medical Practice* standards for the conduct of doctors have been set by the GMC. These play a pivotal role not only in clinical medicine and revalidation, but also during interactions with external agencies when addressing patient complaints for example. Some of the guidance relevant to those acting as expert witnesses includes the following excerpts from the *Good Medical Practice* document:

- you must be **honest and trustworthy** when writing reports and when completing or signing forms, reports and other documents
- you must always be **honest about your experience, qualifications and position**, particularly when applying for posts
- you must do your best to make sure that any documents you write or sign are **not false or misleading**. This means that you must take reasonable steps to verify the information in the documents, and that you must not deliberately leave out relevant information
- if you have agreed to prepare a report, complete or sign a document or provide evidence, you must do so **without unreasonable delay**
- if you are asked to give evidence or act as a witness in litigation or formal inquiries, you must be honest in all your spoken and written statements. You must **make clear the limits of your knowledge** or competence.

It is also worth noting that 'serious or persistent failure to follow this guidance will put your registration at risk.'

Acting as an Expert Medical Witness (2008)

Guidance on the role of the expert witness has been provided by the GMC. It states that:

> The role of an expert witness is to assist the court on specialist or technical matters within their expertise. The expert's duty to the court overrides any obligation to the person who is instructing or paying them. This means that you have a duty to act independently and not be influenced by the party who retains you.

On giving expert advice and evidence:

> ensure that you **understand exactly** what questions you are being asked to answer…seek clarification. If you cannot obtain sufficiently clear instructions, you should not provide expert advice or opinion
>
> evidence or writing reports…restrict your statements to areas in which you **have relevant knowledge or direct experience**…be aware of the standards and nature of practice at the time
>
> only deal with matters, and express opinions, that fall **within the limits of your professional competence**…if outside, make this clear. In the event that you are ordered by the court to answer a

question, regardless of your expertise, you should answer to the best of your ability but make clear that you consider the matter to be outside your competence

give a **balanced opinion**…be able to state the facts or assumptions on which it is based. If you do not have enough information on which to reach a conclusion on a particular point, or your opinion is otherwise qualified, you must make this clear

any report that you write, or evidence that you give, is **accurate** and is not misleading…must take reasonable steps to verify any information you provide, and you must not deliberately leave out relevant information

you are asked to give advice or opinion about an individual without the opportunity to consult with or examine them…**explain any limitations** that this may place on your advice or opinion

your advice and evidence will be relied upon for decision-making purposes by people who do not come from a medical background. Wherever…possible…use language and terminology that will be **readily understood**…explain any abbreviations and medical or other technical terminology

if…you **change your view** on any material matter, you have a duty to ensure that those instructing you, the opposing party and the judge are made aware of this without delay

you must be **honest, trustworthy, objective and impartial**. You must not allow your views about any individual's age, colour, culture, disability, ethnic or national origin, gender, lifestyle, marital or parental status, race, religion or beliefs, sex, sexual orientation or social or economic status to prejudice the evidence or advice that you give.

On keeping up to date:

keep **up to date** in your specialist area of practice…ensure that you understand, and **adhere to, the laws and codes** of practice that affect your work as an expert witness…make sure that you understand:

how to construct a court-compliant report

how to give oral evidence

the specific framework of law and procedure within which you are working.

On information security and disclosure:

you must take all reasonable steps to access all relevant evidence materials and maintain their **integrity and security** whilst in your possession

if…**appropriate consent for disclosure** of information has not been obtained (from the patient or client, or from any third party to whom their medical records refer) you should return the information to the person instructing you and seek clarification

you should **not disclose confidential information** other than to the parties to proceedings, unless:

the subject consents (and there are no other restrictions or prohibitions on disclosure)

you are obliged to do so by law

you are ordered to do so by a court or tribunal

your overriding duty to the court and the administration of justice demands that you disclose information.

On conflicts of interest:

potential conflict of interest, such as any **prior involvement** with one of the parties, or a **personal interest**, you must follow the guidance on disclosure…you may continue to act as an expert witness only if the court decides that the conflict is not material to the case.

The British Medical Association (BMA)

The BMA provides guidance in the form of a document called *British Medical Association Expert Witness Guidance* (October 2007). This document assimilates much of the information provided above from the Ministry of Justice and the CPS, as well as the GMC, and is also very useful for explaining the differences in the legal processes and requirements in England and Wales, Scotland and Northern Ireland.

Under the role of the expert doctor it states that 'the opinion must both be and be seen to be independent, objective and unbiased. It is liable to be tested in cross-examination. The independence of thought of an expert witness must be jealously guarded'.

The Royal College of Anaesthetists (RCA)

Although there is no dedicated RCA guidance on acting as an expert witness, the recently published document, *The Good Anaesthetist* (February 2010), outlines the standards of practice for career grade anaesthetists.

It states in Domain 4 (maintaining trust), attribute 12 (act with honesty and integrity) that: 'An anaesthetist must be honest in any formal statement or report, whether written or oral, making clear the limits of your knowledge or competence.' There is also reference to the 2008 GMC document, *Acting as an Expert witness*.

Other organizations

A number of professional organizations, which register and provide directories of experts in various fields, advise on the process and responsibilities of being an expert witness and look after their interests. Some prominent examples include the following.

The Academy of Experts

This professional body for experts was established in 1987. The Academy of Experts states that its aims include promoting the use of independent experts, promoting a forum for experts and members of the legal profession, maintaining codes of practice, organizing education and training, providing advice, assistance and information, maintaining directories of members, ensuring awareness of the quality of its members and liaising with other bodies, including judicial, legal and government relating to expert advice (the Academy had involvement in the preparation of the Civil Justice Council protocol mentioned above).

Expert Witness Institute

Established in 1996, the Expert Witness Institute states that its objectives include being the voice of expert witnesses, supporting both expert witnesses and the lawyers who make use of them, encouraging training and maintaining standards and consulting with other professional bodies as well as the government (e.g. the EWI was consulted by the Civil Justice Council during the preparation of its protocol above).

The Society of Expert Witnesses

Founded in 1995, the Society of Expert Witnesses declares its main objective to be the promotion of excellence in all aspects of the service provided by expert witnesses through promotion of training, promoting the elevated standards of the society, assisting members in their expert witness business, participating in suitable promotional activity and by cooperating with like-minded bodies.

The UK Register of Expert Witnesses

This website offers support, guidance and promotion for expert witnesses and claims to contain the UK's largest database of vetted expert witnesses.

What qualities should an expert witness possess?

It is generally accepted that a medical expert witness should have the appropriate current medical registration/licence, qualifications, professional training, knowledge, expertise and experience commensurate with the nature and complexity of the case to allow provision of highly specialized and ethical scientific and medical evidence. The appropriate resources, including ability to adhere to the required timescales, is also important.

Having good communication skills, being concise and clear (in thought and report writing), being quick witted, being flexible and with enough self-confidence to modify opinions when fresh evidence arises, and having the ability to inspire confidence in the courtroom environment have all been put forward as desirable qualities for an expert witness.

Expert witnesses should not: be the treating physician, have any pecuniary interest, have any relationship with either plaintiff or defendant or possess inappropriate training or lack of expertise in the field of the case under scrutiny. Expert witness testimony should also not be a full-time occupation.

Do expert witnesses enjoy immunity from prosecution?

Expert witnesses have historically enjoyed immunity from civil litigation in respect of evidence they give in court and evidence provided as statements. This is not a special dispensation for expert witnesses per se as all witnesses in legal proceedings are protected from claims for damages, the intention being that witnesses have the ability to express themselves freely and without fear of a defamation lawsuit.

Expert witnesses' immunity from claims for damages has increasingly come under the spotlight recently, particularly following Professor Sir Roy Meadow's GMC case. In future, it is likely that there will be increasing accountability and liability placed on expert witnesses.

The case of *Paul Wynne Jones v Sue Kaney* ([2010] EWHC 61 (QB)) raised the issue of the expert witness's 'immunity from suit'. Blake J. stated that 'In my judgment a policy of blanket immunity…may well prove to be too broad to be sustainable and therefore disproportionate'. The case has been referred to the Supreme Court and a decision is awaited.

The GMC states that doctors must not assume that 'just because they are working outside a clinical setting, that their actions are somehow beyond the boundaries of their professional responsibilities.' Also that 'when doctors act as expert witnesses, they are speaking from a position of authority. It is essential that their actions continue to justify the trust which the public, and the legal profession, places in them' and that a doctor's serious or persistent failure to follow guidelines will 'put their registration at risk.'

The Ministry of Justice states that 'experts should be aware that any failure by them to comply with the Civil Procedure Rules or court orders or any excessive delay for which they are responsible may result in the parties who instructed them being penalised in costs and even, in extreme cases, being debarred from placing the experts' and that 'courts may also make orders for costs (under section 51 of the Supreme Court Act 1981) directly against expert witnesses who by their evidence cause significant expense to be incurred, and do so in flagrant and reckless disregard of their duties to the Court.'

Sanctions for poor practice or failure to follow guidelines may range from embarrassment, loss of reputation, undermining of credibility, being dropped from medico-legal work, disciplinary proceedings (usually for gross dereliction of duty) from licensing boards or professional organisations, loss of accreditation, being charged with contempt of court for false statements, paying costs, facing criminal prosecution for perjury or even civil action by the accused.

Of interest is a study carried out by the Committee on Professional Liability of the ASA where 30 pairs of anesthesiologist reviewers were asked to independently and implicitly assess appropriateness of care in 103 closed anaesthesia malpractice claims. The level of agreement in the analysis of the claims revealed that the reviewers agreed on 62% of claims and disagreed on 38%. This highlights that disagreement among experts is common and that divergent expert opinions may easily be found by seeking multiple expert opinions.

Recommendations when considering acting as an expert witness

- Make sure you possess the appropriate status, training and attributes.
- Make sure that no conflicts of interest exist.
- Read the GMC guidance on *Good Medical Practice* and *Acting as an Expert Medical Witness*.
- Consider joining a professional expert witness organization and taking a course.
- Read the Academy of Medical Royal Colleges guidance.
- Consult the BMA.
- Consult your medical indemnity organization.
- Take out professional indemnity insurance; make sure your insurance covers expert witness activities.
- Read the Ministry of Justice's Civil and Criminal Procedure Rules regarding Experts and Assessors (Part 35) and Expert Evidence (Part 33) respectively.
- Be rigorously impartial!

List of further reading

Academy of Medical Royal Colleges. Medical expert witnesses. www.aomrc.org.uk/reports-guidance.html (accessed 15 April 2011).

British Medical Association. Expert witness guidance. www.bma.org.uk/employmentandcontracts/2_expert_witnesses/ (accessed 15 April 2011).

Dyer, C. Regulatory bodies can discipline expert witnesses. *BMJ* 2006; **333**: 933.

Dyer, C. Doctors in court. *BMJ* 2008; **337**: a975.

Friston, M. Roles and responsibilities of medical expert witnesses. *BMJ* 2005; **331**(7512): 305–6.

General Medical Council. Acting as an expert witness. July 2008. www.gmc-uk.org/static/documents/content/Acting_as_an_expert_witness.pdf (accessed 15 April 2011).

Posner, K. L., Caplan, R. A. & Cheney, F. W. Variation in expert opinion in medical malpractice review. *Anesthesiology* 1996; **85**: 1049–54.

Royal College of Anaesthetists. The good anaesthetist: standards of practice for career grade anaesthetists. RCA, 2010. www.aagbi.org/publications/guidelines/docs/good_anaesthetist_2010.pdf (accessed 15 April 2011).

Simon, V. The doctor in the witness-box. *BMJ* 1953; **2**(4826): 1–3.

Index

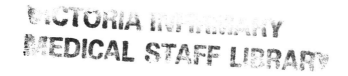